Atlas of PET/MR Imaging in Oncology

Osman Ratib • Markus Schwaiger • Thomas Beyer
Editors

M. Eiber • A.J. Beer • V. Garibotto
O. Rager • C. Tabouret-Viaud • L. Allainmat
Associate Editors

Atlas of PET/MR Imaging in Oncology

Springer

Editors
Osman Ratib
Nuclear Medicine Division
University Hospital of Geneva
Geneva
Switzerland

Markus Schwaiger
Klinikum rechts der Isar
Nuklearmedizinische Klinik u. Poliklinik
Technische Universität München
Munich
Germany

Thomas Beyer
Medical University Vienna
Center for Medical Physics
and Biomedical Engineering
General Hospital Vienna
Waehringer Guertel
Vienna, Austria

Associate Editors
M. Eiber
A.J. Beer
V. Garibotto
O. Rager
C. Tabouret-Viaud
L. Allainmat

ISBN 978-3-662-50995-1 ISBN 978-3-642-31292-2 (eBook)
DOI 10.1007/978-3-642-31292-2
Springer Heidelberg New York Dordrecht London

Softcover reprint of the hardcover 1st edition 2013

Printed on acid-free paper

Springer is part of Springer Science+Business Media (www.springer.com)

Preface

This atlas of early clinical experience from the first two sites to be equipped with a whole-body PET/MR scanner is intended as an introduction to this new hybrid modality and its potential applications in oncology. Written by early adopters of the technique, it highlights the strength of collaboration and combined efforts of expert radiologists and nuclear medicine specialists in developing new diagnostic strategies and imaging protocols that can take full advantage of this innovative technology. The atlas is a testament not only to the efforts of the contributors in optimally applying whole-body PET/MR imaging within their own specific domain but also to their commitment in preparing superb illustrative cases and reference images for the book and further amazing figures and images for the multimedia companion version. This work could not have been achieved without the coordinated efforts of the numerous co-authors of each chapter, each of whom deserves special recognition for their contribution. The authors would also like to thank Dr. A. Baskin for her editorial work and preparation of numerous illustrations and figures and Dr. Benedicte Delattre for her help and valuable technical support in the development of imaging protocols and the preparation of the cases and manuscript for the book. Finally, the authors would like to express their gratitude to Philips Healthcare for providing the support and resources that permitted the development of the interactive multimedia version of the book.

Contents

Part I

Clinical and Technical Principles

Introduction

1

O. Ratib and M. Schwaiger

Contents

O. Ratib (✉)
Department of Medical Imaging and Information Sciences,
Division of Nuclear Medicine and Molecular Imaging,
Geneva University Hospitals, Geneva, Switzerland
e-mail: osman.ratib@hcuge.ch

M. Schwaiger
Klinikum rechts der Isar
Nuklearmedizinische Klinik u. Poliklinik, Technische Universität München, Munich, Germany

PET/MRI in Clinical Practice

Following the path of clinical applications of hybrid PET/CT it would seem logical that PET/MR can provide an innovative and attractive alternative taking full advantage of the superiority of MR over CT in differentiating soft tissue characteristics with a reduction in radiation exposure by replacing CT with MR imaging. The challenges of PET/MR are still numerous both on the technical side as on the practical and clinical side.

From PET/CT to PET/MR

The development of PET/MR started even before the first prototypes of PET/CT were developed. As described in details in the next chapter, the technical challenges were considerable to overcome the interference and cross-talk effects between magnetic field and the photomultipliers of PET detectors. Several alternatives have emerged and lead to the first hybrid devices to appear on the market for clinical applications. Whether it is through a combination of separate coplanar systems or by integrating solid-state PET detectors inside an MRI they provide the means to explore the potential clinical applications of whole-body PET/MR in clinical practice.

Given the broad range of applications of PET imaging, it is oncology that remains today the clinical domain where PET is mostly used. PET imaging was shown to be superior to other imaging techniques in staging and follow-up of numerous specific tumors. The advent of PET/CT has reinforced the clinical utilization of PET by allowing combined PET and CT studies to be acquired quasi-simultaneously with perfect alignment of anatomical and metabolic imaging data. While most clinical studies showed relatively modest improvement in diagnostic accuracy through the sensitivity and specificity of hybrid PET/CT over PET

O. Ratib et al. (eds.), *Atlas of PET/MR Imaging in Oncology*,
DOI 10.1007/978-3-642-31292-2_1, © Springer-Verlag Berlin Heidelberg 2013

and CT performed separately, several studies demonstrated however a significant improvement in diagnostic confidence when both studies were acquired together and images were interpreted with fusion of both modalities. Uncertainties of diagnostic findings that could occur when PET images are interpreted without accurate anatomical localization can be avoided when CT images are co-registered with PET images and provide the necessary anatomical references. Conversely, diagnostic criteria of CT based on structural and morphological observations can be often misleading and subject to difficult interpretation and can be significantly improved when additional metabolic information of PET is provided with combined PET/CT images. While MRI has replaced CT in many clinical applications by providing ability for higher tissue characterization and functional imaging, the added value of PET/MR over PET/CT still remains to be demonstrated in clinical practice. The most immediate application might be in patients that require both PET/CT and MRI in their clinical workup and could benefit from a single study combining PET and MR when CT is of no significant additional value.

Potentials and Challenges of PET/MR

Technical designs of hybrid PET/MR devices differ considerably between different vendors as shown in the next chapter of this book. While integrated system my represent the most logical solution they remain technically more challenging and coplanar systems combining two scanners adjacent to each other provide an alternative that resembles in its design current PET/CT systems where the patient is moved from one to the other modality sequentially. In oncology applications both sequential and simultaneous acquisition of images may provide similar results they differ only on the imaging protocols used.

The remaining challenge of all hybrid PET/MR systems is the calculation of tissue attenuation correction maps similar to those calculated from whole body CT scans in hybrid PET/CT devices. Several techniques of attenuation correction were explored, but the emphasis has been mainly on MR image segmentation for derivation of an attenuation map. Besides image segmentation, other technical challenges for effective attenuation correction in a whole-body PET/MR, including compensation for MR image truncation and correction for RF coils and accessories also need to be implemented. Accurate calculation of tissue attenuation aims mainly toward providing quantitative measurement of PET tracer uptake in tissue. Semi-quantitative calculation of standard tracer uptake (SUV) is the most common technique used today and provides an attractive simple method to estimate the amount of tracer uptake in different tissues. While it can allow for differentiating between benign physiological and potentially pathological tissue tracers uptake, it has only marginal added value in routine clinical practice when PET findings are combined with observations from other imaging modalities such as CT and MR and confronted with multiple other criteria in clinical decision making. It remains however necessary to achieve the best and most accurate correction of tissue attenuation to use PET imaging technology at its full potential and benefit from the added value of quantitative imaging over visual interpretation of PET findings.

The Challenge of Hybrid Imaging Protocols

Depending on the scanner design, imaging protocols can differ significantly depending on the ability to perform sequential or simultaneous acquisitions of both modalities. It remains however that one of the most challenging aspect of hybrid PET/MR is the complexity and heterogeneity of MR protocols that are being used in clinical practice. The wealth of different types of imaging parameters that MRI provides and the diversity and lack of standardization of different imaging protocols have lead to significant differences in protocols used in clinical practice. The general trend is that MR imaging protocols have considerably been extended to include several sequences for better tissue characterization and extraction of functional and physiological parameters of different tissues and organs. The combination for such complex protocols together with additional whole-body imaging sequences of PET and MRI can lead to significantly longer examination time. Therefore, additional efforts and research is needed to optimize hybrid imaging protocols to benefit from the best potential capabilities of each modality while maintaining reasonable imaging time that is compatible with routine clinical practice.

Domains of Clinical Applications of PET/MR

The primary clinical applications of PET/MR that we elected to cover in this book are in oncology. But there are other emerging applications in cardiovascular, in inflammatory and infectious disease as well as in neurodegenerative diseases. MRI has gained a wide adoption in cardiology for the detection of ischemic disease, myocardial viability ad cardiac function. The added value and complementarity of PET in providing a better sensitivity and quantitative analysis of myocardial perfusion and myocardial viability can become good clinical justifications for combined PET/MR studies.

Brain imaging for acute as well as chronic disease often rely on combination of multiple imaging modalities such as PET and MR. In brain imaging however, the rigidity of the head and the easily identifiable skull structures, allow software-based registration technique to provide adequate fusion of different imaging modalities. A wider availability of hybrid PET/MR can however facilitate the use of hybrid imaging for brain studies with more convenience to the patient that does not have to undergo separate studies on different scanners.

Another factor that favors MRI over CT for hybrid imaging is the reduction in radiation exposure. Although for elderly patient and patients under palliative treatment for cancer, radiation exposure may be of minor impact, reduced radiation exposure of PET/MRI compared with PET/CT may be relevant in non-oncological patients and in younger patients with potentially curable disease.

Future of PET/MR in Oncology

This book highlights the potential applications of whole-body hybrid PET/MR in oncology. While it is still a collection of convincing anecdotal cases, it only reflects early observations of two academic centers that were first in adopting this new technique in clinical practice. The diversity of cases and broad scope of clinical domains covered in the different chapters of the book underline the potential applications in oncology but also in other clinical domains. The use of different radiolabeled tracers such as ^{18}F-fluorocholine and ^{18}F-fluorotyrosine show the potential of PET beyond the conventional ^{18}F-FDG tracer in clinical applications of hybrid PET/MR. However this new imaging modality has only been recently introduced for clinical use and will face the same challenges and skepticism that PET/CT technique encountered when it was first introduced. The lack of tangible added value of combined PET/MR over the two examinations acquired separately is the first issue that needs to be addressed both from a clinical perspective and from a medico-economic point of view. It is however foreseeable that increasing demand for objective criteria in determination of adequacy and efficacy of new treatments, in particular in oncology, will drive the development of new tracers and innovative hybrid imaging protocols that take full advantage of complementarity of PET and MR modalities.

Further Reading

Antoch G, Bockisch A (2009) Combined PET/MRI: a new dimension in whole-body oncology imaging? Eur J Nucl Med Mol Imaging 36 Suppl 1:S113–S120

Antoch G, Saoudi N, Kuehl H et al (2004) Accuracy of whole-body dual-modality fluorine-18-2-fluoro-2-deoxy-D-glucose positron emission tomography and computed tomography (FDG-PET/CT) for tumor staging in solid tumors: comparison with CT and PET. J Clin Oncol 22:4357–4368

Bar-Shalom R, Yefremov N, Guralnik L et al (2003) Clinical performance of PET/CT in evaluation of cancer: additional value for diagnostic imaging and patient management. J Nucl Med 44:1200–1209

Beyer T, Pichler B (2009) A decade of combined imaging: from a PET attached to a CT to a PET inside an MR. Eur J Nucl Med Mol Imaging 36 Suppl 1:S1–S2

Beyer T, Weigert M, Quick HH et al (2008) MR-based attenuation correction for torso-PET/MR imaging: pitfalls in mapping MR to CT data. Eur J Nucl Med Mol Imaging 35:1142–1146

Chen W, Jian W, Li HT et al (2010) Whole-body diffusion-weighted imaging vs. FDG-PET for the detection of non-small-cell lung cancer. How do they measure up? Magn Reson Imaging 28:613–620

Collins CD (2007) PET/CT in oncology: for which tumours is it the reference standard? Cancer Imaging 7 Spec No A:S77–S87

Czernin J, Allen-Auerbach M, Schelbert HR (2007) Improvements in cancer staging with PET/CT: literature-based evidence as of September 2006. J Nucl Med 48 Suppl 1:78S–88S

Delso G, Ziegler S (2009) PET/MRI system design. Eur J Nucl Med Mol Imaging 36 Suppl 1:S86–S92

Heusner TA, Kuemmel S, Umutlu L et al (2008) Breast cancer staging in a single session: whole-body PET/CT mammography. J Nucl Med 49:1215–1222

Heusner TA, Kuemmel S, Koeninger A et al (2010) Diagnostic value of diffusion-weighted magnetic resonance imaging (DWI) compared to FDG PET/CT for whole-body breast cancer staging. Eur J Nucl Med Mol Imaging 37(6):1077–1086

Hofmann M, Pichler B, Scholkopf B, Beyer T (2009) Towards quantitative PET/MRI: a review of MR-based attenuation correction techniques. Eur J Nucl Med Mol Imaging 36 Suppl 1:S93–S104

Hu Z, Ojha N, Renisch S et al (2009) MR-based attenuation correction for a whole-body sequential PET/MR system. In: IEEE nuclear science symposium conference record, Orlando, 2009, pp 3508–3512

Lonsdale MN, Beyer T (2010) Dual-modality PET/CT instrumentation-today and tomorrow. Eur J Radiol 73:452–460

Punwani S, Taylor SA, Bainbridge A et al (2010) Pediatric and adolescent lymphoma: comparison of whole-body STIR half-Fourier RARE MR imaging with an enhanced PET/CT reference for initial staging. Radiology 255:182–190

Schmidt GP, Reiser MF, Baur-Melnyk A (2009) Whole-body MRI for the staging and follow-up of patients with metastasis. Eur J Radiol 70:393–400

Shao Y, Cherry SR, Farahani K et al (1997) Simultaneous PET and MR imaging. Phys Med Biol 42:1965–1970

PET/MR Instrumentation

2

T. Beyer, O. Mawlawi, and H.H. Quick

Contents

T. Beyer (✉)
Center for Medical Physics and Biomedical Engineering, General Hospital Vienna, Medical University Vienna, 4L Waehringer Guertel 18-20, 1090 Vienna, Austria
e-mail: thomas.beyer@meduniwien.ac.at

O. Mawlawi
Department of Imaging Physics, MD Anderson Cancer Center, Unit 1352, Houston, TX 77030, USA

H.H. Quick
Institute of Medical Physics (IMP), Friedrich-Alexander-University (FAU) Erlangen-Nürnberg, Henkestr. 91, 91052 Erlangen, Germany

Introduction

Anato-metabolic Imaging

Most people require diagnostic tests during their lifetime in order to detect a suspected malignancy, plan a therapy and follow-up on a treatment. In almost all of these cases diagnostic tests entail a single imaging examination or a series of complementary imaging exams. Non-invasive imaging is central to personalized disease management and includes imaging technologies such as Computed Tomography (CT), Single Photon Emission Computed Tomography (SPECT), Magnetic Resonance Imaging (MRI), Ultrasound (US) or Positron Emission Tomography (PET).

Each of the above imaging tests yields a wealth of information that can be separated generally into anatomical and metabolic information. Anatomical information, such as obtained from CT or US, is represented by a set of sub-mm resolution images that depict gross anatomy for organ and tissue delineation. Malignant disease is typically detected on these images by means of locally altered image contrast or by abnormal deviations from standard human anatomy. It is important to note, that anatomical changes do not necessarily relate to the onset of malignant diseases. In other words, malignant diseases are expressed as abnormal alterations of signaling or metabolic pathways that may lead to detectable anatomical changes. Therefore, anatomical imaging alone may miss diseases frequently or diagnose diseases at an advanced stage only.

PET, as a representative of nuclear medicine imaging methods, has been shown to support accurate diagnosis of malignant disease [1] as well as providing essential information for early diagnosis of neurodegenerative diseases [2] and malfunctions of the cardiovascular system [3]. However, over 90 % of all PET examinations are performed for oncology indications. PET is based on the use of trace amounts of radioactively labeled biomolecules, such as [18F]-FDG, a fluorine-18 labeled analogue to the glucose molecule, that are injected into the patient whereby the distribution of the

O. Ratib et al. (eds.), *Atlas of PET/MR Imaging in Oncology*,
DOI 10.1007/978-3-642-31292-2_2, © Springer-Verlag Berlin Heidelberg 2013

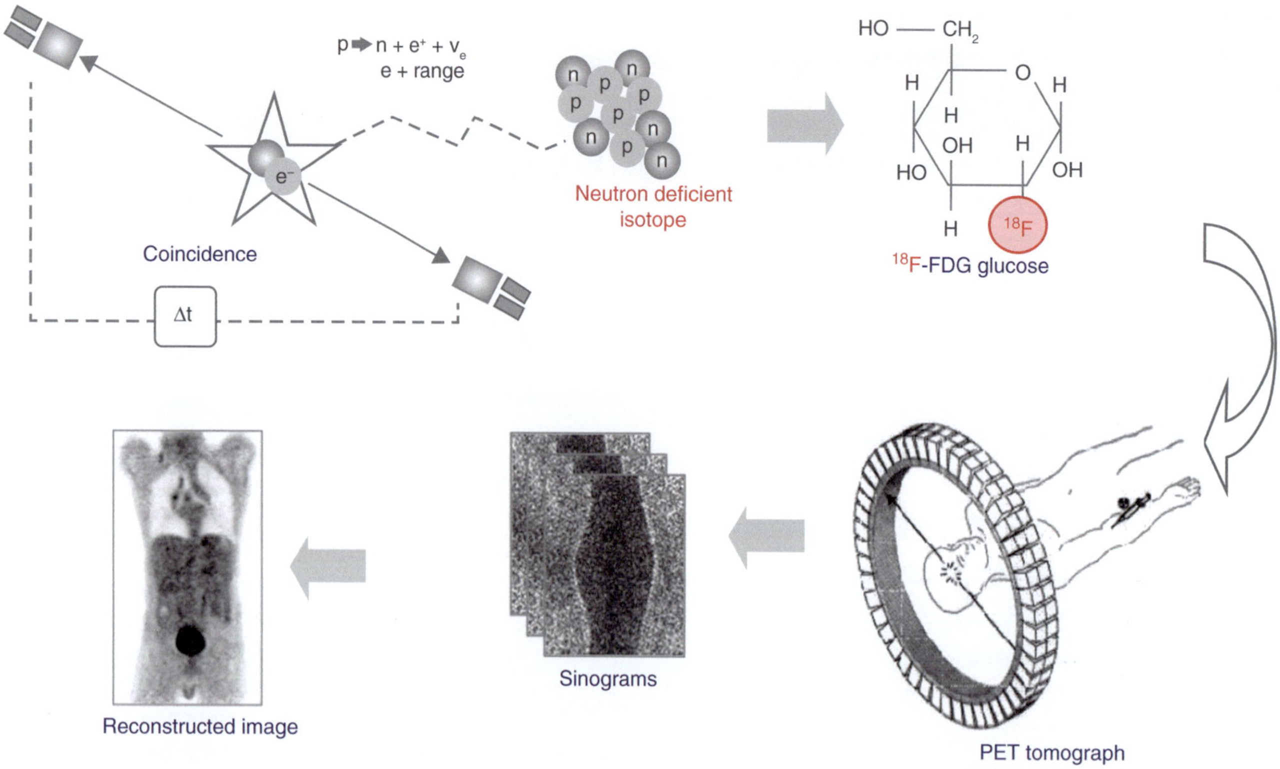

Fig. 2.1 Schematics of PET imaging: a biomolecule is labeled with a positron emitter (e.g., ^{18}F, $T_{1/2}$ ~ 109.8 min) and injected into the patients. The radioactive isotope label decays by emitting a positron, which annihilates with an electron from the surrounding tissue, thus creating two annihilation photons that are emitted back-to-back and detected by a ring of PET detectors. Image reconstruction then follows the same principles as in CT (Courtesy of David W Townsend, Singapore)

tracer is followed by detecting the annihilation photons resulting from the emission and annihilation of the positrons (Fig. 2.1).

In most cases of malignant diseases early diagnosis is key and, therefore, imaging the anatomy of a patient may not suffice in rendering a correct and timely diagnosis. Thus, medical doctors typically employ a combination of imaging techniques during the course of diagnosis and subsequent treatment to monitor their patients. Henceforth, both functional and anatomical information are essential in state-of-the-art patient management. An appreciation for this type of combined information is best illustrated with the introduction of the term "anato-metabolic imaging" [4], in reference to an ideal imaging modality that gathers both anatomical and functional information, preferably within the same examination.

Historically, medical devices to image either anatomical structure or functional processes have developed along somewhat independent paths. The recognition that combining images from different modalities can offer significant diagnostic advantages gave rise to sophisticated software techniques to co-register (aka align, fuse, superimpose) structure and function retrospectively (Fig. 2.2). The usefulness of combining anatomical and functional planar images was evident to physicians as early as in the 1960s [5]. Sophisticated image fusion software was developed from the late 1980s onwards. For relatively rigid objects such as the brain, software can successfully align images from MR, CT and PET, whereas in more flexible environments, such as the rest of the body, accurate spatial alignment is difficult owing to the large number of possible degrees of freedom. Alternatives to software-based fusion have now become available through instrumentation that combines two complementary imaging modalities within a single system, an approach that has since been termed hardware fusion. A combined, or hybrid, tomograph such as PET/CT can acquire co-registered structural and functional information within a single study. The data are complementary allowing CT to accurately localize functional abnormalities and PET to highlight areas of abnormal metabolism.

The advantages of integrated, anato-metabolic imaging are manifold [6]. A single imaging examination provides comprehensive information on the state of a disease. Consequently, functional information is gathered and displayed in an anatomical context. Patients are invited for only one, instead of multiple exams. As shown by several groups, the combination of complementary imaging modalities can yield synergy effects for the acquisition and processing of image data [7, 8]. And, finally, experts in radiology and nuclear medicine are forced to discuss and integrate their knowledge in one report, which will perhaps be more appreciated and considered a benefit in the years to come.

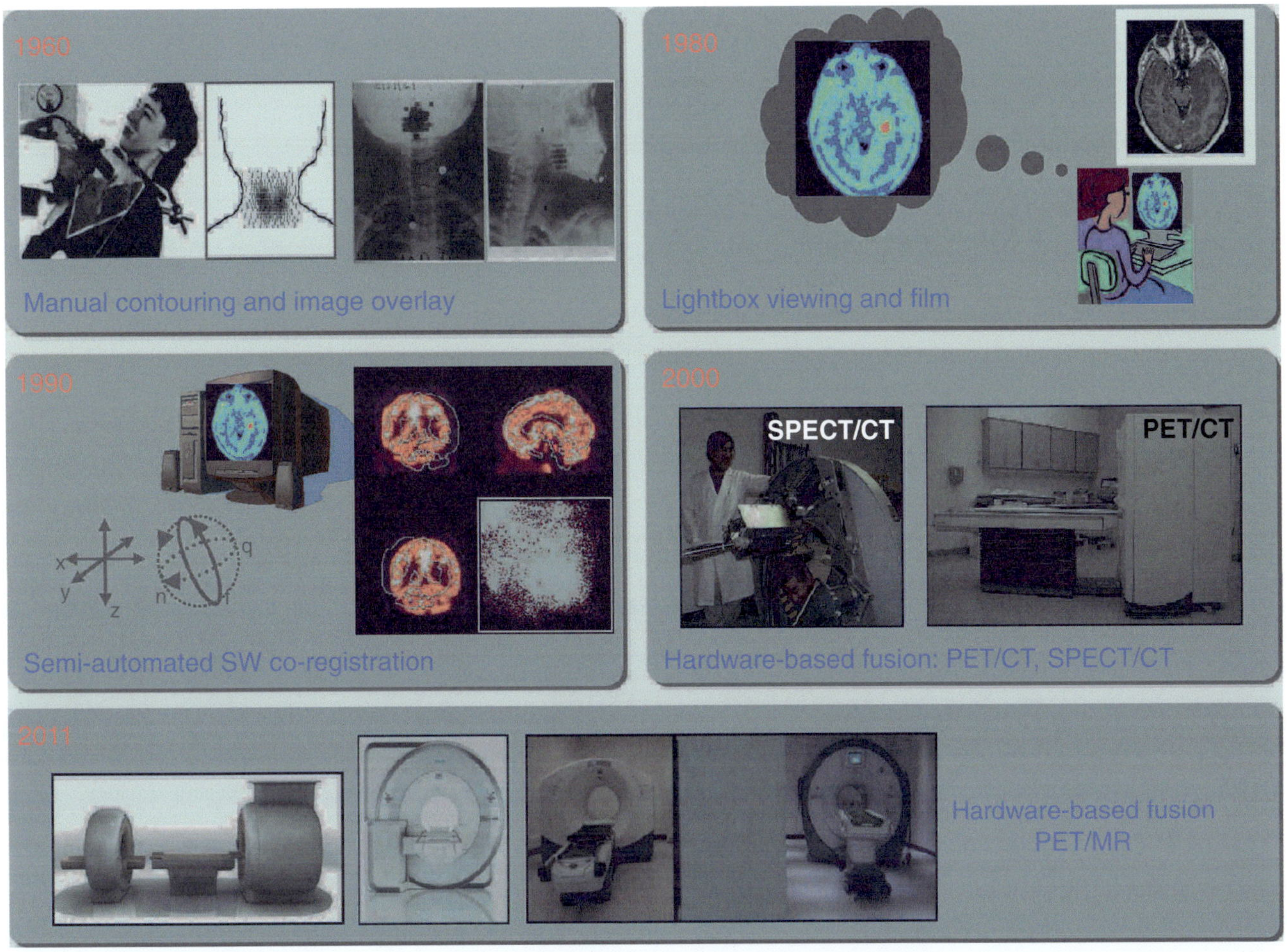

Fig. 2.2 The history of fusion imaging: from the 1960s to the 1990s complementary image information was aligned manually and later with the support of computer-based algorithms. With the introduction of prototype SPECT/CT and PET/CT imaging in the 1990s and PET/MR imaging systems in the mid 2000s the field of hardware image fusion was changed dramatically

PET/CT Imaging

PET imaging has been in clinical practice since the late 1980s, thus providing valuable information in addition to CT imaging in cases where complementary diagnostic information was clinically indicated. However, the lack of fine anatomical detail in PET images may limit the localization of lesions and permit only a poor definition of lesion boundaries. This challenge was overcome by combining high-resolution anatomical CT imaging with PET, thus, providing a hardware combination for "anato-metabolic" imaging [9]. The first proposal to combine PET with CT was made in the early 1990s by Townsend, Nutt and co-workers. The foremost benefit of a PET/CT hardware combination was the intrinsic alignment of complementary image information, further supported by a clinical need at the time. A secondary benefit of this combination came with the ability to use the CT images to derive the required PET attenuation correction factors, one of the pre-requisites for quantitative PET imaging [10]. CT-based attenuation correction has now become the standard in all PET/CT tomographs [11] despite the fact that some assumptions have to be made in order to transform the attenuation values of human tissues at CT energies (e.g. effective CT energies are on the order of 60–90 keV) to attenuation coefficients at the PET energy of 511 keV [12, 13]. Figure 2.3 illustrates the main drivers for PET/CT: anato-metabolic alignment and CT-based attenuation correction.

Following the introduction and validation of the first whole-body PET/CT prototype in 1998 [14] first commercial PET/CT concepts were proposed as of 2001 leading to a breadth of 25 different clinical PET/CT systems offered by six vendors worldwide in 2006. Today, four major vendors offer a range of whole-body PET/CT systems with greatly improved functionalities for both, PET and CT [15]. Table 2.1 summarizes the state-of-the-art PET/CT technology. In brief, all PET/CT systems permit total-body imaging within a single examination while using the available CT image

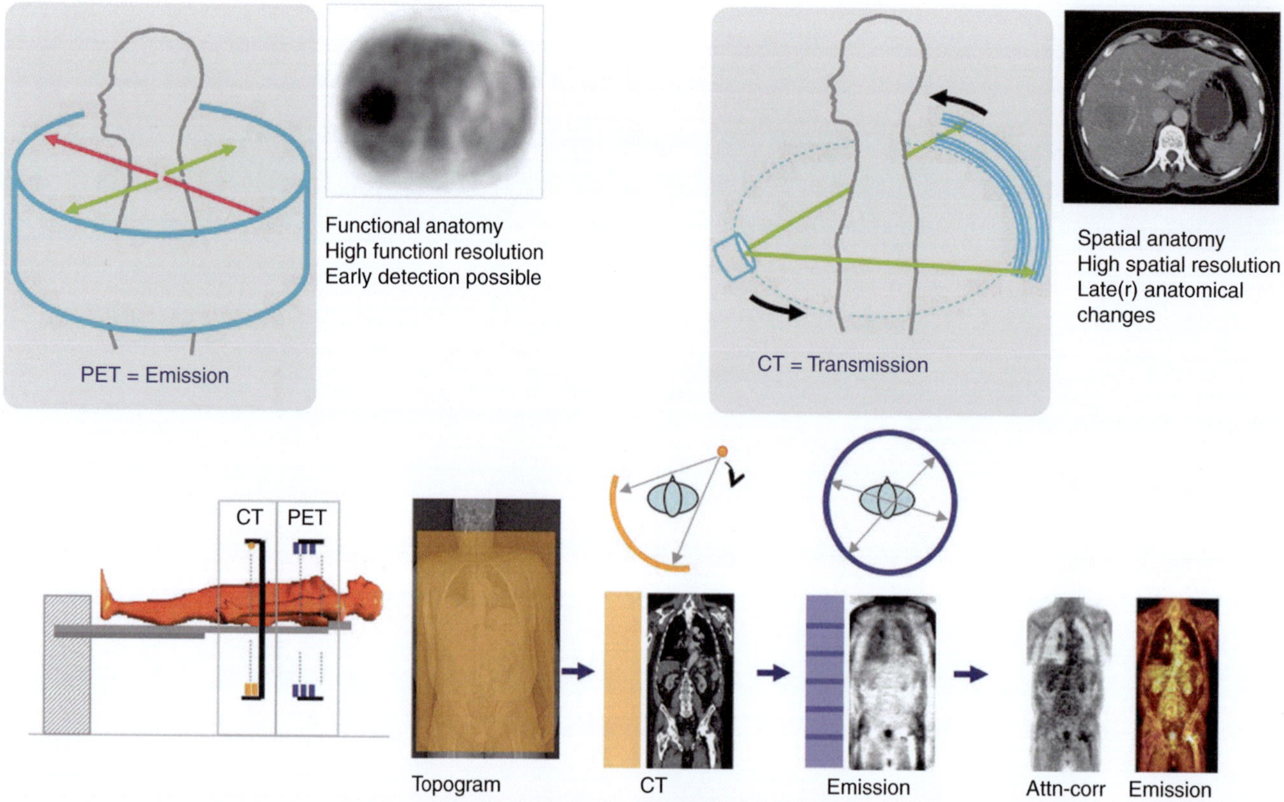

Fig. 2.3 PET and CT can be operated in close spatial proximity without cross-talk degradation of their respective performance parameters. (**a**) PET and CT images provide complementary diagnostic information. (**b**) The use of the CT transmission images for the purpose of noiseless attenuation correction of the emission data comes as a secondary benefit of PET/CT

information for routine attenuation and scatter correction of the PET data [6]. Major technical advances include the incorporation of time-of-flight (TOF) PET acquisition mode [16], the extension of the axial field-of-view (FOV) of the PET [17] and the incorporation of system information, such as the variability of the point spread function across the field-of-view, into the reconstruction process [17].

Time-of-flight-PET was first suggested in the late 1960s in order to improve the signal-to-noise ratio (SNR) of the PET data [18]. In essence, TOF-PET requires the measurement of the arrival time of two annihilation photons arising from a given annihilation; which helps localize the origin of the annihilation (i.e. the tracer) better. TOF-PET requires fast scintillation detectors and advanced detector electronics (see also section "MR-Compatible PET Detectors"). In human studies TOF-PET can help increase the SNR by a factor of 2. Today, still few studies are available that demonstrate a significant diagnostic benefit in routine clinical applications [19, 20], but the options for trading a gain in SNR into reduced injected activities or into shorter emission scan times are available today.

Extending the axial FOV of a PET system comes at the expense of more PET detectors to be added in the axial direction. However, for a given injected activity, more annihilation photon can be detected, thus, increasing the system sensitivity by 80 % for an additional 25 % axial coverage. This gain in sensitivity can be used for reduced emission scan times or activities injected. Despite the required increase in axial bed position overlap, the number of contiguous bed positions required to cover a given co-axial imaging range is reduced in case of PET imaging systems with an extended axial FOV.

Parallax errors arising from depth-of-interaction effects cause the spatial resolution of the PET to be a variant of the spatial location of the annihilation. If the spatial variation of the point-spread-function (PSF) is known a priori, for example, by means of standardized measurements, it can be included in the reconstruction algorithm [17, 21]. The reconstruction process becomes computationally demanding but helps improve the spatial resolution and renders the variations of the PSF in the images uniform across the field-of-view.

Over the years, the above advances have helped improve the quality and reproducibility of PET and PET/CT data (Fig. 2.4) and support a routine examination time for a standard whole-body FDG-PET/CT study of 15 min, or less, a significant advantage when compared to PET/CT imaging from a decade ago.

Table 2.1 State-of-the-art PET/CT imaging systems GE Healthcare, Philips Healthcare, Mediso and Siemens Healthcare (*from left to right*). The figure shows key parameters and performance measures of the PET/CT series

Discovery VCT	Ingenuity TF	AnyScan	Biograph mCT
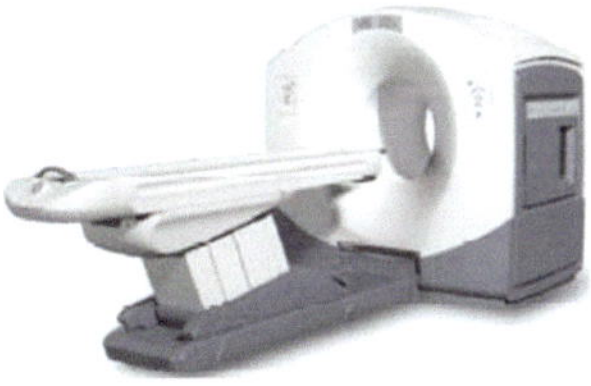	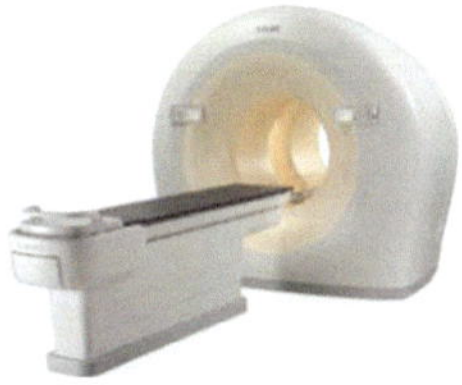	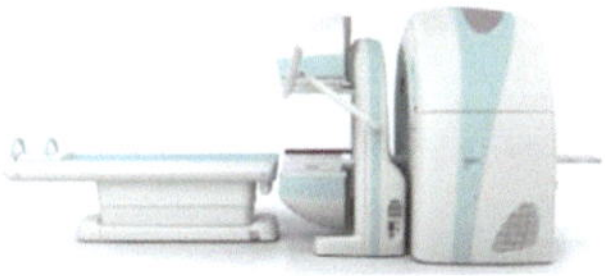	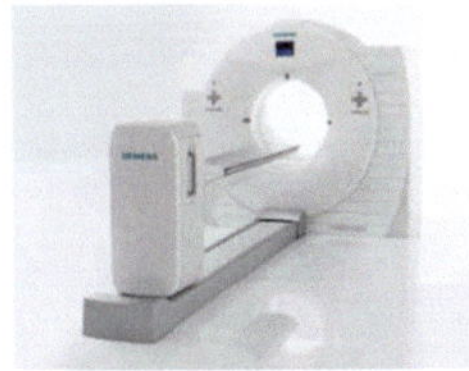
CT: 16-128 slices	CT: 16-128 slices	16-slice CT	CT: 20-128
70 cm patient port	70 cm (85 cm) patient port	70 cm diameter patient port	78 cm patient port
250 kg table weight limit	215 kg table weight limit	250 kg table weight limit	250 kg table weight limit
170 cm co-scan range	190 cm co-scan range	360 cm co-scan range	170 cm co-scan range
24 rings of LYSO(Ce)	44 rings of LYSO(Ce)	24 rings of LYSO(Ce)	52 rings of LSO (Ce) crystals
4.2 x 6.3 x 25 mm^3	4.0 x 4.0 x 22 mm^3	3.9 x 3.9 x 20 mm^3	4.0 x 4.0 x 20 mm^3
Time-of-flight	Time-of-flight		Time-of-flight
15.1 cm axial FOV	18 cm axial coverage	23 cm axial coverage	21.6 cm axial coverage
70 cm transaxial FOV	67 cm transaxial FOV	55 cm transaxial FOV	70 cm transaxial FOV
PET resolution model	PET resolution model		PET resolution model
In-plane resolution: 4.9 mm	In-plane resolution: 4.7 mm	In-plane resolution: 4.1 mm	In-plane resolution: 4.4 mm
Axial resolution: 5.6 mm	Axial resolution: 4.7 mm	Axial resolution: 4.2 mm	Axial resolution: 4.4 mm
3D Sensitivity: 7.0 cps/kBq	3D Sensitivity: 7.0 cps/kBq	3D Sensitivity: 8.1 cps/kBq	3D Sensitivity: 9.7 cps/kBq
Peak NECR: 110 kcps	Peak NECR: 110 kcps	Peak NECR: 150 kcps	Peak NECR: 180 kcps
Scatter: 38% (425 keV)	Scatter: 30% (440 keV)	Scatter: 38% (425 keV)	Scatter: 33% (435 keV)
Coincidence : 4.9 ns	Coincidence : 3.8 ns	Coincidence : 5.0 ns	Coincidence : 4.1 ns
TOF resolution: 549 ps	TOF resolution: 495 ps		TOF resolution: 527 ps

Since 1998, PET/CT imaging has rapidly emerged as an important imaging tool in oncology [22], also supported by above technological advances. There is, mainly for oncology, a growing body of literature that supports the increased accuracy of staging and restaging with PET/CT compared to either CT or PET acquired separately [8]. These improvements are incremental when compared to PET, whereby PET-only demonstrates high levels of sensitivity and specificity for a wide range of disease states already. However, improvement in accuracy of PET/CT compared with PET or CT for staging and restaging is statistically significant and averages 10–15 % over all cancers [8].

Expectations Towards PET/MR

In view of the global success of PET/CT imaging with respect to both diagnostic accuracy and workflow aspects, the expectations for any new combination, such as PET/MR are very high. First and foremost, combinations of PET and MR have been discussed and prototyped since the 1990's, starting at about the same time as PET/CT. However, while PET/CT was conceptualized based on a rather well-defined clinical need to combine functional and anatomical information from PET and CT, respectively, the developments towards an integrated PET/MR system were triggered by pre-clinical research endeavours [23]. In a well-written review of the origins of PET/MR Wehrl and colleagues reason that combined PET/MR has the potential to address major concerns in small animal imaging, such as very high exposure rates from (repeat) CT examinations and unacceptably long anesthesia times of the animals when examining them consecutive in PET and CT, or MR [24].

Almost a decade after the introduction of small animal imaging PET/MR prototype systems, industry took over that idea and presented first design concepts for clinical PET/MR systems as early as 2006. Figure 2.5 presents some key promotional factors for PET/MR in the context of the known benefits and limitations of PET/CT. First, combined PET/MR is appealing because it represents a major technological advancement. Further, assuming technical feasibility, an integrated PET/MR technology could permit simultaneous anato-metabolic

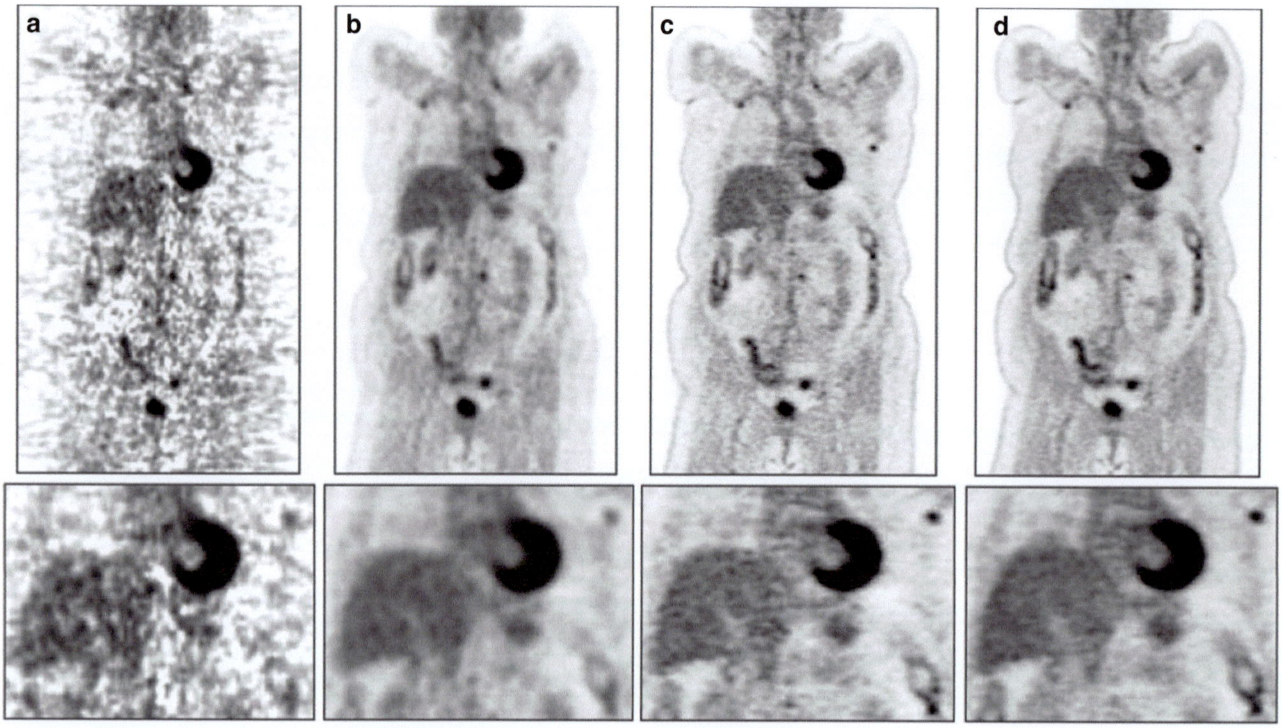

Fig. 2.4 Coronal (*top*) and transaxial (*bottom*) view of an whole-body [18F]-FDG-PET image of a patient with a BMI of 35 acquired in 3D-mode with septa retracted and reconstructed using: (**a**) 3D filtered back-projection algorithm with reprojection (3D-FBRP, 7 mm Gauss), (**b**) clinical reconstruction using FORE rebinning + 2D OSEM (8 subsets, 3 iterations; 5 mm filter), (**c**) 3D Ordinary Poisson (OP)-OSEM with PSF reconstruction (14 subsets, 2 iterations; no smoothing), and (**d**) 3D OP-OSEM with both PSF and Time-of-Flight (TOF) reconstruction (14 subsets, 2 iterations, no smoothing) (Case courtesy of DW Townsend, Singapore)

Fig. 2.5 Expectations for PET/MR in the context of the existing experiences with PET/CT for patient imaging

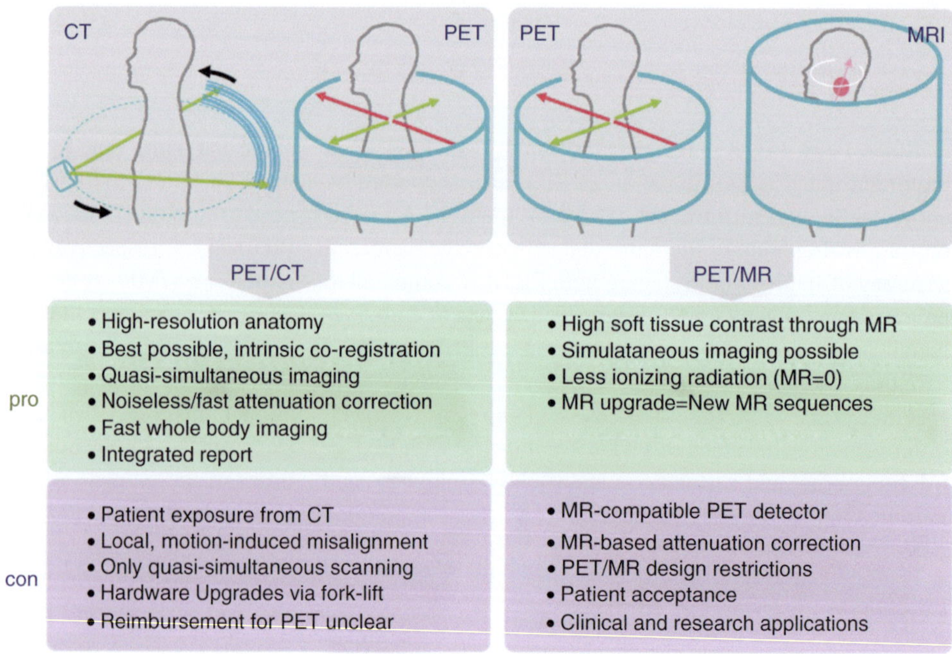

imaging together, with the added potential of MR-based motion correction of the PET data, significantly reduced patient exposure and a increased soft tissue contrast through the use of MR instead of CT, wherever clinically indicated.

Soft tissue enhancement in MR (versus CT) may benefit the imaging of pediatric patients where normally little fatty tissues are present (Fig. 2.6), as well as for studying patients for indications related to the brain, parenchymal organs or the

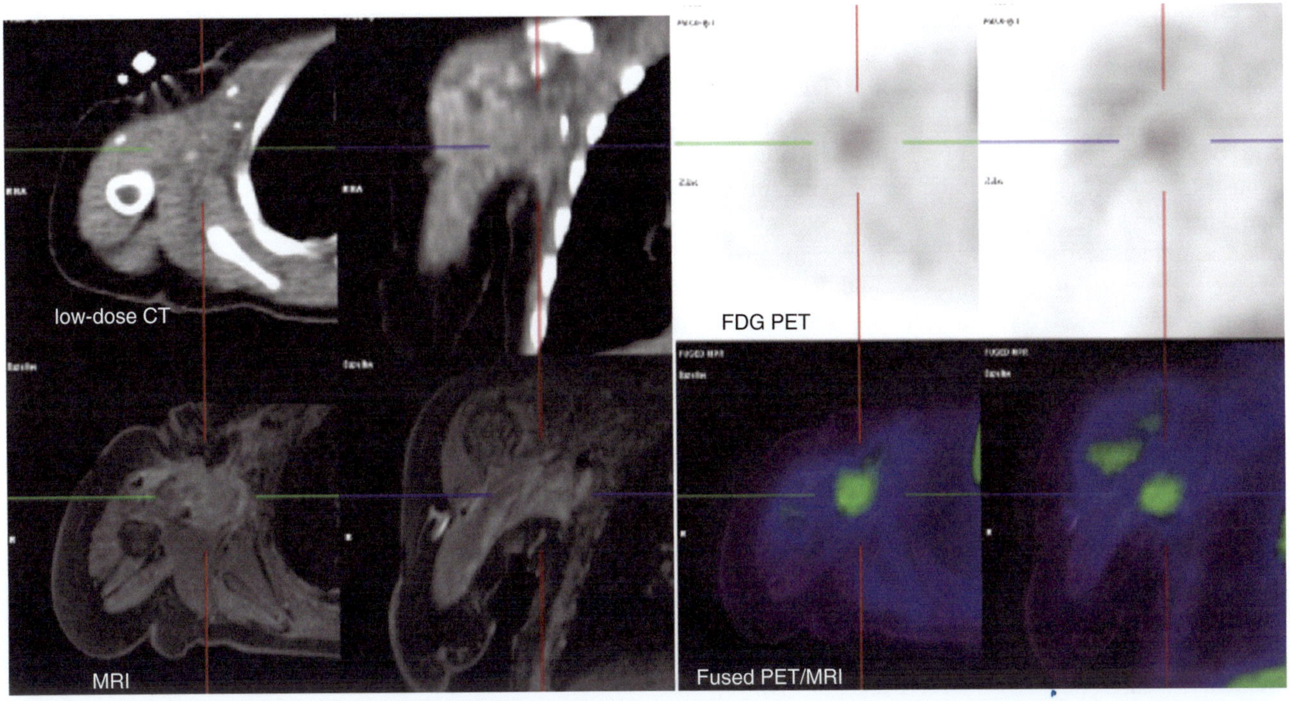

Fig. 2.6 Side-by-side comparison of CT, MR and PET images of a patient with previously irradiated fibrosarcoma. The tumour is poorly visualised on CT but the MRI shows a residual mass. The PET shows residual moderate FDG-avidity, and resection confirmed residual viable tumour. Lack of soft tissue contrast, particularly lack of fat in children compromises anatomical evaluation on CT compared to MRI (Courtesy of Rod Hicks, Peter MacCallum Cancer Centre, Melbourne Australia)

musculoskeletal system. In addition to much improved soft tissue contrast MR is a versatile imaging modality since it provides additional measures of physiologic and metabolic characteristics of human tissue [25]. MRI goes beyond plain anatomical imaging by offering a multitude of endogenous contrasts and a high capability of differentiating soft tissues, as well as many exogenous contrast media ranging from gadolinium-based agents to highly specified cellular markers [26].

MR spectroscopy (MRS), for example, can be used to dissect the molecular composition of tissues by applying selective radiofrequency excitation pulses [27]. Functional processes in living subjects can also be studied via diffusion-weighted (DWI) MRI [28]. Here, a spatially and temporally variant magnetic field, generated by different magnetic field gradients in all three spatial directions, is used to map phase differences in the MRI signal that are caused by diffusing molecules. DWI-MRI has potential clinical applications ranging from diagnosing ischemia in early stroke diagnostics, cancer, multiple sclerosis, or Alzheimer's disease to general fiber tracking via diffusion tensor imaging (DTI) [26, 29, 30], and it is not restricted to the brain [31]. In addition, functional MRI (fMRI) studies can be performed during the same examination. Functional MRI (fMRI) studies are frequently based on the BOLD (blood oxygen level dependent) effect [32]. This effect describes the fact that the magnetic properties of oxygenated and deoxygenated hemoglobin in the blood are different and, therefore, produce different signals when imaged with T2*-sensitive MRI sequences. The BOLD effect also has certain applications in cancer imaging, such as to study tumor angiogenesis, tumor oxygenation and brain activation in eloquent areas prior to surgical resection.

Any of the image information above can be acquired and presented in any direction in space, thus rendering re-orientation of image information in MR similar to a "virtual tilt", that is available in CT-only in directions perpendicular to the main scanner axis, and that are not available in PET/CT imaging.

Similar to CT and PET, MRI has become a whole-body imaging modality thanks, for example, to the advent of parallel imaging techniques and all their derivatives [33–35] and thanks to new whole-body imaging strategies [36, 37]. Image acquisition times have been shortened, thus allowing fast single-contrast MR whole-body coverage from 30 s [36] ranging to multi-contrast, multi-station whole-body MRI examinations to be acquired with high spatial resolution in less than 1 h. Initial results show that whole-body MRI is a promising modality in oncology, especially for the detection of metastases and hematologic malignancies.

Therefore, MRI holds a great potential in replacing CT as the complementary modality to PET in dual-modality tomographs for selected indications where MR outperforms CT already. In theory, MRI seems a perfect anatomical complement to PET.

PET/MR Design Concepts

Following the successful adoption of PET/CT in clinical routine and the ongoing efforts towards combining PET and MRI for pre-clinical research applications [24], industry has quickly adopted the idea of combining PET and MRI for human studies. Figure 2.7 summarizes the main approaches towards PET/MR hardware fusion. In essence, three different design concepts have been proposed: separate PET/CT and MRI systems operated in adjacent rooms (a), PET and MRI systems arranged in the direction of the main scanner axis with a patient handling system mounted in between (b) and a fully integrated PET/MRI system (c).

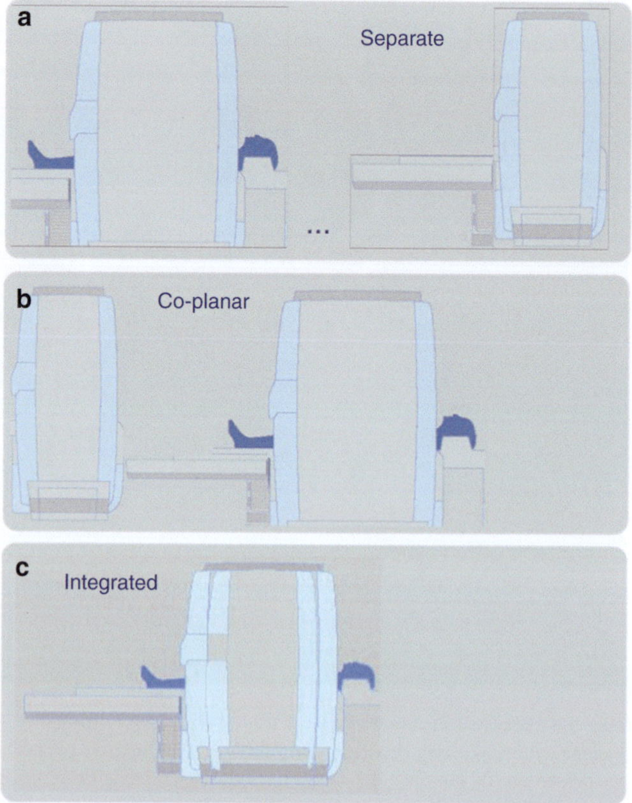

Fig. 2.7 Design concepts for PET/MR: PET/CT and MRI tomographs are operated in adjacent rooms and interlinked with a mobile shuttle system (**a**), a co-planar PET/MR with a whole-body PET and MR operated in close proximity and a combined table platform (**b**), and a fully integrated PET/MR with MR-compatible PET detection system slip-fit into the MR (**c**)

PET/CT-MR Shuttle System

GE Healthcare proposed a straightforward design in late 2010. This design is based on a combination of a dual-modality, whole-body TOF-PET/CT and a 3 T MR system that are operated in adjacent rooms; patients are shuttled from one system to the other without getting off the bed [38]. This approach substitutes the challenges of hardware integration for immense logistical challenges in timing access to the two systems while minimizing patient motion in between examinations. The advantage of this rather simplistic approach to PET/MR is that it is based on existing imaging technologies without significant changes to their hardware components. Patients undergo a PET/CT study leveraging the benefits of time-of-flight PET as discussed before. Following the PET/CT examination patients are then lifted on a mobile docking-table system and shuttled to the MR system where a loco-regional or whole-body MR study is performed depending on the clinical indication. Figure 2.8 illustrates a clinical case from the combined use of PET/CT and MRI using the PET/CT/MR system.

While this design is still available as prototype technology only, it has been argued also as the most cost-effective compared to fully integrated PET/MR based on workflow aspects and machine utilization [39], both of which are site- and operations dependent. Therefore, in practice the clinical and cost efficacy of the separate PET/CT/MR design option (Fig. 2.7a) would be affected by various workflow and installation requirements. For example, both systems need to be installed next to each other and operated within a combined scheduling system. Any deviation from standard protocols would entail extended waiting times with the patients lying on the shuttle system until the next exam can commence. Also, two or even three shuttle systems are required to facilitate a seamless, high-throughput workflow. On the upside this approach does ensure proper attenuation and scatter correction of the PET data based on the available CT information. In turn, the examination time is likely to be the longest of all PET/MR designs and patient convenience is limited by the repositioning in MR or PET/CT using the shuttle system.

Co-planar PET/MR

Philips Healthcare proposed a slightly more integrated approach to PET/MR in 2010 [40]. They also presented the first commercially available PET/MR system for clinical use called the Philips Ingenuity TF PET/MRI. The system (Fig. 2.7b) is based on a co-planar design concept that integrates a whole-body time-of-flight (TOF) PET system and an Achieva 3 T X-series MR system. Both components are joined by a rotating table platform mounted in between [41].

The PET detector and electronics system is based on available Philips PET/CT technology. However, given the proximity of the PET and MR system (about 4 m) some modifications were required to ensure MR-compatibility of the PET system. These modifications include the addition of bulk magnetic shielding of the PET to reduce fringe magnetic fields, the use of higher permeability shields of the photomultiplier tubes

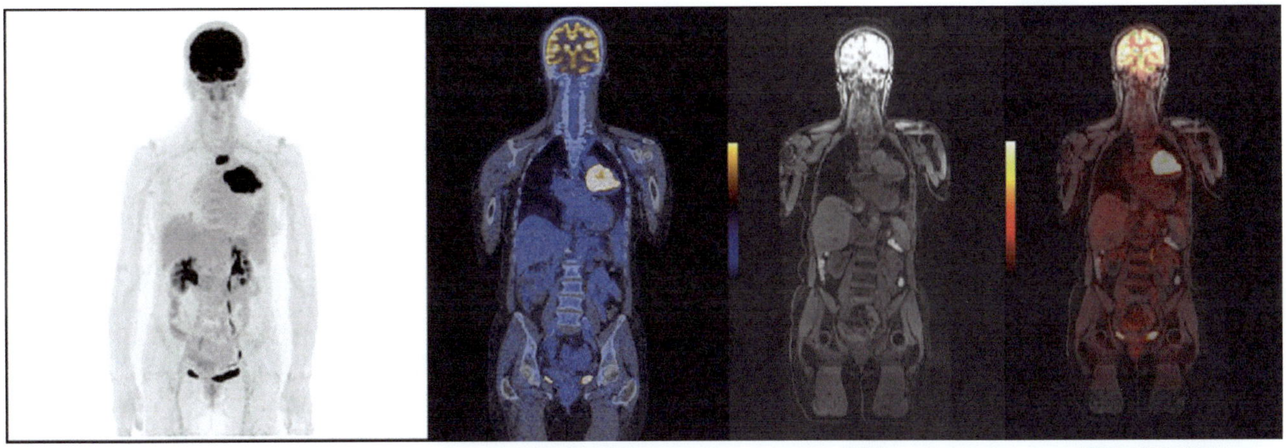

Fig. 2.8 Patient with large left lung lesion undergoing whole-body FDG-PET/CT and whole-body MRI on the separate PET/CT/MR system (Fig. 2.7a). *From left to right*: FDG-PET following CT-based attenuation correction (CT-AC), PET after CT-AC fused with whole-body CT, complementary WB-MR and retrospectively aligned and fused PET(/CT)-MR (Data courtesy of Patrick Veit-Haibach, MD, University Hospital Zürich)

(PMT) inside the PET gantry and the rotation of the cathodes of the PMT's. Further, power and signal cables penetrating the room walls need to be filtered through specially designed radiofrequency (RF) penetration panels to prevent extraneous electromagnetic radiation to enter the scanner room and PET acquisition electronics are enclosed in an RF tight cabinet. These and other modifications are discussed in more detail in [41]. The authors show that despite the modifications to the PET/MRI system components the performance of neither the PET nor of the MR is degraded, and that both systems can be operated in close spatial proximity.

Figure 2.9 illustrates a total-body imaging examination from the co-planar PET/MR system. While this design concept may be regarded as a step closer towards integrated PET/MR (compared to sequential imaging, Fig. 2.7a) it offers sequential PET and MRI imaging with delays that are on the order of those in PET/CT and in sequential PET/CT-MR imaging [42]. It could be argued that co-registration of PET and MR information is slightly better and, perhaps more reproducible, in both modalities compared to the shuttle system in Fig. 2.7a, since patients are not relocated between rooms and repositioned using a mobile patient handling system. However, no study to date has been able to verify this. Unlike with the separate PET/CT-MR system, one modality is idling during co-planar PET/MR imaging, which may be argued to be less cost-effective. However, one should keep in mind that today few indications are clearly defined as key indications for PET/MR, and, therefore, throughput is likely not an issue for the time being. The co-planar PET/MR system offers full MR-flexibility and TOF-PET functionality. Unlike with the separate design, no transmission source is available, thus requiring MR-based attenuation correction methods (see below).

Integrated PET/MR

The first PET/MR design for human use was presented as early as in 2006, representing also the most challenging design concept (Fig. 2.7c) [43]. This PET/MR prototype system (BrainPET, Siemens Healthcare) was intended for brain imaging only and considered a proof-of-concept for a fully integrated PET/MR. The BrainPET system was based on a PET detector ring designed as an insert to a 3T whole-body MR scanner (Magentom Trio, Siemens Healthcare Sector, Erlangen, Germany) with the novelty being the MR-compatible PET detection system that was integrated into the MR system. Here, the PMT were replaced by Avalanche photodiodes (APD), which have been shown to operate in magnetic fields of up to 7 T [44] (see also section "MR-Compatible PET Detectors"). Therefore, in this design LSO (lutetium oxyorthosilicate)-based detector blocks, comprising of a 12 × 12 matrix of 2.5 × 2.5 × 20 mm^3 crystals were directly coupled to a compact 3 × 3 APD array. With this system PET and MRI cover an active co-axial FOV of 19.3 cm simultaneously. The point source sensitivity of the PET system measured with a line source in air was 5.6 % and the spatial resolution was 2.1 mm at the centre of the FOV. No degradation of the MR images was observed due to the presence of the PET detectors and no detrimental effect on the performance of the PET detectors was observed for a number of standard MR pulse sequences [45]. Since 2006 the BrainPET was installed at 4 sites worldwide, with one site operating the PET insert inside a 9.4 T MRI as well. Some preliminary clinical research data are described in [46–48]. Looked upon retrospectively, the clinical test phase of the BrainPET helped pave the road towards whole-body PET/MR, the advanced development of MR-based attenuation

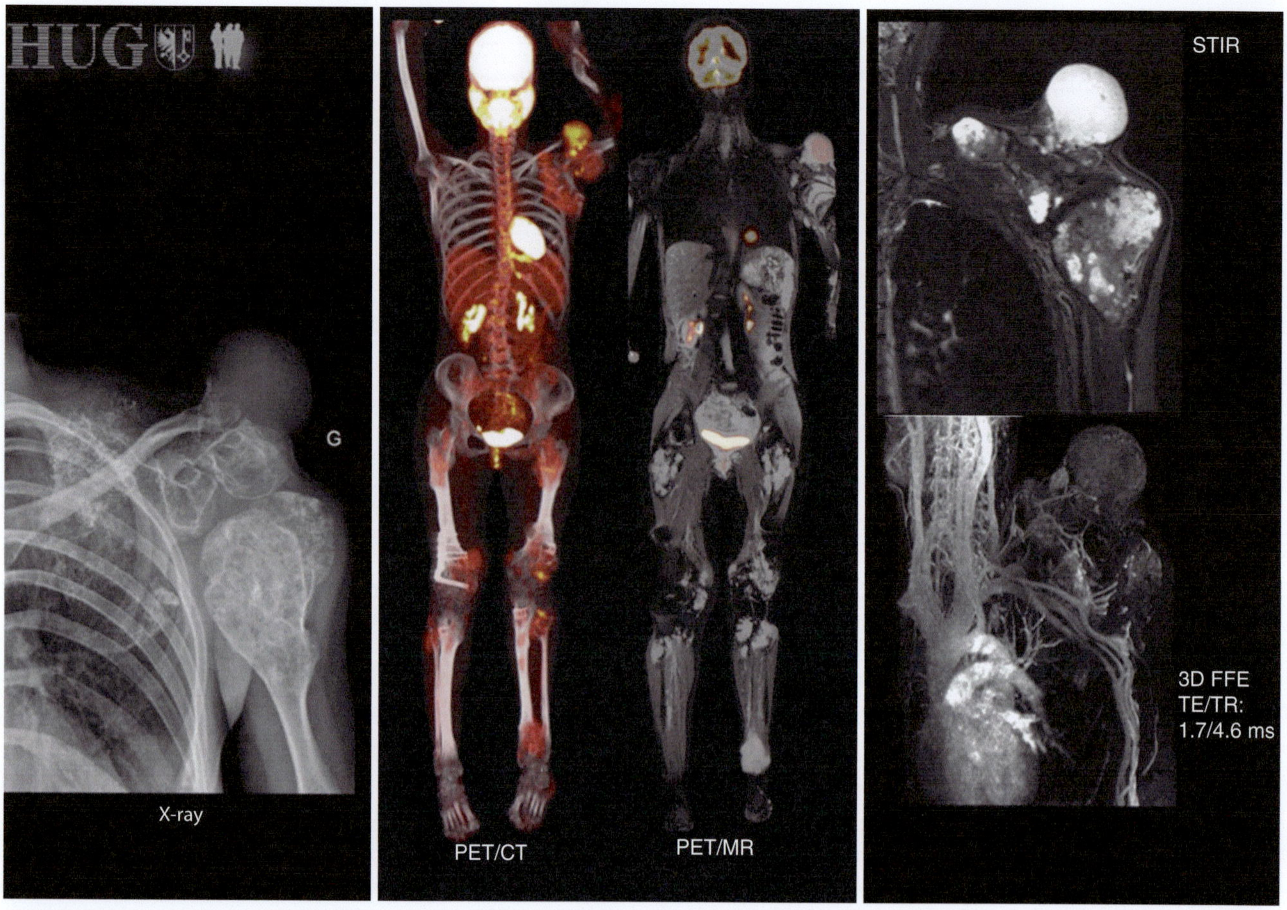

Fig. 2.9 29-y/o female patient with Maffucci syndrome diagnosed in her childhood. This disease is sporadic with multiple enchondromas and hemangiomas. An [18F]-FDG-PET/CT total body study was performed for staging. Subsequent total-body PET/MR, using the same FDG injection, more clearly presents bone involvement and is preferred because of the need of multiple follow-up examinations (Data courtesy of Osman Ratib, MD, University Hospital Geneva)

correction and, perhaps most importantly, an improved communication and closer collaboration of radiologists, nuclear medicine physicians and physicists.

Based on the aforementioned positive BrainPET experiences a further step towards the integrated design concept (Fig. 2.7c) was suggested in late 2010. Then, the first whole-body, integrated PET/MRI system (Biograph mMR, Siemens Healthcare) was proposed. Each PET detector block consists of an 8×8 matrix of LSO crystals coupled to a 3×3 APD-array. The transaxial FOV of the MR is 50 cm, whereas the axial FOV is 45 cm. The PET subsystem consists of 8 rings of 56 blocks with an axial FOV of 25.8 cm and ring diameter of 65.6 cm. Both, the extended axial FOV of the PET and the reduced ring diameter help increase the sensitivity of the PET insert, which in turn could be leveraged, for example, for shorter emission scan times or reduced injected PET activities. Thus, the lack of TOF-capability in APD-based PET systems (see Chap. 3) can be compensated for, in theory, by bringing the PET detectors closer to the centre of the FOV and by extending the axial coverage. A detailed description of the system together with a performance characteristic can be found in [49]. On the downside of the closer integration the integrated PET/MR system, the bore diameter is reduced to 60 cm, which – for the moment – is the reverse trend of PET/CT and MR-only instrumentation with gantry and bore diameters of up to 80 and 70 cm, respectively. Increased gantry and bore diameters help improve patient comfort and compliance and, in addition, leave room for image-guided interventions, if needed.

Perhaps most importantly, the integrated PET/MR design concept allows for simultaneous data acquisition. However, simultaneity of complementary volumetric data acquisition is assured only for a selected MR sequence and emission data that are acquired for the duration of that specific MR sequence. Nonetheless, simultaneous PET/MR is argued to improve the diagnostic accuracy of combined PET/MR over sequential imaging (Fig. 2.7a, b). Figure 2.10 illustrates a case from the Biograph mMR system with very good spatial alignment of PET and MR images in the abdomen.

While the benefit from improved spatio-temporal alignment is immanent to the PET/MR images from integrated PET/MR it is not clear as to how much it is required for clinical

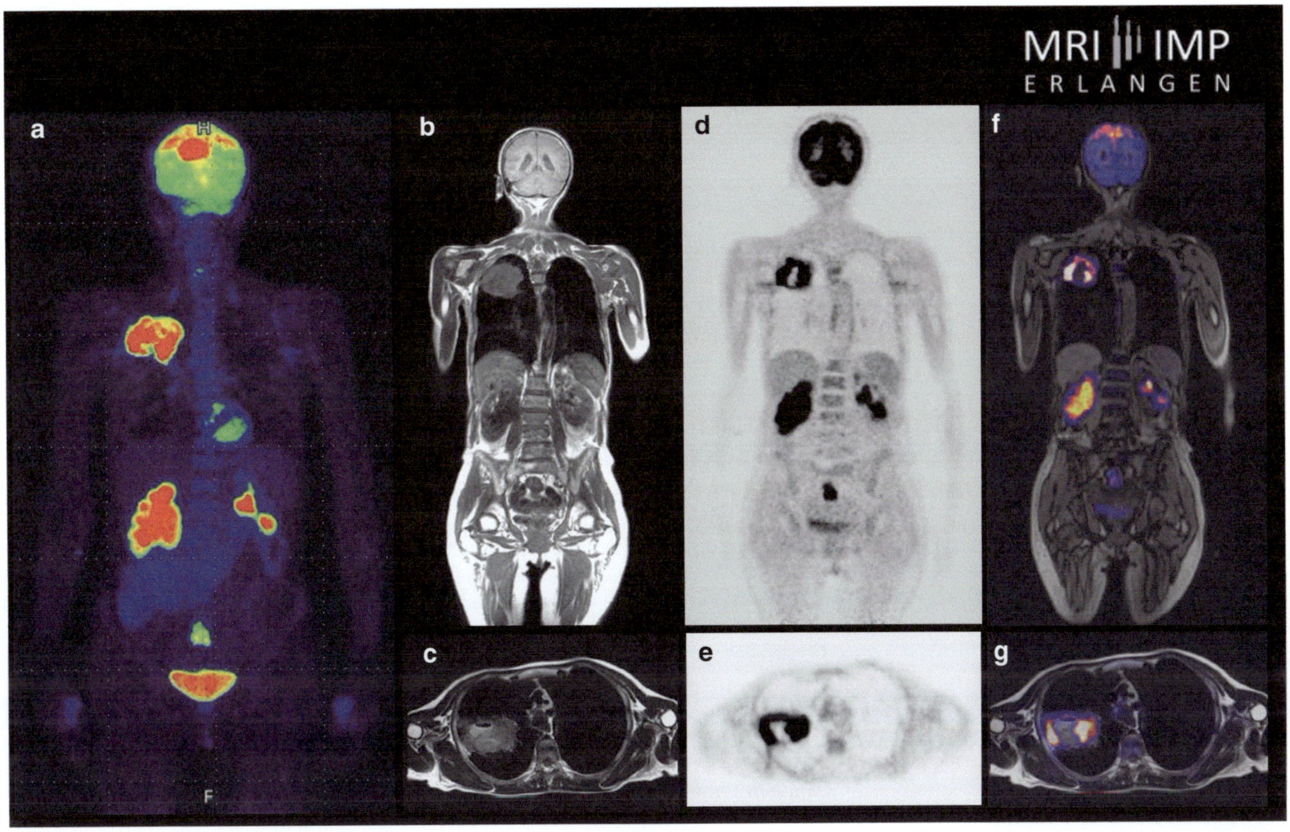

Fig. 2.10 61-y/o female with known squamous cell carcinoma of the lung undergoing [18F]-FDG-PET/MR imaging on an integrated Biograph mMR PET/MR system. (**a**) Increased PET tracer activity synonymous of disseminated disease is depicted in the bronchial carcinoma, frontal lobe metastasis, pancreas and in secondary, metastatic colorectal cancer. Coronal whole-body T1-weighted MR image (**b**), attenuation corrected PET (**d**), and PET/MR image (**f**) and corresponding axial images through the bronchial carcinoma are shown (**c**, **e**, **g**)

routine. Further, PET and MR data are simultaneously acquired only for a limited period of time or for a selected region, or voxel in its extreme. Without a doubt, the closer alignment of PET and MR data in both, an anatomical framework and over various imaging times will help in clinical research, such as when comparing perfusion studies with [15O]-water and arterial spin labeling (ASL) in MR [24]. Also, using integrated PET/MR imaging for shortening combined examination times over those in sequential and co-planar designs is preferred for the well-being of patients with acute diseases, pediatric patients requiring sedation and patients with neurodegenerative diseases. Finally, since MR-based motion detection is conceivable during simultaneous PET/MR imaging, such MR-derived motion vector can potentially be used to correct for motion-induced blurring of the PET emission data [50, 51].

As with the co-planar design, the integrated PET/MR design does not allow for separate transmission imaging and, therefore, PET-based attenuation data must be derived from the available MR information. Thus, a normal workflow starts with the simultaneous acquisition of emission data and a dedicated MR sequence for the purpose of deriving attenuation data. As soon as the short MR-attenuation sequence is complete, additional diagnostic MR sequences can be acquired for the remainder of the pre-defined emission scan. Alternatively, the PET emission data can be acquired in list-mode format and reframed after finishing the MR scan.

Table 2.2 provides an overview of currently available PET/MR systems. All systems support the acquisition of whole-body, if not total-body, examinations. These first PET/MR design concepts vary more widely than the first concepts for PET/CT. This variation can be explained by the complex physical and more demanding technical requirements for a full integration of PET and MR imaging systems, compared to those from a PET/CT integration.

The foremost difference between the PET/MR systems is the type of PET detector. Integrated PET/MR imaging requires a novel PET-based detection system, which will be explained in more detail in Chap. 3. APD-PET does not support TOF-based acquisitions due to the insufficient timing resolution of the APD, thus, only two PET/MR designs offer TOF-capabilities (Table 2.2). Major differences are also seen in the patient table design, which has subsequent effects on the handling of the patients and workflow. Both, the co-planar and the integrated PET/MR require the use of the MR images for human soft tissue attenuation correction, which today is perhaps the biggest challenge for combined PET/MR in the

Table 2.2 State-of-the-art PET/MR imaging systems by GE Healthcare, Philips Healthcare and Siemens Healthcare (*from left to right*). Note, as of 2012 the Philips and Siemens system were FDA-approved and commercially available. The figure shows key parameters and performance measures of the various PET/MR series

Discovery PET/CT-MR	Ingenuity TF	Biograph mMR
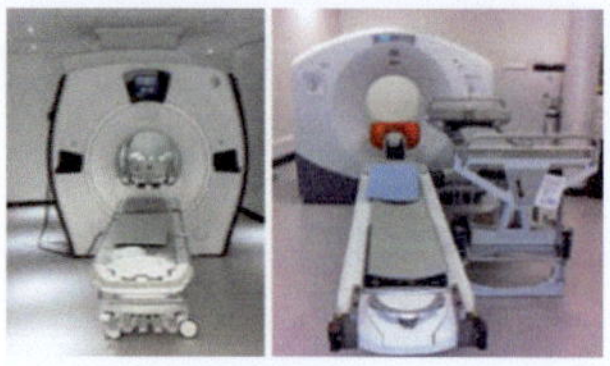	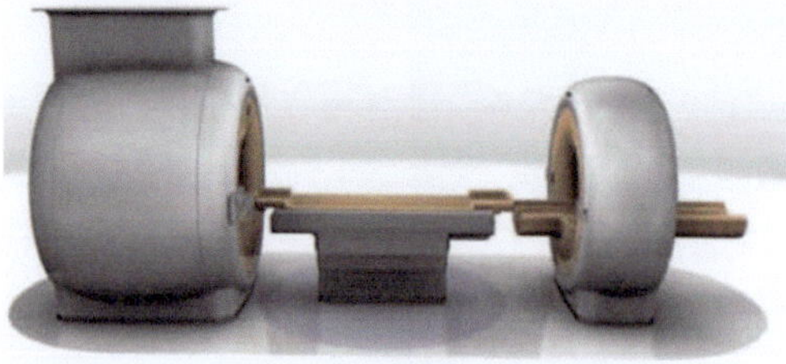	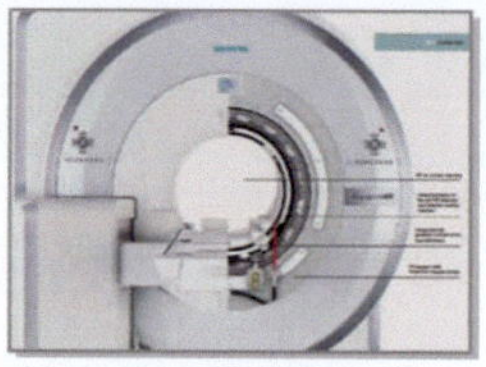
MR	**MR**	**MR**
Discovery MR 750w	Achieva 3T TX	3T (not Verio-based)
70 cm bore diameter	60 cm bore diameter	60 cm bore diameter
50 x 50 x 45 cm FOV	50 x 50 x 45 cm FOV	50 x 50 x 45 cm FOV
16 (32) receive channels	16 (32) receive channels	18 / 32 receive channels
0.5 ppm field homogeneity	0.5 ppm field homogeneity	0.1 ppm field homogeneity
PET	**PET**	**PET**
Discovery PET/CT 690		
4.2 x 6.3 x 25 mm^3 LYSO(Ce)	4.0 x 4.0 x 22 mm^3 LYSO(Ce)	4.0 x 4.0 x 20 mm^3 LSO
81 cm detector ring diameter	90 cm detector ring diameter	66 cm ring diameter
Time-of-flight PET	Time-of-flight PET	No Time-of-flight option
15.7 cm axial coverage	18 cm axial coverage	25.8 cm axial coverage
70 cm bore diameter	70 cm bore diameter	60 cm bore diameter
Patient handling system	**Patient handling system**	**Patient handling system**
Shuttle and docking system	Turning table platform	Integrated table platform
159 kg patient load	200 kg patient load	200 kg patient load
170 cm co-scan range	190 cm co-scan range	140 cm co-scan range
CT-based AC	MR-based AC	MR-based AC
In-plane resolution: 4.9 mm	In-plane resolution: 4.9 mm	In-plane resolution: 4.5 mm
Axial resolution: 5.6 mm	Axial resolution: 4.9 mm	Axial resolution: 4.5 mm
3D Sensitivity: 7.0 cps/kBq	3D Sensitivity: 6.4 cps/kBq (NEMA)	3D Sensitivity: 13.2 cps/kBq
Peak NECR: 130 kcps	Peak NECR: >91kcps @ 16kBq/ml	Peak NECR: 175 kcps
Coincidence : 4.9 ns	Coincidence : 3.8 ns	Coincidence : 5.9 ns
TOF resolution: 549 ps	TOF resolution: 535 ps	No TOF

light of clinically adopted PET/CT imaging when absolute quantification of PET data is considered.

MR-Compatible PET Detectors

Cross-talk effects between PET and MRI may occur when inserting a conventional PET detector and associated electronic components into an existing MR system. This may relate to disruptions of the PET signal cascade as well as to degraded MR imaging. The possible interactions between PET and MR signal generation are manifold. A perfect technical integration of both modalities requires the MR with its electromagnetic environment not to disturb the sensitive PET signals. This encompasses the strong static and homogeneous magnetic field for spin alignment (in the range of several Tesla), the strong spatially (mT/m) and temporally (mT/m/ms) varying electromagnetic gradient fields for spatial signal localization, as well as the pulsed radiofrequency (RF) transmit and receive fields for spin excitation and RF signal reception (MHz range). On the other hand, PET system components must not interfere with any of the above listed electromagnetic fields of the MR system.

Consequently, for a fully-integrated PET/MR system, all PET electronics must be RF shielded in order not to disturb the highly sensitive RF signals detected by the MR components. When shielding the PET components that are located close to the MR gradient coils, the RF shielding has to be designed such that the strong time variant gradient pulses do not produce unwanted Eddy currents in the shielding, which may have a negative effect on the gradient linearity, potentially leading to image distortions [52].

Given the design of standard PET detectors based on photomultiplier tubes (PMTs), a PET/MR configuration is obviously technically more challenging than the combination of PET and CT because phototubes are sensitive even to low

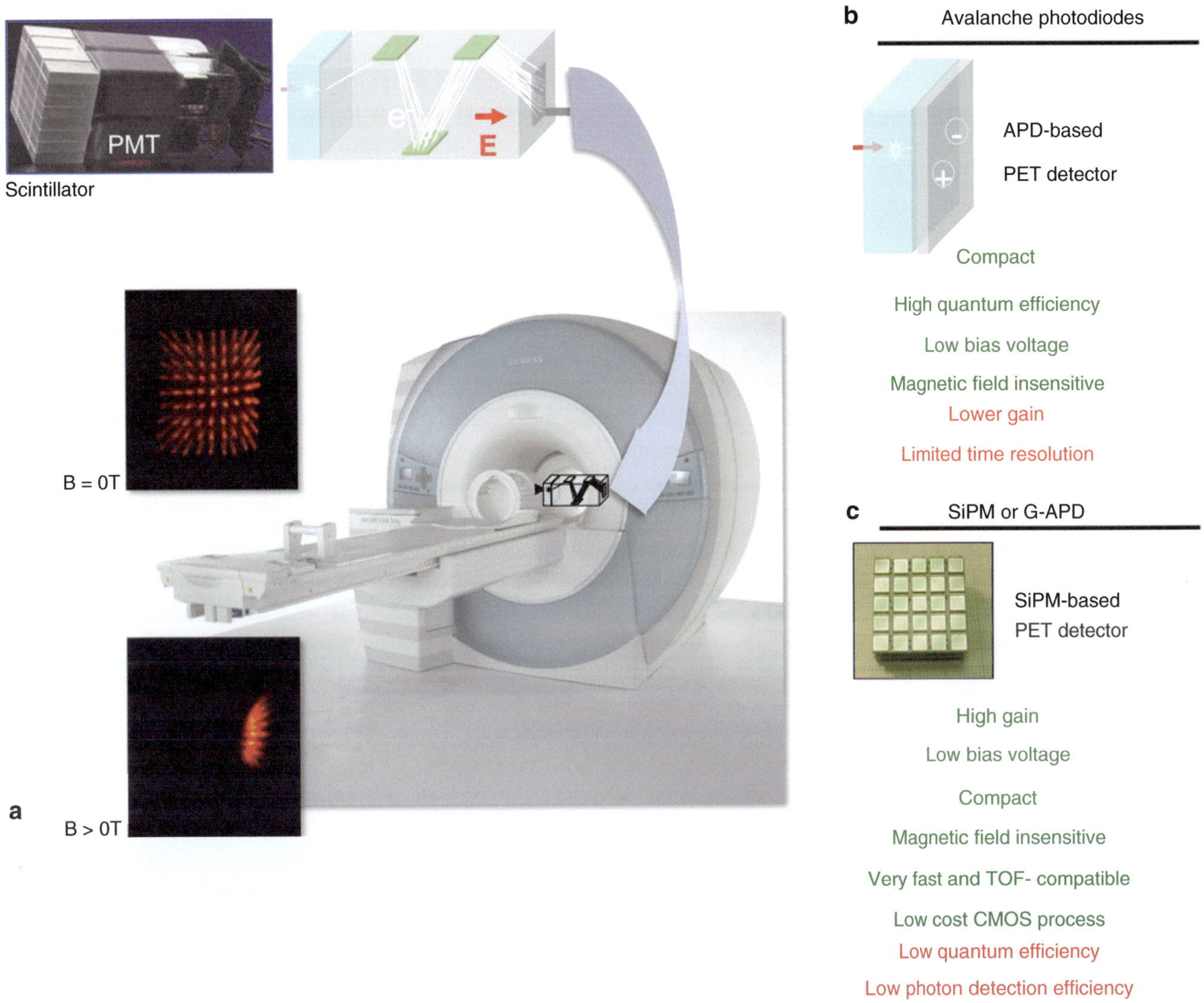

Fig. 2.11 (**a**) Conventional PET detectors using photomultiplier tubes (*PMT*) do not work inside a magnetic field. This is illustrated by the scintillator position profile that is skewed already from fringe fields from a horseshoe magnet placed next to the PET detector/PMR (Courtesy Bernd Pichler, University of Tübingen). New PET detectors (**b**) based on avalanche photodiodes (*APD*) can be made more compact and have been shown to perform in magnetic fields up to 9.4T. Recent developments indicate further improvements for MR-compatible PET detectors based on SiPM, a type of Geiger-APDs (**c**)

magnetic fields (Fig. 2.11). Therefore, early developers of PET/MR concepts, such as Hammer and co-workers, proposed to place only the PET scintillator inside the MR and to use light guides to channel the scintillation light from the detector to the PMT situated outside the primary magnetic field of the MR system [53]. This idea was advanced further by other groups, as discussed by Wehrl in a recent review of the origins of PET/MR [24].

In order to provide PET performance in PET/MR that is similar to PET performance in PET/CT, any MR-compatible PET detector must support accurate 3D positioning and very fast timing information at no cost of volume sensitivity. This, in turn, calls for combinations of scintillators with novel, MR-compatible photodetectors of high granularity such as Avalanche Photodiodes (APD) and Silicon Photomultipliers (SiPM) [54].

Avalanche Photodiodes (APD)

Avalanche photodiodes (APD) are semiconductor devices that transform detected light into an electrical signal following the same principles as ordinary photodiodes. However, unlike ordinary photodiodes, APD's operate exclusively at high electric fields. When an electron–hole pair is generated by photon absorption, the electron (or the hole) accelerate and gain sufficient energy from the high electric field before it collides with the crystal lattice and generates another electron–hole pair while losing some of its kinetic energy in the process (Fig. 2.11b). This process is known as impact ionization. The original as well as the secondary electron (or hole) can then accelerate again under the influence of the high electric field and create more electron hole pairs. This process creates an avalanche of electron hole pairs – hence the name avalanche photodiodes. The rate at which electron–hole pairs are generated by impact ionization is balanced by the rate at which they exit the high-field region and are collected. If the magnitude of the electric field (reverse-bias voltage) is below a value known as the breakdown voltage, the rate of collection exceeds that of electron hole creation and causes the population of electrons and holes to decline and eventually stops.

The number of created electron–hole pairs, referred to as internal gain, is typically in the range of 10^1–10^2 and dependent on the electric field strength (reverse bias voltage). Because the average number of created electron–hole pair is strictly proportional to the incident light photons, this mode of operation is known as linear mode.

Unlike amplification in PMTs, the internal gain of APDs is characterized by fluctuations due to the statistical nature of impact ionization. These gain fluctuations produce excess noise, which increases as the internal gain increases by raising the reverse bias. Other factors that affect the performance of APD include temperature, doping, as well as diode material properties. In addition, APDs are characterized by a relatively long timing resolution (FWHM > 1,000 ps), which limits their use in TOF PET systems. Because of these factors, it is desirable to use APDs at moderate reverse bias voltage and temperature to ensure their stable operation.

On the other hand, APDs are characterized by high quantum efficiency (QE – number of electron or holes created per number of incident scintillation photons) particularly at the wavelengths of PET scintillation detectors. APDs are also immune to after-pulsing, which are spurious pulses generated from electron-holes being trapped by crystal defects and released after a certain delay time, thus, confounding the detection process. Most importantly and contrary to PMTs, APDs are immune to stationary and varying magnetic fields, thus, rendering them suitable for PET/MR systems. APDs typically have a maximum size limited to about 1 cm^2, due to the difficulty of manufacturing large area semiconductor devices, however, the cost of manufacturing APDs is relatively low.

Silicone Photomultipliers (SiPM)

A promising development in photodetection for PET imaging is the introduction of Geiger mode avalanche photodiodes (G-APD, Fig. 2.11c), commonly referred to as silicon photomultiplier (SiPM). This is a novel type of photodetector that is about to reach a performance level that offers significant improvement over APD-based PET.

A SiPM is an APD operated with a reverse bias voltage above the breakdown voltage (~50–60 V above breakdown voltage). In this case, the electron hole pairs generated by photon absorption will multiply by impact ionization faster than they can be extracted, thus, resulting in an exponential growth of electron–hole pairs and their associated photocurrent. This process is known as Geiger discharge. The current flow produced by the Geiger discharge is large and results in a large signal gain (more than 10^5). Following a Geiger discharge, the SiPM is reset by dropping (quenching) the voltage across the photodiode below the breakdown voltage. This will reduce the number of created electron hole pairs and eventually stop the Geiger discharge. The discharge-and-reset cycle is known as the Geiger mode of operation of the photodiode. The turn-on transient of the current discharge is comparatively fast, with several picoseconds while the turn-off transient through quenching is mostly dependent on the SiPM size and is on the order of 100 ns. Quenching can be achieved using active or passive techniques although for high counting capabilities, active quenching is preferred.

One important application of SiPMs is their ability to count photons, which could be used to determine the energy of the incident annihilation photon on a scintillator in a PET system. However, a single SiPM cell has a limitation in that it is essentially either on or off. It cannot distinguish between a single and multiple photons that arrive simultaneously. One only knows that the APD was triggered. This limitation, however, is overcome when using an array of SiPM cells that are connected in parallel. In this case the output of the SiPM array is the sum of the output of each SiPM cell (pixel) in the array. For example, when the photon flux is low and photons arrive at a time interval longer than the recovery time of a pixel, the array will output pulses that equate to a single photoelectron. The generated pulses are then converted to digital pulses and counted. However, when the photon flux is high or the photons arrive in short pulses (pulse width less than the recovery time of the SiPM), the pixel outputs will add up to the equivalent number of incident photons. In this case, the SiPM array behaves in a pseudo-analog manner, because it can measure the incident number of photons per pulse, which is not possible with single photon counting SiPMs.

An important feature of SiPMs is their immunity to excess noise. This is primarily due to the fixed number of electron–hole pairs produced in Geiger mode, which is not defined by the statistics of the impact ionization process as in APDs. Another important feature of SiPMs is their relatively fast rise time, and short time jitter (FWHM = 0.1 ns) defined as the statistical variation of time interval between the photon arrival and the resulting electrical signal from the SiPM – thus, supporting their use in TOF-PET tomographs. Furthermore, the performance of SiPMs (like APDs) is immune to the effects of stationary and temporally varying magnetic fields which allows their use in PET/MR systems.

On the other hand, SiPMs have a relatively low photon detection efficiency (PDE), due to their low QE for scintillation light from PET detectors (40 % at 420 nm). In addition, SiPMs are characterized by high dark count rate, high cross talk and after pulsing as well as a strong temperature and

Table 2.3 Characteristics of photodetectors for PET

	PMT	APD	SiPM
Active area (mm ^{2})	1–2,000 cm^2	1–100 mm^2	1–10 mm^2
Gain	10^5–10^7	10^2	10^5–10^7
Rise time	<1 ns	2–3 ns	~1
Dark current/countrate	<0.1 nA/cm^2	1–10 nA/mm^2	0.1–1 MHz/mm^2
Capacitance (pF/mm^2)	9	2–10	>30
QE @ 420 nm (%)	25	60–80	<40*
Afterpulsing	Yes	No	Yes
Bias voltage (V)	1,000–2,000	~200–1,500	~50
Power consumption	100 mW/ch	10 μW/mm^2	<50 μW/mm^2
Temperature coefficient	<1 %/°C	2–3 %/°C	3–5 %/°C
Bias coefficient	<1 %/V	10 %/V	~100 %/V
Magnetic susceptibility	Very high (mT)	No (up to 9.4 T)	No (up to 15 T)

Information adapted from [54]
*Photon detection efficiency rather than quantum efficiency (QE)

timing dependence on bias, all of which reduce the performance of SiPMs. Table 2.3 shows a comparison between the performance characteristics of APDs, SiPMs, and PMTs.

Recent developments focusing on SiPM intend to create a fully-digital data handling of PET detector signals without employing dedicated read-out, amplifier ASICs, ADCs, etc. Such a fully-digital SiPM (dSiPM) was first presented in 2009 by Frach, Degenhardt and colleagues from Philips Research Aachen [55]. The dSiPM contains over 8,000 G-APDs on a 4×3 mm layer. In a laboratory set-up the coincidence timing resolution using a 22Na source and 3×3×5 mm3 LYSO crystal coupled to dSiPM was 153 ps FWHM and the energy resolution at 511 keV was 10.7 % FWHM. Further advances are expected towards integrating these detection systems in clinical systems, which would certainly be of great benefit for PET/MR systems.

PET/MR Methodological Pitfalls and Technological Challenges

MR-Based Attenuation Correction

In addition to the technical challenges of combining PET and MRI the necessary attenuation correction factors for the PET emission data must be derived from the PET/MR measurements [56]. While in PET/CT PET attenuation data can be derived from transforming available CT transmission images into maps of attenuation coefficients at 511 keV [10], no such transmission data are available in PET/MR. This is primarily due to the lack of physical space to host a transmission source. Secondly, a rotating, metal-encased transmission source, whether X-ray tube, rod or point sources would lead to severe crosstalk with the MR magnetic field. And finally, the available MR images represent, in essence, proton densities that cannot be directly translated into maps of electron densities as obtained from CT transmission measurements. For example, air and cortical bone yield no significantly measurable MR signal, whereas the difference in their photon attenuation properties is 2,500 HU on CT images (Fig. 2.12). Therefore, PET/MR requires novel approaches to MR-based attenuation correction (MR-AC).

Originally, straightforward segmentation-based approaches have been proposed to classify tissues on MR images and to assign respective attenuation coefficients. This approach seems to work well in brain imaging [57]. However, MR-AC in extra-cerebral applications is much more demanding [58]. Therefore, atlas-based approaches have been suggested for MR-AC of brain [59] and torso data [60].

The principle of the atlas approach is to align the MR acquired for the PET/MR study with an average MR image from an atlas comprising pairs of co-registered MR and CT data sets. The same transformation determined from the alignment of the MR of the patient with the MR in the atlas can be applied to the CT volume from the atlas. A combination of the co-registered CT image volume and the patient-specific MR can be used to generate a pseudo CT map of the PET/MR study from which the ACFs can be derived. In view of the absence of an MR bone signal, the bone structures can be extracted from the co-registered atlas CT and combined with an MR image segmented for air and soft tissue. Atlas-based approaches with or without pattern recognition enhancement do account for the presence of bone, but these algorithms are computationally demanding and require a set of aligned CT and MR image volumes for a given PET/MR system [60].

The current implementations of MR-AC of patient tissues are based on a combination of 3D Dixon-VIBE sequences in conjunction with subsequent image segmentation. Here, the gray values provided by the Dixon VIBE sequence are registered to different tissue classes resulting in tissue segmentation. The Dixon technique provides two images with water and fat being 'in phase' and in 'opposed phase'. This allows

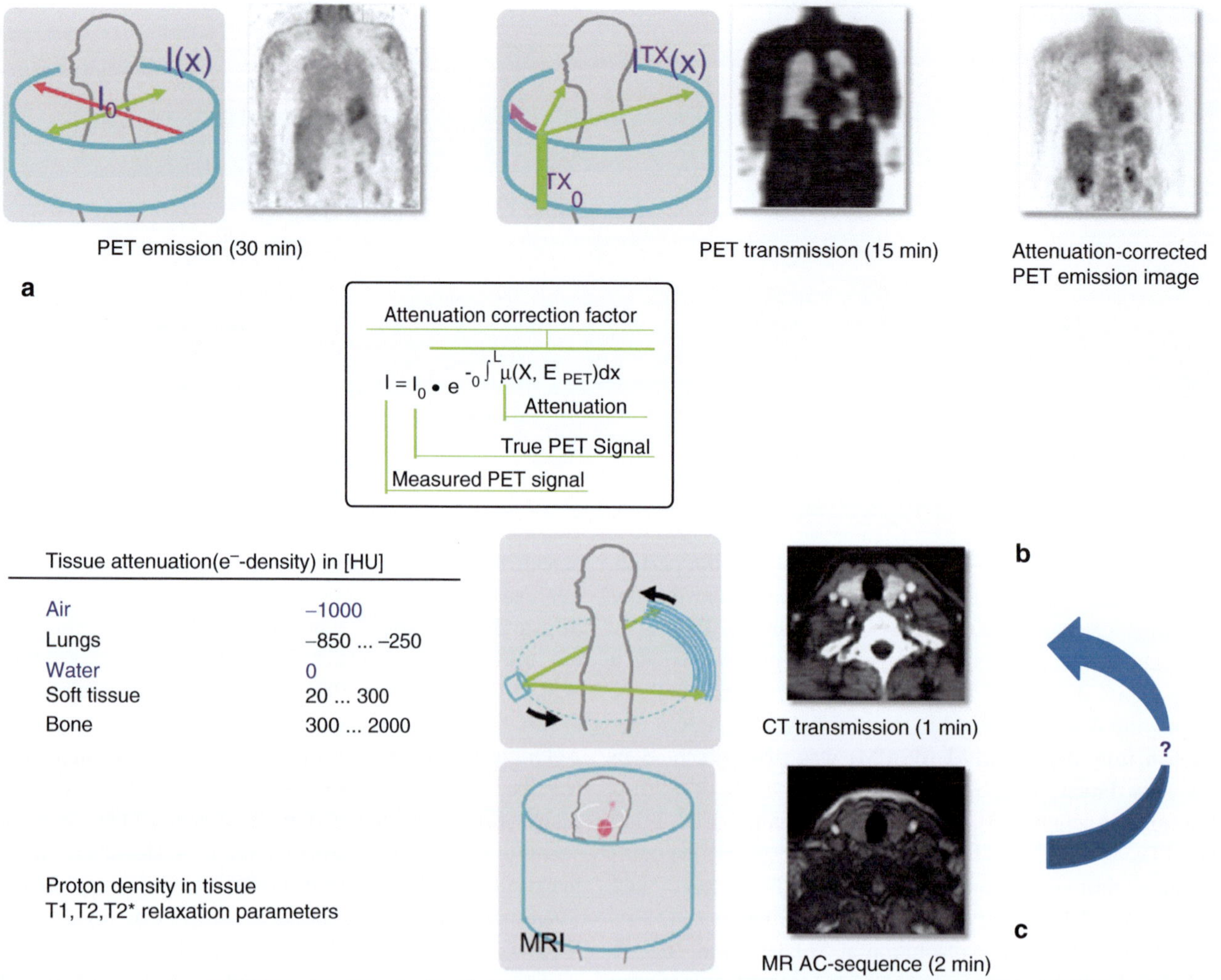

Fig. 2.12 Challenges of MR-based attenuation correction. (**a**) in PET attenuation correction factors can be calculated from separate PET transmission measurements, which take a relatively long time but provide attenuation values at 511 keV. (**b**) in PET/CT CT-based attenuation values, representing a measure of the electron-density, can be used to estimate PET attenuation coefficients. (**c**) In PET/MR no measure of electron density is available and tissue appearance on MR and CT images is markedly different for air and bone. Therefore, no direct measurement is available for MR-based attenuation coefficients

for reconstruction of fat-only, water-only and fat-water images, and results in tissue segmentation of air, fat, muscle, and lungs [61]. Bone is not accounted for in this approach. Initial results in clinical pilot studies have shown that this approach works reliably and provides results that are comparable to corrected images form PET/CT in the same individual. However, further studies are needed to assess the impact of ignoring bone and the overall accuracy of MR-based AC methods on PET quantification.

The Effect of MR Radiofrequency (RF) Coils on MR-AC

In addition to the general transformation of suitable MR image information of patient tissues, other, hardware-related attenuators must be considered during the transformation. This relates to the patient table, transmit and receive radiofrequency (RF) coils as well as positioning aids. The fact that the RF coils are located inside the FOV of the PET system (Fig. 2.7b, c) is a challenge and has only started to be addressed. For brain scans, the head coil is rigid and its attenuation values can be estimated from a reference CT-based attenuation map. Subsequently for any PET/MR study only the relative position of the head coil inside the PET/MR system would be required. Additional work has been directed towards reducing the amount of attenuating materials in MR coils used in PET/CT as exemplified in a modified brain coil for integrated PET/MR imaging [62, 63].

For extra-cranial examinations the situation is more demanding. MR surface coils are required to achieve optimal signal-to-noise-ratio (SNR) and high quality MR images. Surface RF coils may contain elastic components and hence their individual position on the patient cannot easily be

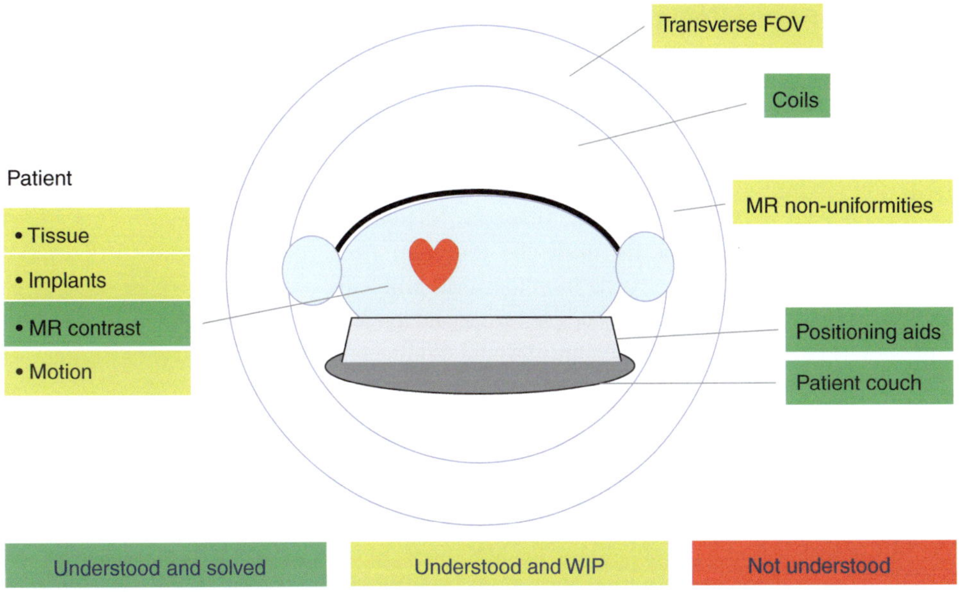

Fig. 2.13 Contributors to attenuation and image distortions in PET/MR. Topics marked as *green* are resolved and addressed, those marked in *yellow* are known but solutions are work-in-progress

predicted. The effect of flexible body coils on overall PET attenuation was recently estimated by Tellmann and colleagues [64]. The authors report a maximum bias of 4 % in attenuation-corrected torso PET if surface coils are not accounted for during AC. This bias is negligible compared to the respective bias in head studies when ignoring dedicated, rigid head RF coils (up to 20 %). MacDonald and colleagues report similar results [65].

All PET/MR vendors today offer CT-based attenuation templates for rigid coils as well as for the patient bed that are seamlessly integrated during the attenuation correction. Nonetheless, clinical studies are required to further study the effect of misaligned RF coil templates and missing templates for accurate representation of flexible coils on PET quantification.

The Presence of MR Contrast Agents

MR-based AC could potentially be biased from the presence of MR contrast materials, which are typically made up of iron oxide and Gd-chelates for oral and intravenous (IV) application, respectively. It is known from the development of CT-based AC that the presence of contrast materials with atomic numbers higher than those of water may lead to biased attenuation maps for PET emission data. The same effects may occur with MRCA that are applied during PET/MR imaging. Furthermore, the presence of MR contrast agents may produce changes in the MR signal intensity that yield biased attenuation maps. First studies indicate no negative effect from MR contrast on PET quantification following MR-based attenuation correction [66, 67].

Limited FOV and Truncation Effects

Given the reduced bore diameter and the relatively long examination times in PET/MR compared to clinical PET/CT, most patients are positioned in the more comfortable position with their arms down. Thus, the patient anatomy may well extend beyond the transverse FOV of the MR (typically 50 cm), whereby the arms or the trunk of the patient are not fully covered by the MR images used for MR-AC. This may yield an underestimation of the reconstructed, attenuation-corrected emission activity concentration. Truncation artifacts were described for PET/CT imaging [68] and have been reviewed for PET/MR [69]. It was shown that with the arms extending beyond the FOV of the MR the PET activity following MR-AC was biased by up to 14 % in the area of truncation. The underestimated activity concentration could be recovered to within 2 % of the nominal concentration following simple, manual extension of the attenuation map.

An alternative solution would be to use the uncorrected PET image to estimate the patient cross-section in those areas outside the measured FOV where no – or only geometrically distorted – MR information is available [70, 71]. The clinical feasibility of this approach still needs to be validated. Particularly, in imaging scenarios with highly specific tracers the arms may be difficult to segment automatically in the uncorrected PET images.

Figure 2.13 summarizes the challenges and the status of MR-based attenuation corrections in PET/MR. Most challenges are understood with some being addressed sufficiently and some awaiting further optimization, validation and clinical adoption.

MR-Based Partial Volume Correction

As early as 1991, Leahy et al. suggested that PET reconstruction could be improved by using anatomical MR images from the same patient as prior information [72]. It is common clinical practice today for neurology patients with a PET-indication to also undergo an MR examination. However, MR-guided PET reconstruction has not yet made the transition from research into clinical routine. Aside from logistical problems associated with the retrieval of the complementary image sets, sub-optimal retrospective image alignment would significantly deteriorate the quality of the PET data [73]. However, in combined PET/MR imaging systems, the spatial (and temporal) alignment accuracy could be improved, thus, helping to promote the concept of MR-guided PET image reconstruction.

Even if the PET image is reconstructed independently of the MR image, it is still possible to use the MR image of the patient as an aid for improved quantification. In particular MR-guided partial volume correction (PVC) was suggested as early as in 1990 [74, 75]. Again PET and MR images from combined PET/MR examinations may facilitate improvements in MR-based PET quantification through the use of MR-based PVC.

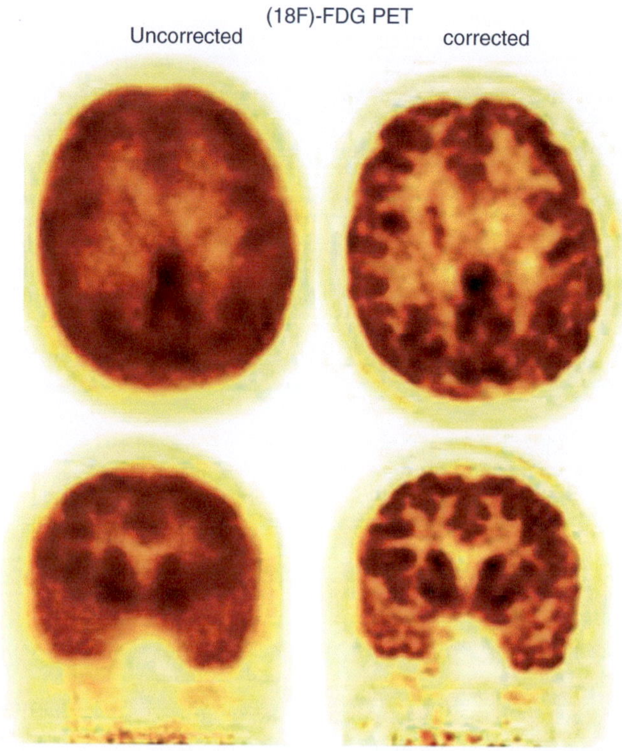

Fig. 2.14 FDG-PET images following attenuation correction (*left*) and motion + attenuation correction (*right*) clearly demonstrate the potentially improved quality of the data from lengthy examinations (Courtesy of J Scheins and H Herzog, Research Centre Jülich)

MR-Based Motion Correction

Patient motion, from involuntary movements, and cardiac as well as respiratory cycles, is a major contribution to degraded PET image quality. In addition, patient motion will lead to local or extended mis-alignment of complementary anato-metabolic image information. In PET/CT, for example, the PET image is acquired over several minutes, while the CT scan is a matter of seconds and frequently acquired during a single breath hold. As a result, patient motion typically causes local misalignment between the PET and CT images and may lead to serious artifacts for AC, for example near the diaphragm. Dedicated breathing instructions have been shown to help reduce misalignment in the thorax and upper abdomen [76, 77]. Other authors have recommended 4D PET/CT acquisition and AC, however, this involves a substantially higher patient radiation dose [78–80].

Respiration is expected to generate misalignment and blurring in PET/MR images, too. As MR scans generally take much longer than CT scans, patients spend an even longer time in the PET/MR compared to PET/CT, and consequently patient motion is likely to cause even more severe artifacts. However, integrated PET/MR system technology offers a promising solution to the problem (Fig. 2.14). Various MRI motion-tracking techniques are available in clinical settings, including but not limited to cloverleaf navigators [81]. Such techniques have been tested with the BrainPET system with promising results from estimating and correcting involuntary head motion as a result of relaxation of neck muscles. Using 3D Hoffman brain phantom and human volunteer studies, Catana et al. reported that high- temporal-resolution MRI-derived motion estimates acquired simultaneously on the hybrid BrainPET system (Siemens Healthcare) can be used to improve PET image quality, thus increasing its reliability, reproducibility, and quantitative accuracy [50].

Likewise, novel 3D cine sequences are under development to track spatio-temporal deformation of organs such as the heart and the thorax. Subsequently, deformation fields are generated and incorporated into the PET reconstruction [51, 82–85].

Thus, the use of periodic MR navigator signals in conjunction with a 4D model of the human torso may help to correct for motion-induced image degeneration in PET/MR data following 4D-MR-AC, which would be a major advantage over CT-AC.

PET/MR Safety

Combined PET/CT has been clinically very successful and may well serve as a benchmark for the development of PET/MR. However, despite the success of PET/CT there are also shortcomings in the use of CT as the anatomical complement to PET. As such, CT uses a source of ionizing radiation for imaging and, therefore, adds significant radiation dose to the overall examination. Brix et al. have shown that the diagnostic CT contributes up to 75 % of the effective dose in patients undergoing whole-body FDG-PET/CT examinations for oncology indications leading to a total of about 25 mSv effective dose [86]. These dose levels may raise concern in selected population like adolescents and females. Figure 2.15a illustrates the relative contribution to patient exposure from the individual steps in a combined PET/CT examination.

In PET/MR examinations, overall patient exposure is reduced significantly by replacing the CT imaging step with an MR imaging sequence (Fig. 2.15b). In addition, MR provides advanced functional imaging information, such as DWI or MRS, without adding to the overall radiation exposure burden. Nonetheless, staff exposure is expected to increase slightly in PET/MR, given the complexity of the patient set-up when employing a range of surface RF body coils. However, no valid data are available as of yet.

Long-term experience and hundreds of millions of routinely and safely performed MR examinations confirm that MRI is a safe imaging modality. Nevertheless, a number of safety concerns do apply to PET/MR as discussed by Brix et al. [87], of which all are all associated with the general safety issues known from MR-only imaging. The strong static magnetic field associated with MR systems potentially can attract ferromagnetic equipment as well as some patient implants, and accelerate these towards the strongest magnetic field in the isocentre of the PET/MR system. In some patients the strong and fast switching gradient fields may lead to peripheral nerve stimulation that are harmless but nevertheless disturbing. Finally, the strong-pulsed RF fields for MR signal excitation can cause tissue heating. As with all other RF transmitting devices, the RF power in MR imaging is limited to harmless values of the specific absorption rate (SAR) not leading to critical tissue heating. Some electric conducting metal implants, however, potentially may increase the local SAR values during an MR examination above the allowed SAR limits. To reduce all associated potential risks of MR imaging, patient questionnaires and patient screening and selection procedures have to be established and used in daily routine.

Accordingly, MR and PET/MR examinations of patients with passive implants (e.g., vascular clips and clamps, intravascular stents and filters, vascular access ports and catheters, heart valve prostheses, orthopedic prostheses, sheets and screws, intrauterine contraceptive devices), active implants (e.g., cardiac pace-makers and defibrillators, cochlear implants, electronic drug infusion pumps) or other objects of ferromagnetic or unknown material (pellets, bullets) are always associated with a potential risk. Careful pre-examination interviews of the patients regarding the presence or absence of passive implants, which may interfere with the MR imaging protocol, or deter the patient from this examination all together is mandatory [87].

Summary and Conclusion

Multi-modality imaging instrumentation has evolved dramatically during the past decade. Combined SPECT/CT, PET/CT and, lately, PET/MR have revolutionized imaging and medical diagnosis. In these times of limited resources in healthcare and rapidly increasing radiation awareness, any predictions for future developments of PET/MR technology must take into account a variety of aspects, ranging from cost-effectiveness to overall radiation dose. While technological innovation, such as PET/MR, always pairs with enthusiasm and public interest, subsequent commercial systems must be affordable and strategies for their clinical implementation must be assessed for their health benefit to justify their pursuit within a local or global healthcare system [88]. The impressive advances in imaging technology of the past decade came at a cost, but at what point do these advances become cost-effective? Whole-body PET examinations that took 1 h at the start of the last decade now take 5 min on PET/CT; the actual imaging takes only a fraction of the time needed for patient preparation and positioning or reporting the study. Does the increased wealth of available information from the MR make up for the increased examination time?

The radiation dose to the patient incurred by PET/CT is clearly an issue. Although the ALARA (as low as reasonably achievable) principle is sound advice, there are clearly groups of cancer-sufferers such as those in children and young adults where the probability of inducing a second, radiation-associated cancer exceeds the benefits that can be accrued from the study. Different imaging strategies should then be adopted, such as MRI, optical imaging or ultrasound.

The commendable drive to reduce radiation exposure to patients has fostered an interest in a combination of PET with MRI. However, it is fair to assume that as long as diseases such as cancer and dementia remain primarily diseases of the elderly, the benefits of nuclear and X-ray imaging will largely outweigh the risks.

Will the coming decade witness the replacement of PET/CT by PET/MRI? Some believe it will, just as in the 1980s there were those who predicted that MRI would replace CT within 5 years. Of course that never happened, as both techniques have strengths and weaknesses and they have each found their niche in the medical imaging armamentarium. The same is likely true of PET/CT and PET/MRI—the technical challenges will be solved and simultaneous acquisition of MRI and PET will undoubtedly open new doors in clinical research and eventually also in the clinic.

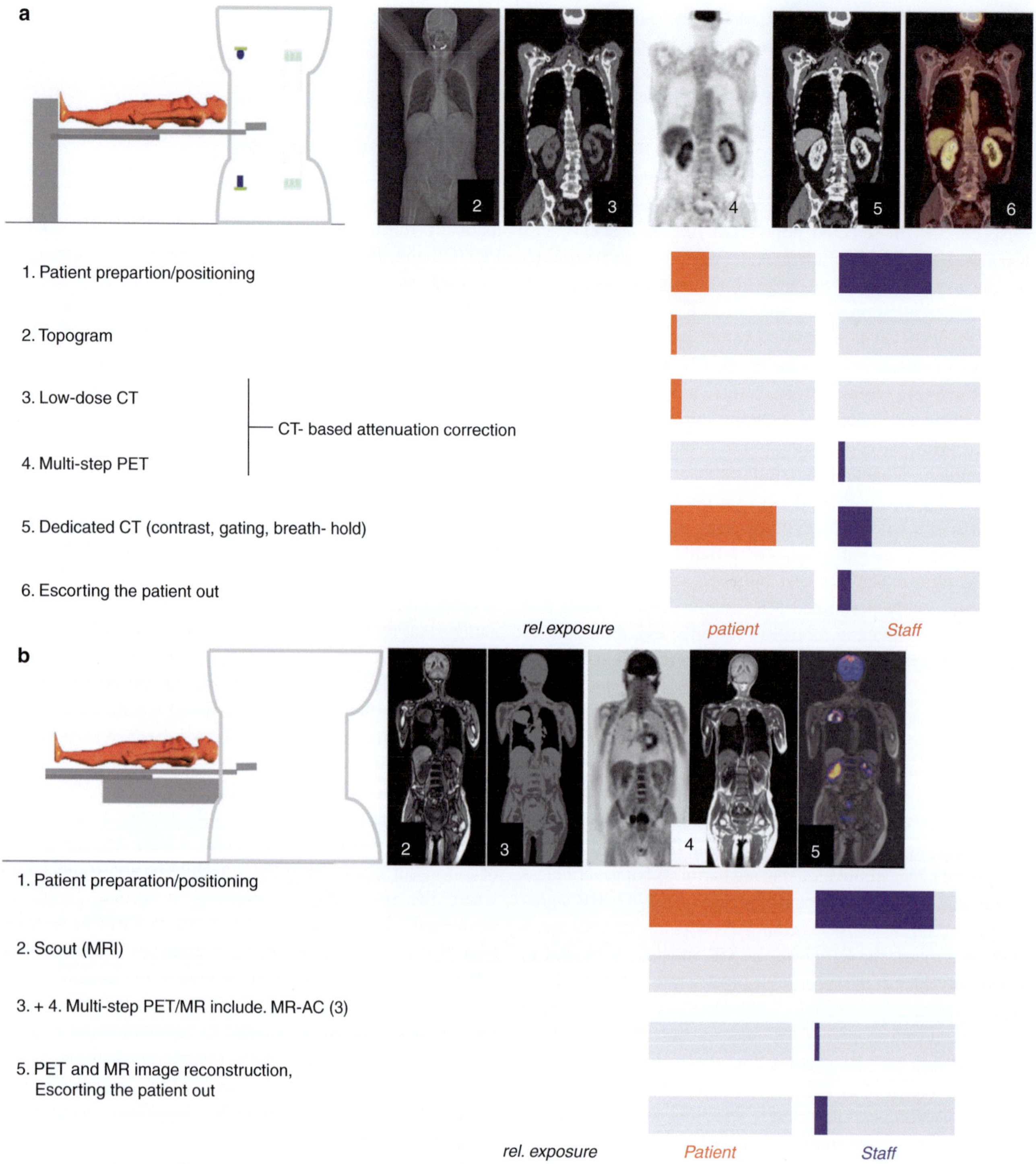

Fig. 2.15 Relative contributions to patient and staff exposure during a whole-body oncology examination in PET/CT (**a**) and PET/MR (**b**). The amount of radioactivity injected into the patient for a PET/CT (**a**, step 1) and PET/MR (**a**, step 1) is assumed to be identical. Note, patient set-up in PET/MR is more elaborate and, therefore, relative and potentially total staff exposures are expected to be higher than those in PET/CT

Acknowledgement We are indebted to Gaspar Delso (GEHC), Hans Herzog (Research Centre Jülich), Jens-Christoph Georgi (Siemens Healthcare), Antonis Kalemis (Philips Healthcare), Bernd Pichler (University of Tübingen), Nina Schwenzer (University of Tübingen), Jürgen Scheins (Research Centre Jülich), Holger Schmidt (University of Tübingen), David W Townsend (Singapore), Rainer Veigel (Philips Healthcare), Patrick Veit-Haibach (Zurich) for helpful discussions and the provision of support materials.

References

1. Gambhir SS et al (2001) A tabulated summary of the FDG PET literature. J Nucl Med 42(5 suppl):1S–93S
2. Herholz K, Heiss W-D (2004) Positron emission tomography in clinical neurology. Mol Imaging Biol 6(4):239–269
3. Knuuti J (2004) Clinical cardiac PET in the future. Eur J Nucl Med 31(4):467–468
4. Wahl RL et al (1993) "Anatometabolic" tumor imaging: fusion of FDG PET with CT or MRI to localize foci of increased activity. J Nucl Med 34:1190–1197
5. Wagner HN (1998) A brief history of positron emission tomography. Semin Nucl Med XXVIII(3):213–220
6. Townsend D (2008) Multimodality imaging of structure and function. Phys Med Biol 53(4):R1–R39
7. von Schulthess GK (2000) Cost considerations regarding an integrated CT-PET system. Eur Radiol 10(suppl 3):S377–S380
8. Czernin J, Allen-Auerbach M, Schelbert H (2007) Improvements in cancer staging with PET/CT: literature-based evidence as of September 2006. J Nucl Med 48(1 suppl):78S–88S
9. Lonsdale M, Beyer T (2010) Dual-modality PET/CT instrumentation-today and tomorrow. Eur J Radiol 73(3):452–460
10. Kinahan P, Hasegawa B, Beyer T (2003) X-ray based attenuation correction for PET/CT scanners. Semin Nucl Med XXXIII(3): 166–179
11. von Schulthess GK, Steinert HC, Hany TF (2006) Integrated PET/CT: current applications and future directions. Radiology 238(2):405–422
12. Kinahan PE et al (1998) Attenuation correction for a combined 3D PET/CT scanner. Med Phys 25(10):2046–2053
13. Burger C et al (2002) PET attenuation coefficients from CT images: experimental evaluation of the transformation of CT into PET 511-keV attenuation coefficients. Eur J Nucl Med 29(7):922–927
14. Beyer T et al (2000) A combined PET/CT tomograph for clinical oncology. J Nucl Med 41(8):1369–1379
15. Beyer T et al (2011) The future of hybrid imaging – part 2: PET/CT. Insights Imaging 2(3):225–234
16. Karp J et al (2008) Benefit of time-of-flight in PET: experimental and clinical results. J Nucl Med 49(3):462–470
17. Jakoby B et al (2009) Performance characteristics of a new LSO PET/CT scanner with extended axial field-of-view and PSF reconstruction. IEEE Trans Nucl Sci 56(3):633–639
18. Budinger T (1983) Time-of-flight positron emission tomography: status relative to conventional PET. J Nucl Med 24(1):73–78
19. Kadrmas D et al (2009) Impact of time-of-flight on PET tumor detection. J Nucl Med 50(8):1315–1323
20. Lois C et al (2010) An assessment of the impact of incorporating time-of-flight information into clinical PET/CT imaging. J Nucl Med 51(2):237–245
21. Goffin K et al (2010) Anatomy-based reconstruction of FDG-PET images with implicit partial volume correction improves detection of hypometabolic regions in patients with epilepsy due to focal cortical dysplasia diagnosed on MRI. Eur J Nucl Med Mol Imaging 37(6):1148–1155
22. Fletcher J et al (2008) Recommendations on the Use of 18F-FDG PET in oncology. J Nucl Med 49(3):480–508
23. Pichler B et al (2010) PET/MRI: paving the way for the next generation of clinical multimodality imaging applications. J Nucl Med 51(3):333–336
24. Wehrl H et al (2009) Pre-clinical PET/MR: technological advances and new perspectives in biomedical research. Eur J Nucl Med Mol Imaging 36(suppl 1):S56–S68
25. Padhani A, Miles K (2010) Multiparametric imaging of tumor response to therapy. Radiology 256(2):348–364
26. Moser E et al (2009) Magnetic resonance imaging methodology. Eur J Nucl Med Mol Imaging 36(suppl 1):S30–S41
27. Porter D, Smith M (1988) Magnetic resonance spectroscopy in vivo. J Biomed Eng 10(6):562–568
28. Bammer R (2003) Basic principles of diffusion-weighted imaging. Eur J Radiol 45(3):169–184
29. Basser P et al (2000) In vivo fiber tractography using DT-MRI data. Magn Reson Med 44(4):625–632
30. Golay X et al (2002) High-resolution isotropic 3D diffusion tensor imaging of the human brain. Magn Reson Med 47(5):837–843
31. Padhani A, Koh D, Collins D (2011) Whole-body diffusion-weighted MR imaging in cancer: current status and research directions. Radiology 261(3):700–718
32. Ogawa S et al (1993) Functional brain mapping by blood oxygenation level-dependent contrast magnetic resonance imaging. A comparison of signal characteristics with a biophysical model. Biophys J 64(3):803–812
33. Sodickson D, Manning W (1997) Simultaneous acquisition of spatial harmonics (SMASH): fast imaging with radiofrequency coil arrays. Magn Reson Med 38(4):591–603
34. Pruessmann K et al (1999) SENSE: sensitivity encoding for fast MRI. Magn Reson Med 42(5):952–962
35. Griswold M et al (2002) Generalized autocalibrating partially parallel acquisitions (GRAPPA). Magn Reson Med 47(6):1202–1210
36. Barkhausen J et al (2001) Whole-body MR imaging in 30 seconds with real-time true FISP and a continuously rolling table platform: feasibility study. Radiology 220(1):252–256
37. Quick H et al (2004) High spatial resolution whole-body MR angiography featuring parallel imaging: initial experience. Fortschr Roentgenstr 176(2):163–169
38. Veit-Haibach P et al (2013) PET/MR imaging using a Tri-modality PET/CT – MR system with a dedicated shuttle in clinical routine. MAGMA 26(1):25–35
39. von Schulthess GK, Burger C (2010) Integrating imaging modalities: what makes sense from a workflow perspective? Eur J Nucl Med Mol Imaging 37(5):980–990
40. Kalemis A, Delattre B, Heinzer S (2013) Sequential whole-body PET/MR scanner: concept, clinical use, and optimisation after two years in the clinic. The manufacturer's perspective. MAGMA 26(1):5–23
41. Zaidi H et al (2011) Design and performance evaluation of a whole-body Ingenuity TF PET/MRI system. Phys Med Biol 56(10):3091–3106
42. Kalemis A, Delattre B, Heinzer S (2013) Sequential whole-body PET/MR scanner – concept, clinical use and optimisations after two years in the clinic. The manufacturer's perspective. MAGMA 26(1):5–23
43. Schmand M et al (2007) BrainPET: first human tomograph for simultaneous (functional) PET and MR imaging. J Nucl Med 48(6):45P
44. Pichler B et al (2006) Performance test of an LSO-APD detector in a 7-T MRI scanner for simultaneous PET/MRI. J Nucl Med 47(4):639–647
45. Herzog H et al (2010) The current state, challenges and perspectives of MR-PET. Neuroimage 49(3):2072–2082
46. Schlemmer H et al (2008) Simultaneous MR/PET imaging of the human brain: feasibility study. Radiology 248(3):1028–1035
47. Boss A et al (2010) Hybrid PET/MRI of intracranial masses: initial experiences and comparison to PET/CT. J Nucl Med 51(8):1198–1205
48. Schwenzer N et al (2012) Simultaneous PET/MR imaging in a human brain PET/MR system in 50 patients-current state of image quality. Eur J Radiol 81(11):3472–3478
49. Delso G et al (2011) Performance measurements of the Siemens mMR integrated whole-body PET/MR scanner. J Nucl Med 52(12):1914–1922
50. Catana C et al (2011) MRI-assisted PET motion correction for neurologic studies in an integrated MR-PET scanner. J Nucl Med 52(1):154–161
51. Tsoumpas C et al (2012) Fast generation of 4D PET/MR data from real dynamic MR acquisitions. Phys Med Biol 56(20):6597–6613

52. Truhn D, Kiessling F, Schulz V (2011) Optimized RF shielding techniques for simultaneous PET/MR. Med Phys 38(7):3995–4000
53. Hammer B (1990) NMR-PET scanner apparatus. U.S. Patent, USA, 3 July 1990
54. Lecomte R (2009) Novel detector technology for clinical PET. Eur J Nucl Med Mol Imaging 36(suppl 1):S69–S85
55. Degenhardt C et al (2009) The digital silicon photomultiplier — a novel sensor for the detection of scintillation light. In: IEEE nuclear science symposium conference (NSS/MIC), Orlando, 24 Oct–1 Nov 2009
56. Keereman V et al (2013) Challenges and current methods for attenuation correction in PET/MR. MAGMA 26(1):81–98
57. Zaidi H, Hasegawa B (2003) Determination of the attenuation map in emission tomography. J Nucl Med 44(2):291–315
58. Beyer T et al (2008) MR-based attenuation correction for torso-PET/MR imaging: pitfalls in mapping MR to CT data. Eur J Nucl Med Mol Imaging 35(6):1142–1146
59. Hofmann M et al (2009) Towards quantitative PET/MRI: a review of MR-based attenuation correction techniques. Eur J Nucl Med Mol Imaging 36(suppl 1):S93–S103
60. Hofmann M et al (2011) MRI-based attenuation correction for whole-body PET/MRI: quantitative evaluation of segmentation- and atlas-based methods. J Nucl Med 52(9):1392–1399
61. Martinez-Möller A et al (2009) Tissue classification as a potential approach for attenuation correction in whole-body PET/MRI: evaluation with PET/CT data. J Nucl Med 50(4):520–526
62. Delso G et al (2009) Study of MR head and neck coil for its use in an integrated MR/PET scanner. J Nucl Med 50(suppl 2):294–295P
63. Delso G et al (2010) Evaluation of the attenuation properties of MR equipment for its use in a whole-body PET/MR scanner. Phys Med Biol 55(15):4361–4374
64. Tellmann L et al (2011) The effect of MR coils on PET quantification in whole-body PET/MR: results from a pseudo-PET/MR phantom study. Med Phys 38(5):2795–2805
65. MacDonald L et al (2011) Effetcs of MR surface coils on PET quantification. Med Phys 38(6):2948–2953
66. Lois C et al (2011) Effect of MR contrast agents on quantitative accuracy of PET in combined whole-body PET/MR imaging. Eur J Nucl Med Mol Imaging 38(suppl 2):S156
67. Lee W et al (2011) Effects of MR contrast agents on PET quantitation in PET/MRI study. J Nucl Med 52(suppl 1):53
68. Beyer T et al (2006) Whole-body 18F-FDG PET/CT in the presence of truncation artifacts. J Nucl Med 47(1):91–99
69. Delso G et al (2010) The effect of limited MR field of view in MR/PET attenuation correction. Med Phys 37(6):2804–2812
70. Nuyts J et al (1999) Simultaneous maximum a posteriori reconstruction of attenuation and activity distributions from emission sinograms. IEEE Trans Med Imaging 18(5):393–403
71. Salomon A et al (2009) Iterative generation of attenuation maps in TOF-PET/MR using consistency conditions. J Nucl Med 50(suppl 2):425P
72. Leahy R, Yan X (1991) Incorporation of anatomical MR data for improved functional imaging with PET. In: XIIth IPMI international conference, Wye, 1991
73. Lipinski B et al (1997) Expectation maximization reconstruction of positron emission tomography images using anatomical magnetic resonance information. IEEE Trans Med Imaging 16(2):129–136
74. Meltzer C et al (1990) Correction of PET data for partial volume effects in human cerebral cortex by MR imaging. J Comput Assist Tomogr 14(4):561
75. Meltzer CC et al (1999) Comparative evaluation of MR-based partial-volume correction schemes for PET. J Nucl Med 40(12):2053–2065
76. Beyer T et al (2003) A limited breath-hold technique for improved image quality in multi-slice PET/CT exams. J Nucl Med 44(5):274P–275P
77. Beyer T et al (2003) Dual-modality PET/CT imaging: the effect of respiratory motion on combined image quality in clinical oncology. Eur J Nucl Med 30(4):588–596
78. Nehmeh S et al (2007) Deep-inspiration breath-hold PET/CT of the thorax. J Nucl Med 48(1):22–26
79. Mori S et al (2009) Effective doses in four-dimensional computed tomography for lung radiotherapy planning. Med Dosim 34(1):87–90
80. Chang G et al (2010) Implementation of an automated respiratory amplitude gating technique for PET/CT: clinical evaluation. J Nucl Med 51(1):16–24
81. van der Kouwe A, Benner T, Dale A (2006) Real-time rigid body motion correction and shimming using cloverleaf navigators. Magn Reson Med 56(5):1019–1032
82. Kellman P et al (2008) Fully automatic, retrospective enhancement of real-time acquired cardiac cine MR images using image-based navigators and respiratory motion-corrected averaging. Magn Reson Med 59(4):771–778
83. Tsoumpas C et al (2010) Simultaneous PET/MR acquisition and MR-derived motion fields for correction of non-rigid motion in PET. Ann Nucl Med 24(10):745–750
84. King A et al (2012) Thoracic respiratory motion estimation from MRI using a statistical model and a 2-D image navigator. Med Imaging Anal 16(1):252–264
85. Buerger C et al (2012) Nonrigid motion modeling of the liver from 3-D undersampled self-gated golden-radial phase encoded MRI. IEEE Trans Med Imaging 31(3):805–815
86. Brix G et al (2005) Radiation exposure of patients undergoing whole-body dual-modality FDG-PET/CT examinations. J Nucl Med 46(4):608–613
87. Brix G et al (2009) Risks and safety aspects related to PET/MR examinations. Eur J Nucl Med Mol Imaging 36(suppl 1): S131–S138
88. Goyen M, Debatin J (2009) Healthcare costs for new technologies. Eur J Nucl Med Mol Imaging 36(suppl 1):S139–S143

Technical Principles and Protocols of PET/MR Imaging

3

A. Kalemis

Contents

A. Kalemis
PET/MR, Philips Healthcare,
Guildford Business Park, Guildford, Surrey GU2 8XH, UK
e-mail: antonis.kalemis@philips.com

Introduction

PET and MRI are two well-established medical imaging modalities that are used frequently as diagnostic tools in a wide range of clinical indications providing complementary information [1]. MRI can provide anatomical information with very high spatial resolution, and functional measurements at organ and tissue level with high diagnostic sensitivity. On the other hand, PET images functional processes at cellular and sub-cellular level with very high diagnostic specificity and high tracer detection sensitivity (10^{-11}–10^{-12} mol/l) [2] but with a spatial resolution inferior to MRI. This complementary matching of capabilities renders both PET(/CT) and MRI necessary in several disease pathways, particularly in oncology and neurology. A significant workflow limitation, when both modalities are needed, is the physical and organisational separation of the two systems [3]. Patients who need both PET and MR imaging are often referred for such scans independently and, often, they are scanned with a significant time difference. This renders the fusion of information from both examinations difficult or even impossible due to disease status changes or several other technical and organisational factors [4]. Hence, when MRI is the preferred imaging modality versus CT, PET/MR should be more clinically useful than PET/CT and a combined single examination could provide significant benefits to both the patient and the hospital.

Today, there are two different designs for combined PET/MR systems; positioning PET inside the MRI magnet or in tandem, similar to PET/CT [5]. Both philosophies attempt to balance clinical utility, user flexibility in developing clinically-relevant PET/MR-dedicated imaging protocols, potential sacrifices in relation to stand-alone state-of-the-art PET and MRI imaging capabilities and cost. Irrespectively, of the design and technical differences with the stand-alone systems, PET/MR, as a novel imaging option, requires significant innovation at various levels in order to surpass current concerns and scepticism. The latter are of clinical, organisational and technological nature. Questions about how it compares with PET/CT, under which clinical

O. Ratib et al. (eds.), *Atlas of PET/MR Imaging in Oncology*,
DOI 10.1007/978-3-642-31292-2_3, © Springer-Verlag Berlin Heidelberg 2013

scenarios either of them should be used, patient throughput, ease of workflow, building and running costs, ownership of device and staff (between different departments), reliability of new the technology and image quality in comparison to stand-alone systems are common discussion points.

Operational Requirements

It is common in healthcare for radical new technologies to require a second innovation wave, in the area of its structure and organisation, in order to optimise their contribution in disease management and patient pathway [6]. An organisation wishing to adopt PET/MR, in particular, has to overcome its complicated logistics, often the single-modality trained technical personnel, the staffing requirement from two different departments and the excessive scanning time required to acquire both PET and MR scans, which raises significantly the cost of each scan. At this level, institutions are requested to innovate in order to successfully adopt this novel technology.

At infrastructure level, some degree of cross-departmental collaboration and in some cases even restructuring is necessary to bring the Nuclear Medicine (NM) and Radiology staff much closer. Dual-training of the technical personnel is essential in order to operate the scanner while another long-term consideration is the need to cross-train Radiologists and Nuclear Medicine physicians from both modalities [7]. However, such needs are not straightforward due several factors, amongst others the existing territorial and protective practices in many healthcare facilities and the variations in the legal frameworks for imaging technologists [8]. In many hospitals Radiology and NM departments are far from each other creating further complications in staff allocation and/or logistics of the new scanners. Therefore, a successful model needs to be devised for the placement of the scanner considering its heavy needs for MR, PET and Radiochemistry expert support while residing within a controlled area for radiation and high magnetic fields.

Innovation is also needed in defining new imaging procedures that consider the extra time and find workarounds. Depending on the patient population of the institution, the staff and the other medical imaging scanners, a different departmental (or cross-departmental) workflow may be necessary to optimise the use of all systems and personnel. A sound business case that demonstrates the added value of PET/MR in comparison to PET/CT, MRI or concurrent referrals to both modalities (i.e. the current clinical practice) [9] is also necessary to demonstrate a favourable cost/benefits balance, to these other alternatives [10, 11]. Competition is not just in the area of clinical use; procurement for PET/MR will also compete against PET/CT and MRI due to limitations in funding, space within hospitals, personnel and attracting research grants. Therefore, in order to succeed, the new modality must demonstrate better qualities than its rivals. From the system perspective, these qualities translate into superior diagnostic accuracy, a feasible workflow, adequate patient throughput and comfort, as well as imaging protocol flexibility that facilitates optimisation.

PET/MR Applications

It is still uncertain whether PET/MR will become a routine clinical imaging modality. The lack of solid evidence for its benefits on specific clinical indications, compared with PET/CT and MRI entails, at the time this book was written, the absence of any reimbursement framework for joint PET/MR scans. Therefore, the first and foremost need is the identification of those clinical indications that PET/MR excels over 'conventional' imaging in diagnostic accuracy, workflow or reduction of overall costs to an extend that referring physicians consider sending their patients for scans and healthcare regulatory authorities provide the appropriate reimbursement for such procedures. However, the experience with PET/CT shows that even when validated clinical applications are found, they will require further time to gain patient referrals and receive reimbursement [9].

Several editorials and review papers have been published, the last few years, discussing potential applications for PET/MR, based on current experience from PET(/CT) and MRI [1, 3, 4, 12–16]; while many groups use the stand-alone modalities in investigational studies and assess the benefits of combining multi-modal information in staging, therapy monitoring and disease follow-up. Recently, the first studies on clinical use have started to appear in scientific literature.

One of the potential applications that PET/MR could have an impact is on brain imaging. PET has several attractive features such as high sensitivity and specificity in detecting biochemical and molecular tracers, while its inherent poor spatial resolution can be improved by recent advances in image reconstruction that incorporate resolution recovery approaches [17, 18]. Even more importantly, however, fusing quantitative PET images with high-resolution MR anatomical images can enhance the information extracted from both modalities, while at the same time advanced MR techniques, such as diffusion weighted imaging (DWI), perfusion with MR contrast agents, functional activation (fMRI), MR spectroscopy (MRS) or Diffusion Tensor Imaging (DTI), may yield complementary to PET information [12]. In Table 3.1, a thorough list of the biological properties that can be assessed by MRI and PET is presented.

So far, very limited work has been published in brain imaging using integrated PET/MR systems. In Neuro-Oncology, two groups performed feasibility studies in

Table 3.1 Biological properties that can be assessed by PET and MRI

MRI	PET
Morphology	Flow ($H_2{}^{15}O$)
Water motion in tissue (DWI)	Metabolism (^{18}F-FDG)
Vascular anatomy (MRA)	Blood volume ($C^{15}O$)
Perfusion (PWI, DCE-MRI)	Oxygen consumption (^{15}O)
Tissue metabolites (MRS for ^{1}H, ^{13}C, ^{23}Na, ^{31}P)	Vascular permeability (labelled AA)
Functional activation (fMRI)	Nucleic acid synthesis (^{18}F-FLT)
Cerebral fibre tracts (DTI)	Transmitters (e.g. DOPA)
Oxygen consumption (^{17}O)	Receptors (e.g. Raclopride)
Migration of cells (Fe labelling)	Enzymatic activity (e.g. MP4A)
	Angiogenesis (e.g. ^{18}F-RGB)
	Tracer & drugs (labelled compounds) distribution & kinetics
	Enzymatic activity in transfected cells

Adapted from Heiss [12]

patients with intracranial masses using different PET tracers (^{18}F-FDG, ^{11}C-methionine, ^{68}Ga-DOTATOC) combined with anatomical-MR, DTI, arterial spin labelling (ASL) and/or proton-spectroscopy [19, 20]. A different study also found that DTI-MR/PET provided important information for the treatment planning of brain tumours in four patients [21]. Neuner et al. have also demonstrated the use of ^{18}F-FET and ^{11}C-Methionine in combination with anatomical MRI, DTI, MRS and fMRI in PET/MR [22]. Finally, several groups have also shown the benefits of combined PET and MR information using stand-alone systems. Some of such applications include glioma staging [15], therapy planning [23, 24] and differential diagnosis from inflammatory demyelination [25]; therapy response of glioblastomas [26] and meningiomas [27]; as well as in image-guided neurosurgery for brain tumours [28, 29]. Apart from neuro-oncology, PET/MR may be useful in the assessment of damage inflicted by stroke [30], or as shown recently in neurodegenerative diseases [31–34], as well as epilepsy [35–37]. Furthermore, there are literature reports of combined PET and MRI use for various research studies, amongst others, in schizophrenia [38, 39], addictions [40], autism [41], aphasia [42] and multiple sclerosis [43].

Today, all the commercial PET/MR tomographs are designed with whole-body imaging capabilities, as this is necessary in order to perform oncological and cardiac scans. Advanced cardiovascular imaging is expected to be another opportunity for PET/MR given the excellent attributes of cardiac MRI and PET's absolute quantification [44]. Publications that demonstrate the successful combination of PET and MR imaging already exist in cardiomyopathy [45], evaluation of myocardial infarction [46] and its response to different therapy schemes [47, 48] and evaluation of carotid artery stenosis [49]. Therefore, although clinical evidence using integrated systems is still under way, PET/MR is expected to be a very useful modality for cardiovascular imaging [44].

Oncology is the main application of PET with highest volumes of scans globally and one of the areas with the biggest procedures growth for MRI. Moreover, the combination of these two modalities exhibit complementary advantages such as enhanced accuracy in the staging of primarily disease as well as in the assessment of local lymph node involvement and distant metastases [50]. Pilot studies with integrated systems have already shown the feasibility [51] of oncological PET/MR and potential clinical benefits in head and neck cancer [52], and lung cancer [53]; while its use was also showcased in single case studies for indications such as paediatric oncology [16], prostate [54, 55] and therapy follow up for malignancies of the liver [56]. Extensive discussions of the expected benefits of PET/MR in oncology can be found in literature [50, 57, 58].

Clinical Protocols and Workflow Considerations

An important concern for PET/MR scans is time. Both PET and MRI require long acquisition times for a comprehensive examination. Extended scan times have an impact on patient comfort (and increase of drop-out rates) and throughput, increasing the cost per scan. Therefore, some consideration on how to reduce acquisition time without losing important information is necessary for the various applications and the two system designs. Imaging acquisitions can be classified in two groups initially: single-organ imaging and imaging over several bed positions (e.g. whole- and total-body imaging). Each of the two categories may comprise scans for very different indications; however, patient set-up and imaging order can be similar.

Single-Organ Imaging

Single organ imaging is often performed within one (e.g. for brain) or more than one (e.g. for lungs) bed-positions, depending on the organ size and the scanner's field-of-view (FOV), to study organ function (e.g. brain, heart, liver) or regional disease (e.g. tumour, carotid plaques) in detail. They often require dynamic, gated or longer PET and/or MR acquisitions. Most of the times, MRI requires the longest acquisition times, due to the several pulse sequences and further functional information that may be necessary for a comprehensive diagnosis. In scanners with simultaneous acquisition capabilities, the required acquisition time for diagnostic MR and the extra sequences required for MR-based PET attenuation correction (MRAC) will define the total acquisition time.

It is common for research brain PET imaging to require dynamic acquisitions for studying tracer kinetics. These are long scans in order to capture both early and late phases of the tracer uptake. In these cases simultaneous PET/MR acquisition is prefered, from the workflow perspective, as MR scans can be acquired at the same time. One example is given in Fig. 3.1 for an application in neuro-oncology [22].

In clinical practice, shorter, static scans are more common. The most predominant brain PET indications include assessment of dementia with FDG or Amyloid imaging, surgical planning for focal epilepsy with FDG and to a lesser extent Parkinson's disease with ^{18}F-DOPA. Neuro-oncology uses tracers for metabolic assessment, receptor imaging and hypoxia as, and in addition to the list in Table 3.1. Most of these scans are static and, although shorter than many dynamic acquisitions, are still longer than the individual bed-position duration in whole-body protocols, requiring still 15-20 min as a crude average. In these cases, diagnostic MR may require longer acquisitions, again due to several different contrasts that may be required. Two generic imaging protocols for such scans are illustrated in Fig. 3.2 for simultaneous and sequential acquisitions. In both cases, the MR scans can start before or after PET depending on the workflow of the department and, in some occasions, MR scans may start during the radiotracer's uptake time [59].

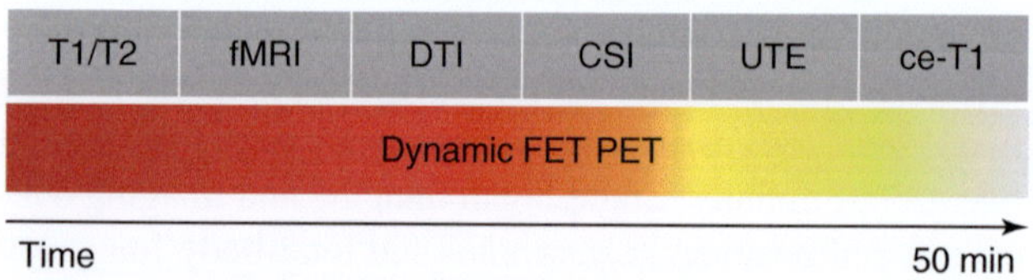

Fig. 3.1 Example protocol for PET/MR scan in neuro-oncology, comprising a dynamic ^{18}F-FET PET and several MR acquisitions, where *CSI* Chemical Shift Imaging, *UTE* Ultra-Short Time Echo, *ce* contrast enhanced scan (Adapted from Neuner et al. [22])

As indicated earlier, another promising area for PET/MR use is in cardiovascular imaging [44]. Imaging of myocardial viability, e.g. after acute myocardial infarction, or identifying vulnerable plaques in the carotid arteries also require single-bed acquisitions. Myocardial imaging often requires motion compensation for heart movement, which is performed through cardiac gating. Such gating in PET/MR can be done either using image-derived information from MRI, to gate both PET and MRI data in a simultaneous acquisition system, or via external triggering of both modalities in sequential acquisition systems. Figure 3.3 illustrates cardiac-gated exams acquired using the two different gating approaches.

Cardiac imaging protocols may have similar forms to those in Fig. 3.2. Depending on the amount and type of MR sequences needed, as well as the scanner's technology, but they are often faster than brain scans. An example of a comprehensive cardiac gated protocol and acquisition times, using a sequential system, is presented in Table 3.2 [59].

Whole-Body Imaging

For whole-body (i.e. eyes-to-thighs) or total-body (i.e. head-to-toes) imaging, several bed positions are acquired and merged. Modern PET systems require between 1 and 3 min per bed position, and the amount of bed positions needed is defined by the length of the required scan and the axial size of PET FOV. The latter in the current PET/MR scanners vary between 18 and 25.8 cm with overlap up to 50 % [60, 61]. On the other hand, diagnostic MR protocols may easily surpass 60 min of total acquisition time. The type of acquisition for both subsystems can vary significantly and, on some occasions, the protocols may need modifications in light of new data arising from one of the two modalities. For example, in a staging examination, both local disease and possible distant metastases, need to be assessed. In that case MRAC/localisation scan, followed by the FDG-PET acquisition is performed first and findings may indicate the distant regions with sus-

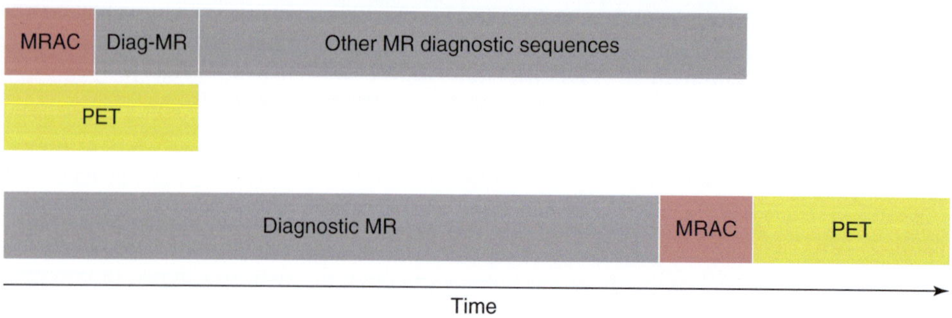

Fig. 3.2 Simultaneous and sequential PET/MR scans for a single-bed/station image acquisition

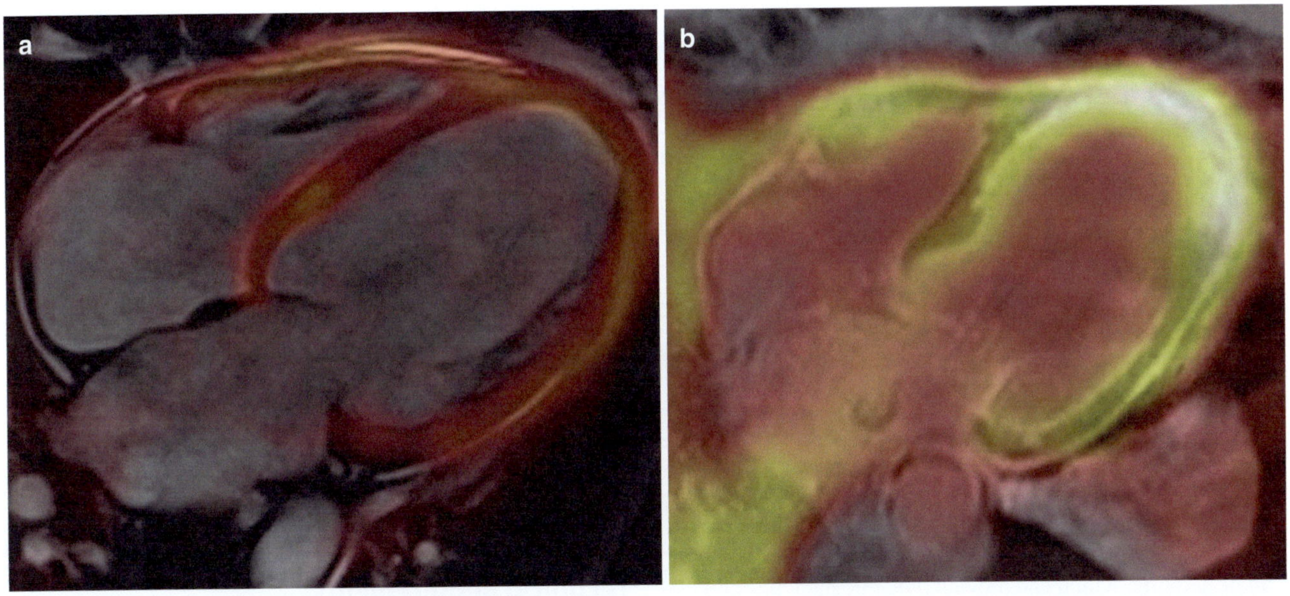

Fig. 3.3 Gated PET/MR studies acquired (**a**) on a simultaneous acquisition system with MR image-derived gating (Image courtesy of Siemens Healthcare) and (**b**) on a sequential acquisition system with independent external ECG triggering (Image courtesy of Dr R Nkoulou & Prof JP Vallée, HUG)

Table 3.2 Comprehensive sequential PET/MR imaging protocol for assessing myocardial viability

Heart protocol	Acq. time (min)	Effective acq. time (min)[a]	Acq. res (mm)	Rec. res. (mm)	TR/TE (ms)
M2D-B-TFE	00:00:09	00:01:00	2.07/1.85/10.0	0.61/0.61/10.0	2.8/1.40
B-TFE 2 chamber (LV)	00:00:09	00:01:00	2.01/1.79/8.00	1.16/1.16/8.00	3.2/1.60
B-TFE 2 chambers (RV)	00:00:11	00:01:00	2.01/1.79/8.00	1.16/1.16/8.00	3.2/1.66
B-TFE 4 chambers	00:00:11	00:01:00	2.01/1.82/8.00	1.16/1.16/8.00	3.3/1.66
B-TFE short axis (×8 to cover all LV)	00:01:15	00:08:00	2.01/1.82/8.00	1.16/1.16/8.00	3.3/1.66
Dynamic sTFE 3 slices	00:00:59	00:00:59	2.98/3.03/10.0	1.28/1.28/10.0	2.5/1.27
PSIR-TFE-2 chambers	00:00:06	00:01:00	1.60/2.29/10.0	0.61/0.61/10.0	6.1/3.0 (TI=90)
PSIR-TFE-4 chambers	00:00:06	00:01:00	1.60/2.29/10.0	0.61/0.61/10.0	6.1/3.0 (TI=90)
PSIR-TFE-short axis	00:00:06	00:01:00	1.60/2.29/10.0	0.61/0.61/10.0	6.1/3.0 (TI=90)
IR-TFE-LL	00:00:10	00:01:00	2.73/2.78/10.0	1.37/1.37/10.0	8.0/3.2
3D-IRTFE 4 chambers	00:00:09	00:01:00	2.01/2.01/10.0	1.16/1.16/5.00	3.5/1.13
3D-IRTFE 2 chambers	00:00:09	00:01:00	2.01/2.01/10.0	1.16/1.16/5.00	3.5/1.13
3D-IRTFE short axis	00:00:09	00:01:00	2.01/2.01/10.0	1.16/1.16/5.00	3.5/1.13
atMR cardiac	00:01:06	00:01:06	3.00/3.00/6.00	1.88/1.88/6.00	4.1/2.3
Gated FDG-PET (10 cardiac phases)	00:10:00	00:10:00		4.00/4.00/4.00	
Total time	**00:14:45**	**00:22:59**			

Courtesy of Prof JP Vallée, Dr R Nkoulou, Prof O Ratib, HUG
In Italics are all the PET/specific components
[a]Counting breathold time and recuperation, each sequence is performed in ~1 min

pected metastasis to be interrogated later on by the localised diagnostic MR contrasts (e.g. in breast cancer staging).

On a PET/MR tomograph with simultaneous acquisition capabilities, PET acquisitions run for 2–6 min per bed position [62, 63] and, during this time, MR also acquires data for MRAC (19 s/bed) as well as other relevant for each examination, sequences. Often, specific body areas require longer MR acquisitions, e.g. for the complete assessment of primary tumours. Depending on the clinical indication, PET tracer and processes of the department, these extra MR sequences can be performed before or after the simultaneous PET/MR acquisition. When the additional MR scans are performed prior to PET/MR acquisition, and for PET agents such as FDG, the patient may be scanned during the uptake period after the tracer injection. For FDG, however, consideration should be given in minimising potential FDG uptake in muscles [64]. Alternatively, when the additional MR scans are performed after simultaneous PET/MR, an additional PET acquisition

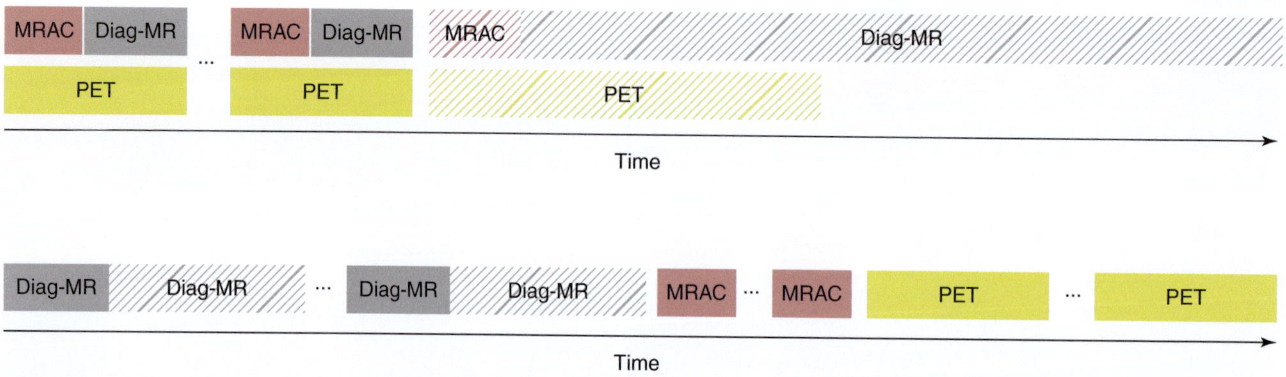

Fig. 3.4 Generalised simultaneous (*top*) and sequential (*bottom*) PET/MR whole-body imaging protocols. Diag-MR and MRAC indicate diagnostic MR acquisitions and MR sequences for attenuation correction and PET localisation, respectively. *Solid bars* indicate the minimum required acquisitions while hatched bars are extra imaging required by specific imaging protocols and their relative positions. The two time axes do not suggest equal acquisition time between the two protocols

can be acquired which can provide dynamic data [62] or a late acquisition which for agents such as FDG it is shown to provide more or different information than early scans [65–68].

On the other hand, in a different scanner with sequential acquisition capabilities, one option would be to perform all the diagnostic MR acquisitions at the beginning, followed by MRAC dedicated sequences and then PET. A clinical indication which would use such a protocol (Fig. 3.4) is to assess response to treatment or in Head/Neck cancer surgery planning [59]. Workflow optimisation is even more necessary for sequential acquisition settings, since the luxury of PET acquisition during MR is not present. Hence, current sequential scanner designs are trying to leverage technologies from both modalities such as Time-of-Flight (TOF) PET and multiple transmission MRI in order to minimise the required imaging time. The MRAC whole-body scan requires approximately 4–6 min [69], while a TOF PET scan is shown to be performed as fast as 30s/bed position [70, 71] but times between 1-2 min/bed are more common. The decision for how long to acquire PET data depends on the site preferences and experience with TOF-PET systems. Examples in literature exist which demonstrate the use of PET with short acquisition protocols for FDG [72] and other radio-tracers [73].

One improvement in the area of high-field MR is brought by the introduction of parallel transmission, which reduces the local Specific Absorption Rate (SAR), resulting in shorter pulse repetition time and, hence, faster acquisitions [74, 75]. Gains in acquisition time, though, vary depending on the pulse sequences used. From comparisons with standard high-field MR in literature it was found to accelerate lumbar spine imaging by 50 % for T2 sagittal and 18 % for T1 sagittal sequences; while in the pelvis, T2 fast spin-echo sequences could be acquired with a time gain of 33 % [76]. Finally, the average expected acquisition time improvement from multi-transmit was found to be 31 % across 77 clinically tested MR sequences [77].

Technical Requirements

The necessary technology for building a PET/MR scanner is already described in detail in a different chapter of this book. The current section attempts to link specific clinical and/or workflow needs for PET/MRI and the main technological requirements which may address these needs. The two main such needs is the reduction of scan time and the equivalence of image quality as well as quantification of PET/MR in comparison with stand-alone MRI and PET/CT.

Scan Time

As it became apparent so far in the discussion, one major consideration is the PET/MR acquisition time. Shorter exam times ensure patient comfort and faster throughput (implying reduced cost per exam). However, faster throughput should be considered together with the fact that radiation exposure to staff might be higher in PET/MR than in PET/CT due to longer patient setting-up times that MRI scans require, and the current lack of formalised reimbursement framework for PET/MR scans. These two parameters may limit anyhow the patient availability per day for PET/MR scans.

On the other hand, both PET and MRI have limitations with respect to their signal detection efficiency. For PET imaging, only a certain amount of radiotracer can be administered according to national and local health and safety regulations, while the tomograph itself has a significantly low detection efficiency, despite its ability for absolute quantification [78]. MRI has also low sensitivity, due to the inherent low macroscopic magnetisation of the human body [79]. Therefore, the longer the acquisition time, the better the quantification and image quality can be achieved by for both modalities.

The scanner design and several technologies can improve the above compromise. From the PET side, the straightforward approach is to increase the solid angle of the detector exposed to radioactivity with direct effect on system sensitivity [80]. This can be achieved by increasing the axial FOV and/or placing the detector closer to the body. This has already been successfully employed by one system design [61]. In the last 6 years, advancements in scintillation crystals, electronics and reconstruction algorithms have enabled PET systems to compute with higher accuracy the origin of each registered event using Time-of-Flight (TOF) and significantly improving the signal-to-noise (SNR) ratio in images [81] at levels higher than expected for the given sensitivity of the scanner [82] and keeping all other imaging parameters equal. This route has also been exploited by another system design [60].

From the MRI side, several techniques have been attempted in order to reduce the acquisition time. Fast pulse sequences have been developed, sometimes at the expense of spatial resolution or SNR [83]. The use of 3T MRI despite its excellent spatial resolution and contrast that introduced it made acquisitions longer due to the need to account for increased levels of local Specific Absorption Rate (SAR) by increasing Repetition Times (TR) in the pulse sequences [84]. Two other MRI technologies, that lead to a reduction in scan time, is parallel acquisition with multiple coil elements [85], and parallel transmission [86]. Parallel acquisition uses multiple receiver coil channels that provide additional spatial information for the reconstruction of the under-sampled K-space in the phase encoding direction [87]. Parallel acquisition algorithms work either with the acquired aliased images (e.g. SENSE [88]) or by reconstructing the missing K-space data (e.g. GRAPPA [89]). A more recent technology, parallel transmission utilizes multiple transmission channels and RF sources to adjust the power, amplitude, phase and waveform for optimal excitation and homogeneous receive fields for each specific patient anatomy [76]. The latter has as a result homogeneous fat suppression [90] and better image quality for difficult regions such as spine [77], breast [91], heart [92] and pelvis [76]. In addition, parallel transmission benefits PET/MR through the reduction of local SAR, allowing for significant increases in scanning speed [76].

Image Quality and Quantification

A major advantage for PET/MR versus MRI is the high specificity of PET as well as its relative and absolute quantification of the radiotracer bio-distribution. This becomes possible after the implementation of several corrections on the PET data related to ionising radiation measurements; namely, radioactive decay, the attenuation and scatter of photons in matter and random registered coincidences resulting into faulty estimated events [93]. For PET/MR, most of these corrections are estimated using identical or similar procedures to stand-alone PET and PET/CT. However, this is not true for attenuation correction [94] and scatter correction may also be problematic in certain clinical applications.

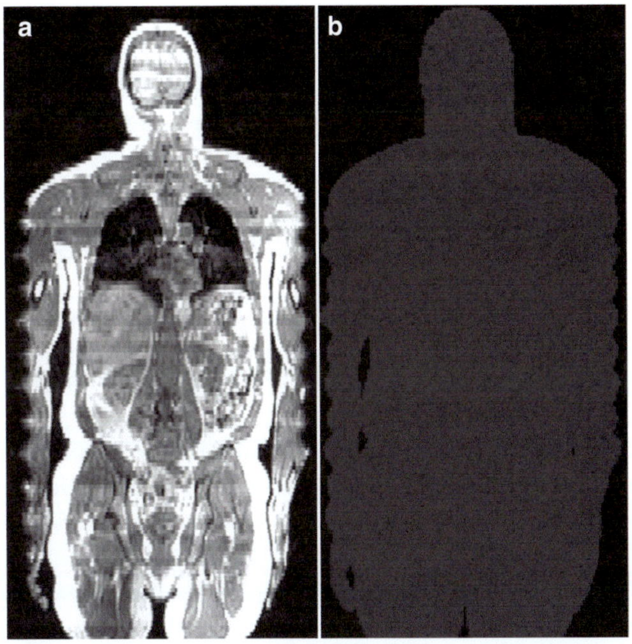

Fig. 3.5 Example of (**a**) the MR FOV truncation, and (**b**) the maximum intensity projection of the resulting MRAC map demonstrating the truncation effect

Attenuation correction in stand-alone PET is performed by acquiring a transmission scan using rotating ^{68}Ge or ^{137}Cs sources or, in modern PET/CTs, a low-dose CT scan (CTAC) is used (Fig. 2.12). In contrast to CT, MRI does not provide the electron density information of the scanned object, the primary cause of photon attenuation. Therefore, MR images require further manipulation to derive attenuation coefficients. Several MR-based attenuation correction (MRAC) methods exist in literature, based on anatomical atlases [95], segmentation of images obtained with specific MR sequences [96–98] or a combination of both [99]. Two further requirements for such methodology are to use MR images that can be acquired in a clinically feasible time (as a significant amount of PET/MR applications are expected to require whole-body imaging) and are able to provide useful clinical information for whole-body disease assessment. Currently, the methods implemented on the commercial systems use specific MR-sequences and segmentation of three [69] or four [97] different classes of attenuating media.

Another important concern for MRAC is the smaller MRI transverse FOV versus that of PET. This difference frequently results in truncation of hands and shoulders in the MR image of a number of patients (Fig. 3.5a). The result is a truncated MRAC map (Fig. 3.5b) causing bias in quantification and image artefacts in PET [100, 101]. The currently implemented truncation compensated methods on the two commercial systems use two different approaches. The missing parts of the attenuation maps are estimated in the first case by a modified iterative reconstruction algorithm using the emission PET data [102], while the second utilises an edge-detection algorithm operating on the reconstructed non-attenuated PET image and using prior knowledge of the scanner design [100].

The first implemented MRAC methods do not take into account cortical bone [97, 103], the highest attenuating material in the human body. Although currently published data from both commercially implemented methods do not show any clinically relevant quantitative inaccuracies [69, 97, 104], a different study showed that MRAC without a bone class underestimates SUVs in certain areas such as spine and pelvis [105]. Another study, using CTAC maps processed in such a way to mimic MRAC, found SUV_{mean} underestimated by 11 % for total bone lesions with femur being the highest (17 %) [106]. These findings indicate that, depending on the clinical application, more thorough studies may identify quantification concerns for first generation MRAC methods.

Since the transverse relaxation time (T2) of cortical bone is very short [107], the signal from bone has decayed at the time of image acquisition in classical MR sequences. Thus, a separation of air and bone is not possible on the acquired MR images. To obtain a bone signal, Ultra-short Echo Time (UTE) sequences, in particular, have been used [108, 109] for MR attenuation correction. UTE sequences sample the free induction decay (FID) directly after the excitation of the spins, yielding signal from bone and all other tissue, while an echo signal is acquired in the same sequence, where the bone signal has already decayed. Attenuation maps are then derived by segmenting the images into air, tissue and bone components [59]. Unfortunately, such sequences require long acquisition time [108] while the resulting images do not have clinically relevant information for most examinations. This is an on-going area of research and several academic and industry groups are trying to improve MRAC with clinically sensible MR acquisition times.

Another area of concern regarding MRAC the presence of magnetically susceptible materials (e.g. metal implants or medical devices) in the MR FOV, will result into susceptibility artefacts, i.e. signal void areas and bright signals in the tissues surrounding the implants [110]. Such artefacts propagate in the MRAC map in a relatively arbitrary fashion, depending on the location and extent of the artefact (Fig. 3.6). Metal artefact reduction sequences (MARS) can be used to reduce the size and intensity of susceptibility artefacts from magnetic field distortion [111]. However, currently only manual corrections may be available.

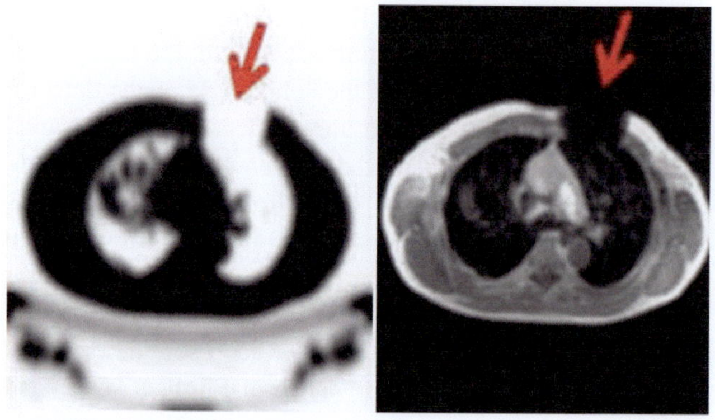

Fig. 3.6 Example of MR artefacts in the acquired image due a cardiac stent, as propagated in the MRAC (Image courtesy of Philips Healthcare)

Apart from attenuation correction, scatter correction may also need some consideration in PET/MR. Although the standard methodology performs very well for most clinical situations, on certain clinical settings when patient set-up may differ from PET/CT, this difference may impact on scatter correction accuracy. For example, in breast cancer, MR patient set-up is different from PET/CT, prone vs. supine positioning, respectively. The main benefit for prone imaging is that the breast tissues are extended by gravity providing higher spatial resolution than in supine position. When prone positioning is selected in PET/MR, occasionally certain parts of the body exhibit extremely low radiotracer uptake, such as the area behind the breast. This causes the scatter correction to fail, impacting both image quality and quantification. To address the incorporation of a priori information from the MR scan in the scatter correction has been investigated [112]. One such example is illustrated in Fig. 3.7.

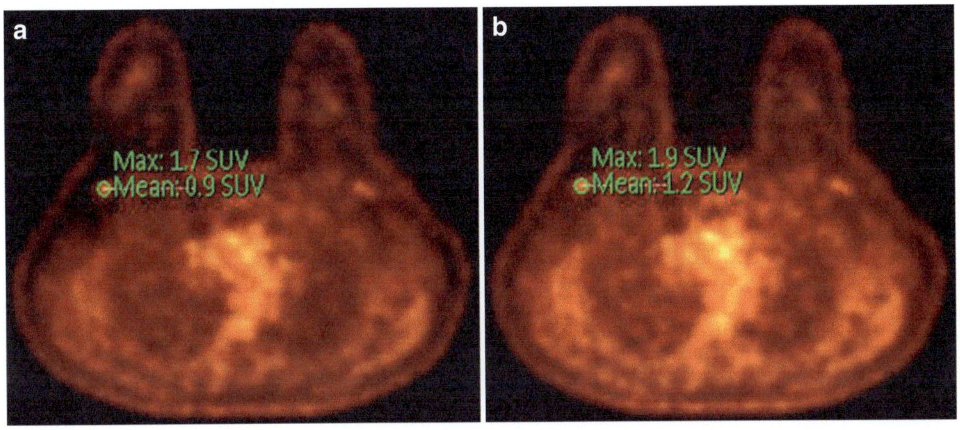

Fig. 3.7 FDG-PET image of a patient in prone position with scatter artefacts impacting on the image quality and quantification in the area behind the right breast (**a**). The same PET image with a modified scatter correction, incorporating information from the MR scan, shows higher SUV uptake, but not enough to indicate malignancy, and higher consistency with the background contrast (**b**) (Images from Kalemis et al. [59])

Conclusions

This chapter has presented generic forms of PET/MR protocols, as been reported by users in literature, and the impact that current technologies have on such imaging protocols. By the time this book was published, whole-body PET/MR had already been in the clinic for two and a half years. During this period a lot of effort was devoted into proving that the new modality performs equally well with stand-alone modalities and PET/CT. For most cases this is already proven but efforts are still underway for improving technologies such as MR-based attenuation correction and motion correction/compensation. The clinical exposure of PET/MR identifies important areas for improvement and accordingly, technology is still expected to improve in capabilities and performance, and system designs to mature. Judging from PET/CT, most probably we are still several years away from fully-optimised technologies.

Although, the period where image quality comparison between PET/CT vs. PET/MR slowly comes to an end and the next phase of investigating the clinical benefits of the new technology has already started. The optimisation of imaging protocols is an inherent part of streamlining workflows and improving the acquisition of diagnostic information and a two-way impact is expected between the implementation of novel technology and testing of new imaging protocols. Even preliminary results from this phase are of paramount importance for the establishment and acceptance rate of the new modality. Obviously, only time can tell the future of PET/MR; however, judging from the interest, motivation and the investment already made for this novel imaging technology one may say that its chances are quite high. The following chapters will give an idea of future PET/MR clinical applications.

References

1. Ratib O, Beyer T (2011) Whole-body hybrid PET/MRI: ready for clinical use? Eur J Nucl Med Mol Imaging 38(6):992–995
2. Jones T (2002) Molecular imaging with PET – the future challenges. Br J Radiol 75 Spec No:S6–S15
3. Pichler BJ, Kolb A, Nagele T, Schlemmer HP (2010) PET/MRI: paving the way for the next generation of clinical multimodality imaging applications. J Nucl Med 51(3):333–336
4. Schiepers C, Dahlbom M (2011) Molecular imaging in oncology: the acceptance of PET/CT and the emergence of MR/PET imaging. Eur Radiol 21(3):548–554
5. Zaidi H, Del Guerra A (2011) An outlook on future design of hybrid PET/MRI systems. Med Phys 38(10):5667–5689
6. Kielstra P (2009) Doctor innovation: shaking up the health system. The Economist Intelligence Unit, London
7. Oates ME, Diagnostic Radiology Participants of ACRSNMTF, II (2012) Integrated residency training pathways of the future: diagnostic radiology, nuclear radiology, nuclear medicine, and molecular imaging. J Am Coll Radiol 9(4):239–244
8. Bolus NE, George R, Washington J, Newcomer BR (2009) PET/MRI: the blended-modality choice of the future? J Nucl Med Technol 37(2):63–71; quiz 72–63
9. Hicks RJ, Lau EW (2009) PET/MRI: a different spin from under the rim. Eur J Nucl Med Mol Imaging 36(Suppl 1):S10–S14
10. Goyen M, Debatin JF (2009) Healthcare costs for new technologies. Eur J Nucl Med Mol Imaging 36(Suppl 1):S139–S143
11. von Schulthess GK, Schlemmer HP (2009) A look ahead: PET/MR versus PET/CT. Eur J Nucl Med Mol Imaging 36(Suppl 1):S3–S9
12. Heiss WD (2009) The potential of PET/MR for brain imaging. Eur J Nucl Med Mol Imaging 36(Suppl 1):S105–S112
13. Saraste A, Knuuti J (2012) Cardiac PET, CT, and MR: what are the advantages of hybrid imaging? Curr Cardiol Rep 14(1):24–31
14. Herzog H, Langen K-J, Kaffanke J, Weirich C, Neuner I, Stoffels G, Kops ER, Scheins J, Tellmann L, Shah NJ (2010) MR-PET opens new horizons in neuroimaging. Future Neurol 5(6):807–815
15. Jansen NL, Graute V, Armbruster L, Suchorska B, Lutz J, Eigenbrod S, Cumming P, Bartenstein P, Tonn JC, Kreth FW, la Fougere C (2012) MRI-suspected low-grade glioma: is there a need to perform dynamic FET PET? Eur J Nucl Med Mol Imaging 39(6):1021–1029
16. Beuthien-Baumann B, Platzek I, Lauterbach I, van den Hoff J, Schramm G, Zophel K, Laniado M, Kotzerke J (2012) Improved anatomic visualization of a glomus caroticum tumour within the carotic bifurcation with combined 68 Ga-DOTATATE PET/MRI. Eur J Nucl Med Mol Imaging 39(6):1087–1088

17. Cui J, Pratx G, Prevrhal S, Zhang B, Shao L, Levin CS (2011) Measurement-based spatially-varying point spread function for list-mode PET reconstruction on GPU. In: IEEE nuclear science symposium and medical imaging conference (NSS/MIC), 2011 IEEE, 23–29 Oct 2011, Valencia, pp 2593–2596
18. Panin VY, Kehren F, Rothfuss H, Hu D, Michel C, Casey ME (2006) PET reconstruction with system matrix derived from point source measurements. Nucl Sci IEEE Trans 53(1):152–159
19. Schwenzer NF, Stegger L, Bisdas S, Schraml C, Kolb A, Boss A, Muller M, Reimold M, Ernemann U, Claussen CD, Pfannenberg C, Schmidt H (2012) Simultaneous PET/MR imaging in a human brain PET/MR system in 50 patients – current state of image quality. Eur J Radiol. doi:10.1016/j.ejrad.2011.12.027
20. Boss A, Bisdas S, Kolb A, Hofmann M, Ernemann U, Claussen CD, Pfannenberg C, Pichler BJ, Reimold M, Stegger L (2010) Hybrid PET/MRI of intracranial masses: initial experiences and comparison to PET/CT. J Nucl Med 51(8):1198–1205
21. Boss A, Kolb A, Hofmann M, Bisdas S, Nagele T, Ernemann U, Stegger L, Rossi C, Schlemmer HP, Pfannenberg C, Reimold M, Claussen CD, Pichler BJ, Klose U (2010) Diffusion tensor imaging in a human PET/MR hybrid system. Invest Radiol 45(5):270–274
22. Neuner I, Kaffanke JB, Langen KJ, Kops ER, Tellmann L, Stoffels G, Weirich C, Filss C, Scheins J, Herzog H, Shah NJ (2012) Multimodal imaging utilising integrated MR-PET for human brain tumour assessment. Eur Radiol 22(12):2568–2580
23. Arbizu J, Tejada S, Marti-Climent JM, Diez-Valle R, Prieto E, Quincoces G, Vigil C, Idoate MA, Zubieta JL, Penuelas I, Richter JA (2012) Quantitative volumetric analysis of gliomas with sequential MRI and (11)C-methionine PET assessment: patterns of integration in therapy planning. Eur J Nucl Med Mol Imaging 39(5):771–781
24. Heinzel A, Stock S, Langen K-J, Müller D (2012) Cost-effectiveness analysis of FET PET/guided target selection for the diagnosis of gliomas. Eur J Nucl Med Mol Imaging 39(7):1089–1096
25. Takenaka S, Shinoda J, Asano Y, Aki T, Miwa K, Ito T, Yokoyama K, Iwama T (2011) Metabolic assessment of monofocal acute inflammatory demyelination using MR spectroscopy and (11) C-methionine-, (11)C-choline-, and (18)F-fluorodeoxyglucose-PET. Brain Tumor Pathol 28(3):229–238
26. Galldiks N, Langen KJ, Holy R, Pinkawa M, Stoffels G, Nolte KW, Kaiser HJ, Filss CP, Fink GR, Coenen HH, Eble MJ, Piroth MD (2012) Assessment of treatment response in patients with glioblastoma using O-(2-18F-fluoroethyl)-L-tyrosine PET in comparison to MRI. J Nucl Med 53(7):1048–1057
27. Thorwarth D, Henke G, Muller AC, Reimold M, Beyer T, Boss A, Kolb A, Pichler B, Pfannenberg C (2011) Simultaneous 68Ga-DOTATOC-PET/MRI for IMRT treatment planning for meningioma: first experience. Int J Radiat Oncol Biol Phys 81(1):277–283
28. Pirotte B, Goldman S, Dewitte O, Massager N, Wikler D, Lefranc F, Ben Taib NO, Rorive S, David P, Brotchi J, Levivier M (2006) Integrated positron emission tomography and magnetic resonance imaging-guided resection of brain tumors: a report of 103 consecutive procedures. J Neurosurg 104(2):238–253
29. Pirotte B, Goldman S, Van Bogaert P, David P, Wikler D, Rorive S, Brotchi J, Levivier M (2005) Integration of [11C]methionine-positron emission tomographic and magnetic resonance imaging for image-guided surgical resection of infiltrative low-grade brain tumors in children. Neurosurgery 57(1 Suppl):128–139; discussion 128–139
30. Garibotto V, Vargas MI, Lovblad KO, Ratib O (2011) A PET/MRI case of corticocerebellar diaschisis after stroke. Clin Nucl Med 36(9):821–825
31. Brockmann K, Reimold M, Globas C, Hauser TK, Walter U, Machulla HJ, Rolfs A, Schols L (2012) PET and MRI reveal early evidence of neurodegeneration in spinocerebellar ataxia type 17. J Nucl Med 53(7):1074–1080
32. Drzezga A, Becker JA, Van Dijk KR, Sreenivasan A, Talukdar T, Sullivan C, Schultz AP, Sepulcre J, Putcha D, Greve D, Johnson KA, Sperling RA (2011) Neuronal dysfunction and disconnection of cortical hubs in non-demented subjects with elevated amyloid burden. Brain 134(Pt 6):1635–1646
33. Kanda T, Ishii K, Uemura T, Miyamoto N, Yoshikawa T, Kono AK, Mori E (2008) Comparison of grey matter and metabolic reductions in frontotemporal dementia using FDG-PET and voxel-based morphometric MR studies. Eur J Nucl Med Mol Imaging 35(12):2227–2234
34. Karow DS, McEvoy LK, Fennema-Notestine C, Hagler DJ Jr, Jennings RG, Brewer JB, Hoh CK, Dale AM, Alzheimer's Disease Neuroimaging I (2010) Relative capability of MR imaging and FDG PET to depict changes associated with prodromal and early Alzheimer disease. Radiology 256(3):932–942
35. Brodbeck V, Spinelli L, Lascano AM, Wissmeier M, Vargas M-I, Vulliemoz S, Pollo C, Schaller K, Michel CM, Seeck M (2011) Electroencephalographic source imaging: a prospective study of 152 operated epileptic patients. Brain 134(10):2887–2897
36. Carne R, O'Brien T, Kilpatrick C, MacGregor L, Litewka L, Hicks R, Cook M (2007) 'MRI-negative PET/positive' temporal lobe epilepsy (TLE) and mesial TLE differ with quantitative MRI and PET: a case control study. BMC Neurol 7(1):16
37. Rubi S, Setoain X, Donaire A, Bargallo N, Sanmarti F, Carreno M, Rumia J, Calvo A, Aparicio J, Campistol J, Pons F (2011) Validation of FDG-PET/MRI coregistration in nonlesional refractory childhood epilepsy. Epilepsia 52(12):2216–2224
38. Buchsbaum MS, Buchsbaum BR, Hazlett EA, Haznedar MM, Newmark R, Tang CY, Hof PR (2007) Relative glucose metabolic rate higher in white matter in patients with schizophrenia. Am J Psychiatry 164(7):1072–1081
39. Buchsbaum MS, Haznedar MM, Aronowitz J, Brickman AM, Newmark RE, Bloom R, Brand J, Goldstein KE, Heath D, Starson M, Hazlett EA (2007) FDG-PET in never-previously medicated psychotic adolescents treated with olanzapine or haloperidol. Schizophr Res 94(1–3):293–305
40. Chang L, Alicata D, Ernst T, Volkow N (2007) Structural and metabolic brain changes in the striatum associated with methamphetamine abuse. Addiction 102(Suppl 1):16–32
41. Haznedar MM, Buchsbaum MS, Hazlett EA, LiCalzi EM, Cartwright C, Hollander E (2006) Volumetric analysis and three-dimensional glucose metabolic mapping of the striatum and thalamus in patients with autism spectrum disorders. Am J Psychiatry 163(7):1252–1263
42. Uttner I, Mottaghy FM, Schreiber H, Riecker A, Ludolph AC, Kassubek J (2006) Primary progressive aphasia accompanied by environmental sound agnosia: a neuropsychological, MRI and PET study. Psychiatry Res 146(2):191–197
43. Versijpt J, Debruyne JC, Van Laere KJ, De Vos F, Keppens J, Strijckmans K, Achten E, Slegers G, Dierckx RA, Korf J, De Reuck JL (2005) Microglial imaging with positron emission tomography and atrophy measurements with magnetic resonance imaging in multiple sclerosis: a correlative study. Mult Scler 11(2): 127–134
44. Nekolla SG, Martinez-Moeller A, Saraste A (2009) PET and MRI in cardiac imaging: from validation studies to integrated applications. Eur J Nucl Med Mol Imaging 36(Suppl 1):S121–S130
45. Knaapen P, Gotte MJ, Paulus WJ, Zwanenburg JJ, Dijkmans PA, Boellaard R, Marcus JT, Twisk JW, Visser CA, van Rossum AC, Lammertsma AA, Visser FC (2006) Does myocardial fibrosis hinder contractile function and perfusion in idiopathic dilated cardiomyopathy? PET and MR imaging study. Radiology 240(2): 380–388
46. Slart R, Glauche J, Golestani R, Zeebregts C, Jansen J, Dierckx R, Oudkerk M, Willems T, Glaudemans A, Boersma H, Tio R (2012) PET and MRI for the evaluation of regional myocardial perfusion

and wall thickening after myocardial infarction. Eur J Nucl Med Mol Imaging 39(6):1065–1069

47. Qiao H, Zhang H, Zheng Y, Ponde DE, Shen D, Gao F, Bakken AB, Schmitz A, Kung HF, Ferrari VA, Zhou R (2009) Embryonic stem cell grafting in normal and infarcted myocardium: serial assessment with MR imaging and PET dual detection. Radiology 250(3):821–829
48. Wu YW, Tadamura E, Yamamuro M, Kanao S, Marui A, Tanabara K, Komeda M, Togashi K (2007) Comparison of contrast-enhanced MRI with (18)F-FDG PET/201Tl SPECT in dysfunctional myocardium: relation to early functional outcome after surgical revascularization in chronic ischemic heart disease. J Nucl Med 48(7): 1096–1103
49. Tang TY, Moustafa RR, Howarth SP, Walsh SR, Boyle JR, Li ZY, Baron JC, Gillard JH, Warburton EA (2008) Combined PET/FDG and USPIO-enhanced MR imaging in patients with symptomatic moderate carotid artery stenosis. Eur J Vasc Endovasc Surg 36(1):53–55
50. Antoch G, Bockisch A (2009) Combined PET/MRI: a new dimension in whole-body oncology imaging? Eur J Nucl Med Mol Imaging 36(Suppl 1):S113–S120
51. Drzezga A, Souvatzoglou M, Eiber M, Beer AJ, Furst S, Martinez-Moller A, Nekolla SG, Ziegler S, Ganter C, Rummeny EJ, Schwaiger M (2012) First clinical experience with integrated whole-body PET/MR: comparison to PET/CT in patients with oncologic diagnoses. J Nucl Med 53(6):845–855
52. Boss A, Stegger L, Bisdas S, Kolb A, Schwenzer N, Pfister M, Claussen CD, Pichler BJ, Pfannenberg C (2011) Feasibility of simultaneous PET/MR imaging in the head and upper neck area. Eur Radiol 21(7):1439–1446
53. Schwenzer NF, Schraml C, Muller M, Brendle C, Sauter A, Spengler W, Pfannenberg AC, Claussen CD, Schmidt H (2012) Pulmonary lesion assessment: comparison of whole-body hybrid MR/PET and PET/CT imaging – pilot study. Radiology 264(2):551–558
54. Lord M, Ratib O, Vallee JP (2011) (1)F-Fluorocholine integrated PET/MRI for the initial staging of prostate cancer. Eur J Nucl Med Mol Imaging 38(12):2288
55. Takei T, Souvatzoglou M, Beer AJ, Drzezga A, Ziegler S, Rummeny EJ, Schwaiger M, Eiber M (2012) A case of multimodality multiparametric 11C-choline PET/MR for biopsy targeting in prior biopsy-negative primary prostate cancer. Clin Nucl Med 37(9):918–919
56. Wissmeyer M, Heinzer S, Majno P, Buchegger F, Zaidi H, Garibotto V, Viallon M, Becker CD, Ratib O, Terraz S (2011) ^{90}Y Time-of-flight PET/MR on a hybrid scanner following liver radioembolisation (SIRT). Eur J Nucl Med Mol Imaging 38(9):1744–1745
57. Buchbender C, Heusner TA, Lauenstein TC, Bockisch A, Antoch G (2012) Oncologic PET/MRI, part 1: tumors of the brain, head and neck, chest, abdomen, and pelvis. J Nucl Med 53(6):928–938
58. Buchbender C, Heusner TA, Lauenstein TC, Bockisch A, Antoch G (2012) Oncologic PET/MRI, part 2: bone tumors, soft-tissue tumors, melanoma, and lymphoma. J Nucl Med 53(8):1244–1252
59. Kalemis A, Delattre BM, Heinzer S (2013) Sequential whole-body PET/MR scanner: concept, clinical use, and optimisation after two years in the clinic. The manufacturer's perspective. MAGMA 26(1):5–23
60. Zaidi H, Ojha N, Morich M, Griesmer J, Hu Z, Maniawski P, Ratib O, Izquierdo-Garcia D, Fayad ZA, Shao L (2011) Design and performance evaluation of a whole-body Ingenuity TF PET/MRI system. Phys Med Biol 56(10):3091–3106
61. Delso G, Furst S, Jakoby B, Ladebeck R, Ganter C, Nekolla SG, Schwaiger M, Ziegler SI (2011) Performance measurements of the Siemens mMR integrated whole-body PET/MR scanner. J Nucl Med 52(12):1914–1922
62. Martinez-Moller A, Eiber M, Nekolla SG, Souvatzoglou M, Drzezga A, Ziegler S, Rummeny EJ, Schwaiger M, Beer AJ (2012) Workflow and scan protocol considerations for integrated whole-body PET/MRI in oncology. J Nucl Med 53(9):1415–1426
63. Werner MK, Schmidt H, Schwenzer NF (2012) MR/PET: a new challenge in hybrid imaging. AJR Am J Roentgenol 199(2):272–277
64. Boellaard R, O'Doherty MJ, Weber WA, Mottaghy FM, Lonsdale MN, Stroobants SG, Oyen WJ, Kotzerke J, Hoekstra OS, Pruim J, Marsden PK, Tatsch K, Hoekstra CJ, Visser EP, Arends B, Verzijlbergen FJ, Zijlstra JM, Comans EF, Lammertsma AA, Paans AM, Willemsen AT, Beyer T, Bockisch A, Schaefer-Prokop C, Delbeke D, Baum RP, Chiti A, Krause BJ (2010) FDG PET and PET/CT: EANM procedure guidelines for tumour PET imaging: version 1.0. Eur J Nucl Med Mol Imaging 37(1):181–200
65. Hamada K, Tomita Y, Qiu Y, Tomoeda M, Ueda T, Tamai N, Hashimoto N, Yoshikawa H, Aozasa K, Hatazawa J (2009) (18) F-FDG PET analysis of schwannoma: increase of SUVmax in the delayed scan is correlated with elevated VEGF/VPF expression in the tumors. Skeletal Radiol 38(3):261–266
66. Chen YM, Huang G, Sun XG, Liu JJ, Chen T, Shi YP, Wan LR (2008) Optimizing delayed scan time for FDG PET: comparison of the early and late delayed scan. Nucl Med Commun 29(5):425–430
67. Nakamoto Y, Higashi T, Sakahara H, Tamaki N, Kogire M, Doi R, Hosotani R, Imamura M, Konishi J (2000) Delayed (18)F-fluoro-2-deoxy-D-glucose positron emission tomography scan for differentiation between malignant and benign lesions in the pancreas. Cancer 89(12):2547–2554
68. Laffon E, de Clermont H, Vernejoux JM, Jougon J, Marthan R (2011) Feasibility of assessing [(18)F]FDG lung metabolism with late dynamic PET imaging. Mol Imaging Biol 13(2):378–384
69. Schulz V, Torres-Espallardo I, Renisch S, Hu Z, Ojha N, Bornert P, Perkuhn M, Niendorf T, Schafer WM, Brockmann H, Krohn T, Buhl A, Gunther RW, Mottaghy FM, Krombach GA (2011) Automatic, three-segment, MR-based attenuation correction for whole-body PET/MR data. Eur J Nucl Med Mol Imaging 38(1):138–152
70. Murray I, Kalemis A, Glennon J, Hasan S, Quraishi S, Beyer T, Avril N (2010) Time-of-flight PET/CT using low-activity protocols: potential implications for cancer therapy monitoring. Eur J Nucl Med Mol Imaging 37(9):1643–1653
71. Conti M (2011) Focus on time-of-flight PET: the benefits of improved time resolution. Eur J Nucl Med Mol Imaging 38(6):1147–1157
72. Derlin T, Weber C, Habermann CR, Herrmann J, Wisotzki C, Ayuk F, Wolschke C, Klutmann S, Kroger N (2012) 18F-FDG PET/CT for detection and localization of residual or recurrent disease in patients with multiple myeloma after stem cell transplantation. Eur J Nucl Med Mol Imaging 39(3):493–500
73. Derlin T, Toth Z, Papp L, Wisotzki C, Apostolova I, Habermann CR, Mester J, Klutmann S (2011) Correlation of inflammation assessed by 18F-FDG PET, active mineral deposition assessed by 18F-fluoride PET, and vascular calcification in atherosclerotic plaque: a dual-tracer PET/CT study. J Nucl Med 52(7):1020–1027
74. Zhu Y (2004) Parallel excitation with an array of transmit coils. Magn Reson Med 51(4):775–784
75. Harvey PR, Zhai Z, Morich M, Mens G, van Yperen G, DeMeester G, Graesslin I, Hoogeveen R (2009) SAR behavior during whole-body multitransmit RF shimming at 3.0T. In: Proceedings of the 17th scientific meeting, International Society for Magnetic Resonance in Medicine, Honolulu, 2009, p 4786
76. Willinek WA, Gieseke J, Kukuk GM, Nelles M, Konig R, Morakkabati-Spitz N, Traber F, Thomas D, Kuhl CK, Schild HH (2010) Dual-source parallel radiofrequency excitation body MR imaging compared with standard MR imaging at 3.0 T: initial clinical experience. Radiology 256(3):966–975
77. Nelles M, Konig RS, Gieseke J, Guerand-van Battum MM, Kukuk GM, Schild HH, Willinek WA (2010) Dual-source parallel RF transmission for clinical MR imaging of the spine at 3.0 T: intraindividual comparison with conventional single-source transmission. Radiology 257(3):743–753
78. Bailey DL (2003) Date acquisition and performance characterization in PET. In: Valk PE, Bailey DL, Townsend DW, Maisey MN

(eds) Positron emission tomography; basic science and clinical practice, 2nd edn. Springer, London, pp 69–90
79. Brix G (2008) Physical basics. In: Reiser MF, Semmler W, Hricak H (eds) Magnetic resonance tomography. Springer, Berlin, pp 8–25
80. Budinger TF (1998) PET instrumentation: what are the limits? Semin Nucl Med 28(3):247–267
81. El Fakhri G, Surti S, Trott CM, Scheuermann J, Karp JS (2011) Improvement in lesion detection with whole-body oncologic time-of-flight PET. J Nucl Med 52(3):347–353
82. Budinger TF (1983) Time-of-flight positron emission tomography: status relative to conventional PET. J Nucl Med 24(1):73–78
83. Blake MA, Hochman MG, Edelman R (2003) Basic principles of MRI including fast imaging. In: Zlatkin MB (ed) MRI of the shoulder, 2nd edn. Lippingcott Williams & Wilkins, Philadelphia
84. DeLano MC, Fisher C (2006) 3T MR imaging of the brain. Magn Reson Imaging Clin N Am 14(1):77–88
85. Pruessmann KP (2006) Encoding and reconstruction in parallel MRI. NMR Biomed 19(3):288–299
86. Katscher U, Börnert P, Leussler C, van den Brink JS (2003) Transmit SENSE. Magn Reson Med 49(1):144–150
87. Deshmane A, Gulani V, Griswold MA, Seiberlich N (2012) Parallel MR imaging. J Magn Reson Imaging 36(1):55–72
88. Pruessmann KP, Weiger M, Scheidegger MB, Boesiger P (1999) SENSE: sensitivity encoding for fast MRI. Magn Reson Med 42(5):952–962
89. Griswold MA, Jakob PM, Heidemann RM, Nittka M, Jellus V, Wang J, Kiefer B, Haase A (2002) Generalized autocalibrating partially parallel acquisitions (GRAPPA). Magn Reson Med 47(6):1202–1210
90. Heilman JA, Derakhshan JD, Riffe MJ, Gudino N, Tkach J, Flask CA, Duerk JL, Griswold MA (2012) Parallel excitation for B-field insensitive fat-saturation preparation. Magn Reson Med. doi:10.1002/mrm.23238
91. Rahbar H, Partridge SC, Demartini WB, Gutierrez RL, Parsian S, Lehman CD (2012) Improved B(1) homogeneity of 3 tesla breast MRI using dual-source parallel radiofrequency excitation. J Magn Reson Imaging 35(5):1222–1226
92. Mueller A, Kouwenhoven M, Naehle CP, Gieseke J, Strach K, Willinek WA, Schild HH, Thomas D (2012) Dual-source radiofrequency transmission with patient-adaptive local radiofrequency shimming for 3.0-T cardiac MR imaging: initial experience. Radiology 263(1):77–85
93. Bailey DL, Karp JS, Surti S (2003) Physics and instrumentation in PET. In: Valk PE, Bailey DL, Townsend DW, Maisey MN (eds) Positron emission tomography; basic science and clinical practice, 2nd edn. Springer, London, pp 41–67
94. Hofmann M, Pichler B, Scholkopf B, Beyer T (2009) Towards quantitative PET/MRI: a review of MR-based attenuation correction techniques. Eur J Nucl Med Mol Imaging 36(Suppl 1): S93–S104
95. Schreibmann E, Nye JA, Schuster DM, Martin DR, Votaw J, Fox T (2010) MR-based attenuation correction for hybrid PET/MR brain imaging systems using deformable image registration. Med Phys 37(5):2101–2109
96. Keereman V, Vandenberghe S, De Deene Y, Luypaert R, Broux T, Lemahieu I (2008) MR-based attenuation correction for PET using an Ultrashort Echo Time (UTE) sequence. In: IEEE nuclear science symposium conference record, Dresden, 19–25 Oct 2008, pp 4656–4661
97. Martinez-Moller A, Souvatzoglou M, Delso G, Bundschuh RA, Chefd'hotel C, Ziegler SI, Navab N, Schwaiger M, Nekolla SG (2009) Tissue classification as a potential approach for attenuation correction in whole-body PET/MRI: evaluation with PET/CT data. J Nucl Med 50(4):520–526
98. Johansson A, Karlsson M, Nyholm T (2011) CT substitute derived from MRI sequences with ultrashort echo time. Med Phys 38(5):2708–2714
99. Hofmann M, Steinke F, Scheel V, Charpiat G, Farquhar J, Aschoff P, Brady M, Scholkopf B, Pichler BJ (2008) MRI-based attenuation correction for PET/MRI: a novel approach combining pattern recognition and atlas registration. J Nucl Med 49(11):1875–1883
100. Hu Z, Renisch S, Schweizer B, Blaffert T, Ojha N, Guo T, Tang J, Tung C, Kaste J, Schulz V, Torres I, Shao L (2010) MR-based attenuation correction for whole-body PET/MR system. In: IEEE nuclear science symposium conference record (NSS/MIC), Knoxville, 30 Oct–6 Nov 2010, pp 2119–2122
101. Delso G, Martinez-Moller A, Bundschuh RA, Nekolla SG, Ziegler SI (2010) The effect of limited MR field of view in MR/PET attenuation correction. Med Phys 37(6):2804–2812
102. Nuyts J, Michel C, Fenchel M, Bal G, Watson C (2010) Completion of a truncated attenuation image from the attenuated PET emission data. In: Nuclear science symposium conference record (NSS/MIC), 2010 IEEE, Knoxville, 30 Oct–6 Nov 2010, pp 2123–2127
103. Hu Z, Ojha N, Renisch S, Schulz V, Torres I, Buhl A, Pal D, Muswick G, Penatzer J, Guo T, Bönert P, Tung C, Kaste J, Morich M, HAVENS T, Maniawski P, Schäfer W, Günther RW, Krombach GA, Shao L (2009) MR-based attenuation correction for a whole-body sequential PET/MR system. In: IEEE nuclear science symposium conference record (NSS/MIC), Orlando, pp 3508–3512
104. Eiber M, Martinez-Moller A, Souvatzoglou M, Holzapfel K, Pickhard A, Loffelbein D, Santi I, Rummeny EJ, Ziegler S, Schwaiger M, Nekolla SG, Beer AJ (2011) Value of a Dixon-based MR/PET attenuation correction sequence for the localization and evaluation of PET/positive lesions. Eur J Nucl Med Mol Imaging 38(9):1691–1701
105. Hofmann M, Bezrukov I, Mantlik F, Aschoff P, Steinke F, Beyer T, Pichler BJ, Scholkopf B (2011) MRI-based attenuation correction for whole-body PET/MRI: quantitative evaluation of segmentation- and atlas-based methods. J Nucl Med 52(9):1392–1399
106. Samarin A, Burger C, Wollenweber SD, Crook DW, Burger IA, Schmid DT, von Schulthess GK, Kuhn FP (2012) PET/MR imaging of bone lesions – implications for PET quantification from imperfect attenuation correction. Eur J Nucl Med Mol Imaging 39(7):1154–1160
107. Du J, Hamilton G, Takahashi A, Bydder M, Chung CB (2007) Ultrashort echo time spectroscopic imaging (UTESI) of cortical bone. Magn Reson Med 58(5):1001–1009
108. Keereman V, Fierens Y, Broux T, De Deene Y, Lonneux M, Vandenberghe S (2010) MRI-based attenuation correction for PET/MRI using ultrashort echo time sequences. J Nucl Med 51(5):812–818
109. Catana C, van der Kouwe A, Benner T, Michel CJ, Hamm M, Fenchel M, Fischl B, Rosen B, Schmand M, Sorensen AG (2010) Toward implementing an MRI-based PET attenuation-correction method for neurologic studies on the MR-PET brain prototype. J Nucl Med 51(9):1431–1438
110. Bagheri MH, Hosseini MM, Emami MJ, Foroughi AA (2012) Metallic artifact in MRI after removal of orthopedic implants. Eur J Radiol 81(3):584–590
111. Olsen RV, Munk PL, Lee MJ, Janzen DL, MacKay AL, Xiang QS, Masri B (2000) Metal artifact reduction sequence: early clinical applications. Radiographics 20(3):699–712
112. Hu Z, Ye J, Hsieh Y-L, Renisch S, Blaffert T, Heinzer S, Loubeyre P, Maniawski P, Shao L, Ratib O (2012) Technical optimization of breast imaging on a combined PET/MR system. J Nucl Med Meet Abstr 53(1_MeetingAbstracts):369

Part II

PET/MR Atlas of Clinical Cases in Oncology

Head and Neck Cancers

4

O. Rager, M. Becker, and A.J. Beer

Contents

Head and Neck Cancers

Head and neck cancers comprise about 5.5 % of all cancers worldwide. More than 90 % of head and neck malignancies are squamous cell carcinomas (HNSCC) mainly caused by tobacco and alcohol consumption. However, HNSCC caused by infection with the Human Papilloma Virus (HPV) type 16 and 18 are increasingly seen in younger adults, particularly in the oropharynx. These tumors are usually smaller and their prognosis is slightly better as compared to non HPV-related cancers.

Due to the rich lymphatic drainage, lymph node metastases are common and may even be seen in early tumors. The prevalence of lymph node metastases at initial presentation depends on the site of tumor origin and its presence affects overall survival considerably. A particular feature of HNSCC is the high rate of synchronous or metachronous second tumors, which are most often seen in the lung or esophagus.

Treatment of HNSCC includes surgery, radiation therapy ± chemotherapy or a combination of the two.

Because of its excellent soft tissue resolution, MRI is often used as a first line imaging modality for the assessment of loco-regional disease, whereas PET/CT is mainly used for the assessment of lymph node metastases, distant disease and for the detection of tumor recurrence after treatment. PET/MRI combines the advantages of both modalities and contributes to the diagnostic work up of these tumors.

O. Rager (✉)
Department of Imaging, Division of Nuclear Medicine and Molecular Imaging, Geneva University Hospital, Geneva, Switzerland
e-mail: olivier.rager@hcuge.ch

M. Becker
Department of Imaging, Division of Radiology, Geneva University Hospital, Geneva, Switzerland
e-mail: minerva.becker@hcuge.ch

A.J. Beer
Department of Nuclear Medicine, Klinikum Rechts der Isar, Technische Universität München, Munich, Germany

O. Ratib et al. (eds.), *Atlas of PET/MR Imaging in Oncology*,
DOI 10.1007/978-3-642-31292-2_4, © Springer-Verlag Berlin Heidelberg 2013

Squamous Cell Carcinoma of the Larynx

Clinical History

Fifty-three-year-old male. Consults for dysphonia and odynophagia since 5 months.

Tobacco: 120 pack years.

Alcohol: 50 g/day.

Because of increasing dyspnea, the patient underwent tracheotomy 10 days prior to imaging. A tumor lesion was seen endoscopically suggesting a squamous cell carcinoma. Prior to endoscopy, a [18F]FDG-PET/MRI was performed.

Imaging Technique

High-resolution [18F]FDG-PET/MRI with axial T2w SE and T1w SE images before and after injection of intravenous Gadolinium chelates (Gd). Axial high-resolution Dixon sequence after intravenous administration of Gd with sagittal and coronal 2D reformations. The axial MRI sequences were obtained using a 2–3 mm slice thickness, a field of view of 20 × 20 cm and a 512 × 512 matrix. MRI, PET and fused PET MRI images of the head and neck area are provided.

Findings

Hyperintense lesion on T2w images with heterogeneous enhancement after intravenous injection of Gadolinium chelates and with intense hypermetabolism on the PET acquisition. The transglottic mass infiltrates the thyroid cartilage and the pre-laryngeal soft tissues, the left cricoid and the left arythenoid cartilage. Moderate focal uptake around the tracheostomy. Large necrotic lymph node metastases are seen bilaterally in the neck involving levels III and V on the left side and levels II–IV on the right.

Teaching Points

Transglottic laryngeal HNSCC are aggressive tumors involving at least two of the laryngeal regions (supraglottic, glottic and subglottic). They typically invade the thyroid cartilage and may extend into the soft tissues in the neck (stage T4 according to UICC and AJCC guidelines). Tumor spread into the soft tissues in the neck may also occur not only through the cartilages but also through the thyrohyoid membrane.

Transglottic HNSCC often have lymph node metastases at initial presentation. Lymph node metastases are often necrotic. Necrosis is typically seen as hyperintense areas on T2w images and as non-enhancing areas after intravenous injection of Gd. FDG metabolism may be quite variable depending on the degree of necrosis.

Lymph node metastases typically involve several neck levels. If the subglottis is invaded, metastatic lymph nodes should be looked for in the upper mediastinum.

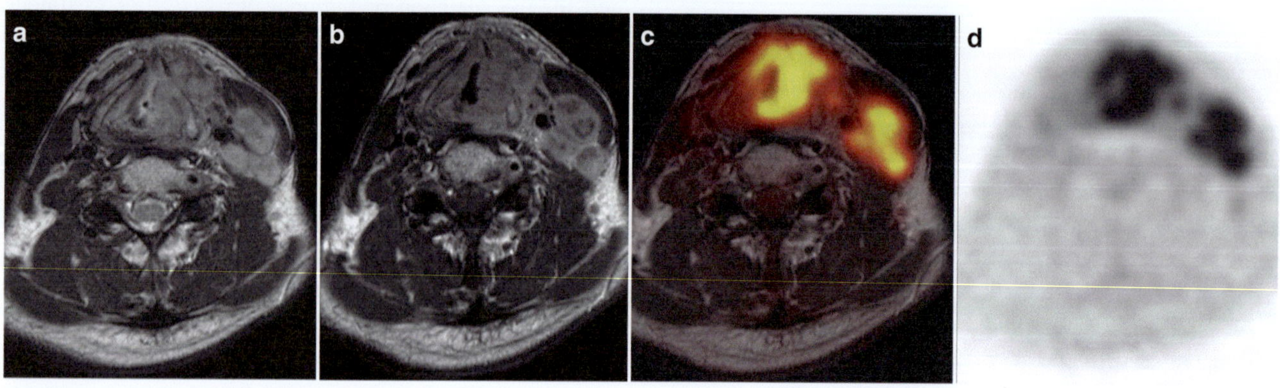

Fig. 4.1 Axial [18F]FDG-PET/MRI images at the level of the tumor: (**a**) T2w, (**b**) T1w+Gd, (**c**) fused T1w+PET, (**d**) PET. [18F]FDG-PET/MRI has the ability to precisely assess tumor spread as described above, in particular invasion of the laryngeal cartilages (thyroid, cricoid and arytenoid), extralaryngeal soft tissues, and submucosal spaces, as well the lymph node status, which is less well possible with PET/CT (Fig. 4.2)

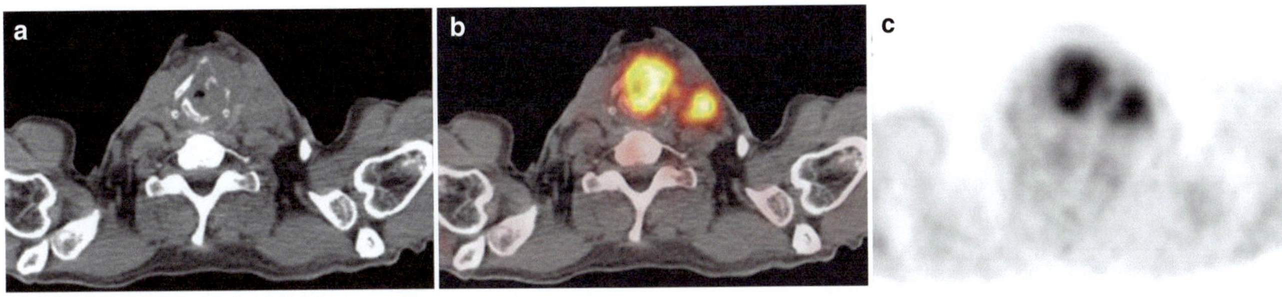

Fig. 4.2 Axial PET/CT obtained in the same patient shows the corresponding images at the level of the tumor: (**a**) CT (**b**) fused PET/CT (**c**) PET alone

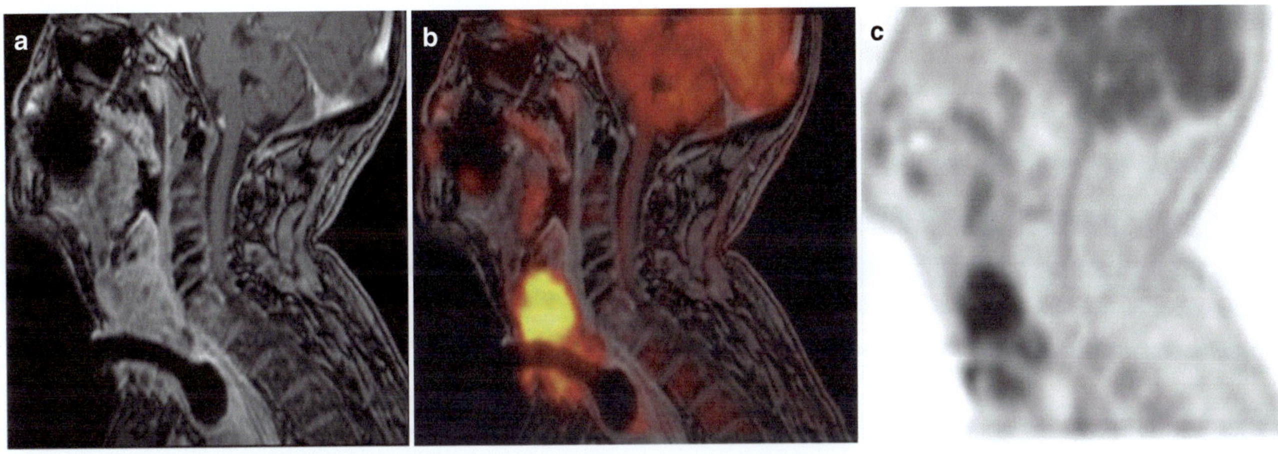

Fig. 4.3 Sagital PET/MR images: (**a**) sagittal 2D reformatted Dixon sequence, (**b**) fused sagittal Dixon images and PET image, (**c**) PET. The transglottic tumor spread is easily seen on these images. Note high metabolic uptake within the tumor and moderate hypermetabolism around tracheostomy corresponding to inflammatory changes

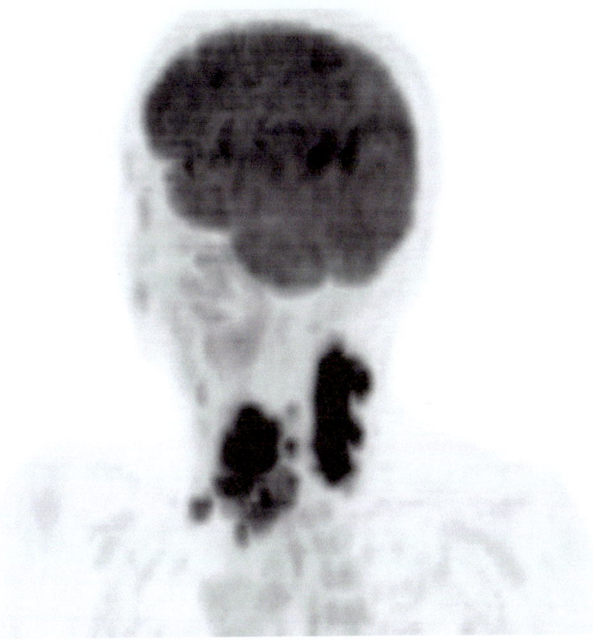

Fig. 4.4 Lateral oblique MIP PET scan showing the laryngeal tumor and bilateral involvement of lymph nodes

Oropharyngeal HNSCC

Clinical History

Fifty-seven years old male referred for restaging of a tonsillar tumor after radiotherapy and chemotherapy.

Smoker since 40 years, 1 package per day. The patient had endarterectomy of the left carotid and is currently treated for hypertension. Tongue pain since 3 months.

Imaging Technique

High-resolution [18F]FDG-PET/MRI with axial T2w SE and T1w SE images before and after injection of intravenous Gadolinium-chelates (Gd). The axial MRI sequences were obtained using a 2–3 mm slice thickness, a field of view of 20×20 cm and a 512×512 matrix. MRI, PET and fused [18F]FDG-PET/MRI images of the head and neck area and chest are provided.

Findings

Ulceration of the left amygdaloglossal sulcus with an area of necrosis seen on T2w images. No enhancing lesion is present after injection of Gd. Based on the MRI findings, the diagnosis is scar tissue. However, the hypermetabolic focus on the PET and on the fused [18F]FDG-PET/MRI images indicates the persistence of tumor. There is also a hypermetabolic lymph node in the left level II and a necrotic lymph node metastasis without hypermetabolism adjacent to it. Note the presence of a second lesion in the lung, which proved to be a synchronous lung tumor. The findings were confirmed surgically. However, the tumor size of the recurrent HNSCC was largely underestimated at [18F]FDG-PET/MRI.

Teaching Points

[18F]FDG-PET/MRI can identify distant metastases and synchronous tumors.

Although it can differentiate scar tissue and necrotic tissue from viable tumor, the size of the detected tumor may be grossly underestimated, as was the case here.

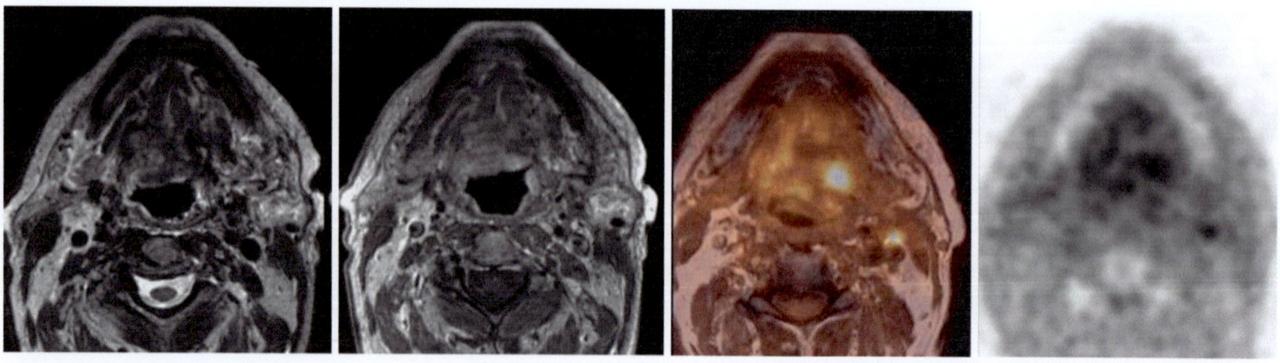

Fig. 4.5 Ulceration of the left amygdaloglossal sulcus with an area of necrosis surrounded by a low signal rim corresponding to scar tissue on T2w MR images. The focal FDG uptake suggested residual tumor

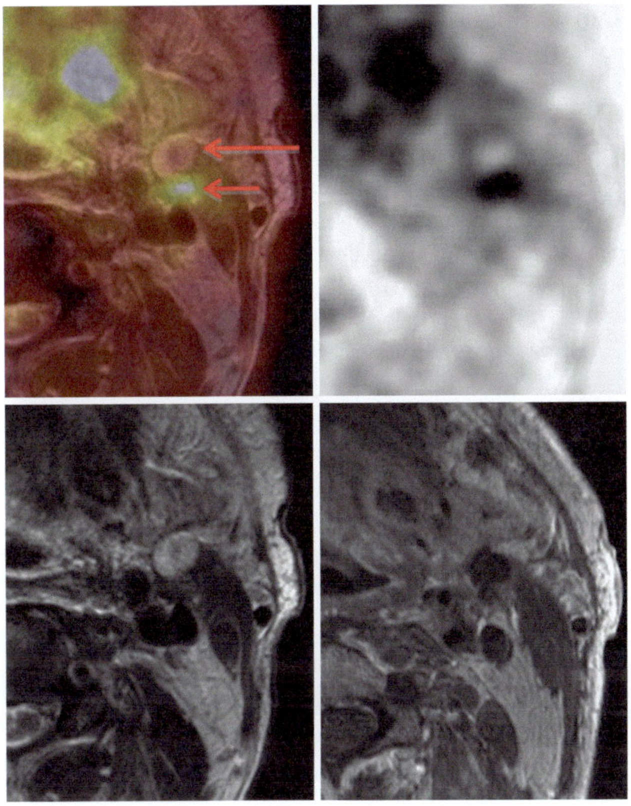

Fig. 4.6 A millimetric lymph node with intense hypermetabolism (shown with a *short red arrow*) and a necrotic lymph node metastasis with a peripheral halo of low metabolism (shown with *long red arrow*). Both lymph nodes were metastatic

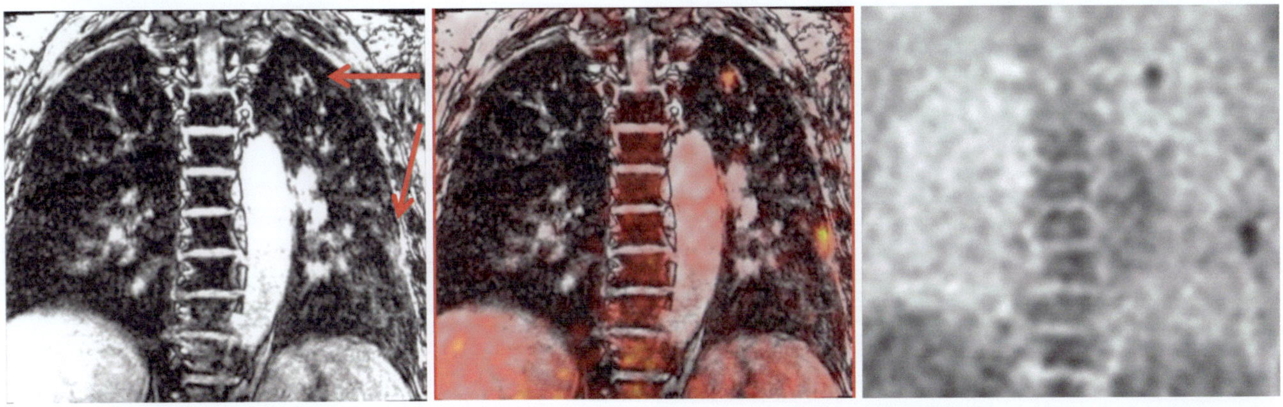

Fig. 4.7 Hypermetabolic lung nodule in the upper left lobe corresponding to a synchronous lung tumor versus a pulmonary metastasis. Biopsy revealed a second primary lung tumor. The focal uptake area in the apical segment of the inferior lobe corresponded to infectious disease

Lymphoma of the Nasal Fossa

Clinical History

Sixty-seven-year-old male in good general health with recent onset of asthenia, stuffy nose and sinusitis slowly progressing over several months. Antibiotic treatment did not improve symptoms. Clinical workup reveals a nasal mass and biopsy reveals a diffuse large B-cell lymphoma.

PET/MRI was performed for pre-treatment staging.

Imaging Technique

PET: 376 MBq 18F-FDG, 70 kg/174 cm patient, 240 min uptake time, 9 beds × 3 min.

MRI: T1w SE, 3DTFE (Act. TR/TE 6.2/3.0, 0.80 × 1.03 × 1.02 mm^3).

Findings

Large hypermetabolic tumor mass of the left nasal cavity displacing and infiltrating the nasal septum and causing obstruction of the osteomeatal complex. Note mucous retention in the left maxillary sinus due to blocked drainage.

Teaching Points

Extranodal lymphomas are rare but may affect all head and neck localizations.

Lymphomatopus masses share common imaging characteristics due to their increased cellularity: low signal on T2-w sequences, low ADC values and high SUVmax values.

Despite their large size, major areas of necrosis are often absent resulting most often in characteristic homogenous enhancement patterns after intravenous administration of Gd.

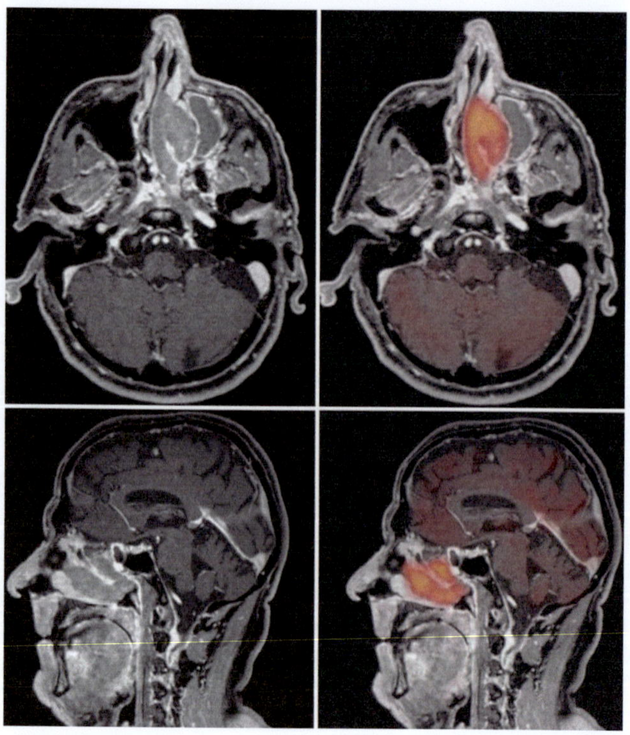

Fig. 4.8 Axial and sagittal 3D T1 TFE MRI images (*left*) and fused PET/MRI images (*right*) showing a large hypermetabolic mass in the left nasal fossa and ethmoid cells infiltrating the nasal septum and causing mucous retention in the left maxillary sinus

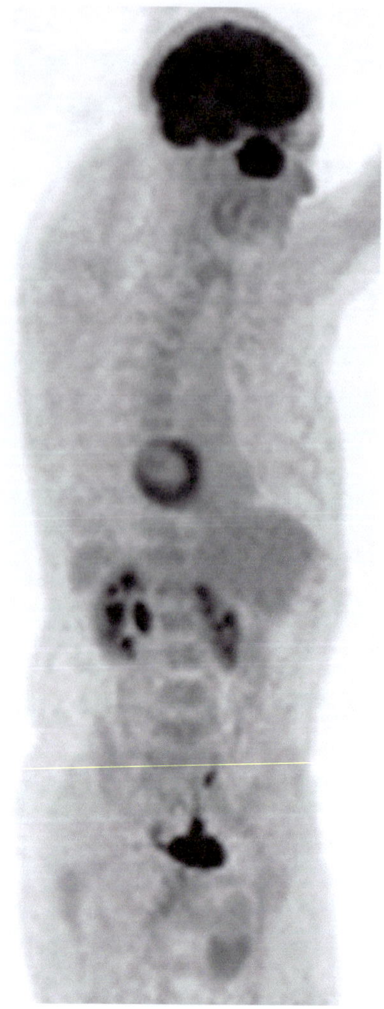

Fig. 4.9 Lateral oblique MIP image of the whole body PET scan showing the hypermetabolic lesion in the nasal fossa but no other distant lesions

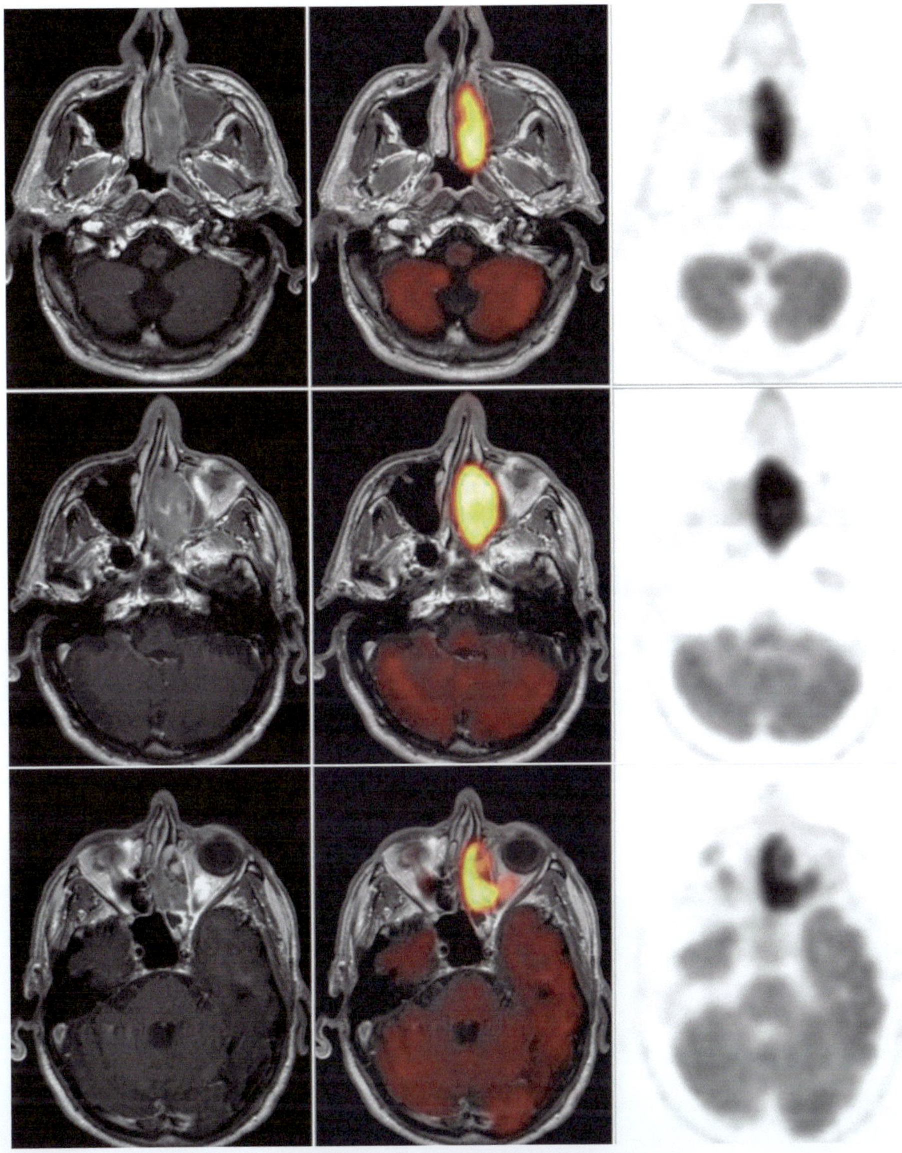

Fig. 4.10 Axial views obtained at three different levels with MRI (*left*) PET (*right*) and fused (*middle*) images

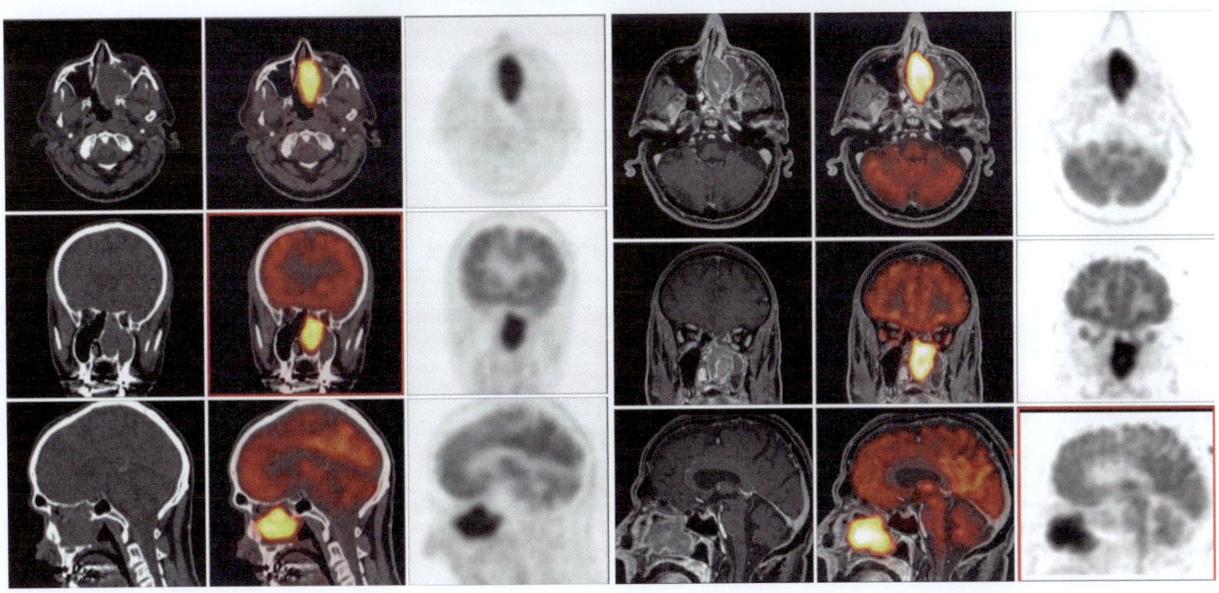

Fig. 4.11 Comparison of three orthogonal views centered around the nasal fossa lesion from PET/CT (*left*), and PET/MRI (*right*)

Retrocricoid Carcinoma

Clinical History

Sixty-two-year-old male with 62 pack years. Alcohol stopped since 1 year. The patient complained of dysphagia since 6 months, fatigue and weight loss of 8 kg. Initial PET/CT showed a retrocricoid tumor with a right-sided nodal metastasis. PET/CT and [18F]FDG-PET/MRI after radio-chemotherapy were performed for pre-operative evaluation.

Imaging Technique

Initial contrast-enhanced PET/CT. Unenhanced PET/CT and Gd-enhanced [18F]FDG-PET/MRI after chemo-radiotherapy. [18F]FDG-PET/MRI with axial T1w and T2w SE images, DWI images and 2D axial, coronal and sagittal 2D reformatted images of a high-resolution Dixon sequence obtained after intravenous administration of Gd.

Findings

PET/CT prior to chemoradiation shows a bulky bilateral retrocricoid tumor with a level III lymph node metastasis on the right. Both PET/CT and [18F]FDG-PET/MRI obtained after chemo-radiotherapy show only partial local response. The right level III lymph node metastasis, however, has disappeared.

Teaching Points

Retrocricoid tumors constitute between 2.5 and 3.5 % of all hypopharyngeal cancers. Tobacco and alcohol consumption are the main etiologic factors followed by the Plummer Vinson syndrome.

Retrocricoid HNSCC are often detected later than piriform sinus cancers because presenting symptoms are vague. Tumors are typically located submucosally and tend to spread downwards into the cervical esophagus. Lymph node metastases are seen in up to 75 % of cases at initial presentation. Cure is difficult to achieve.

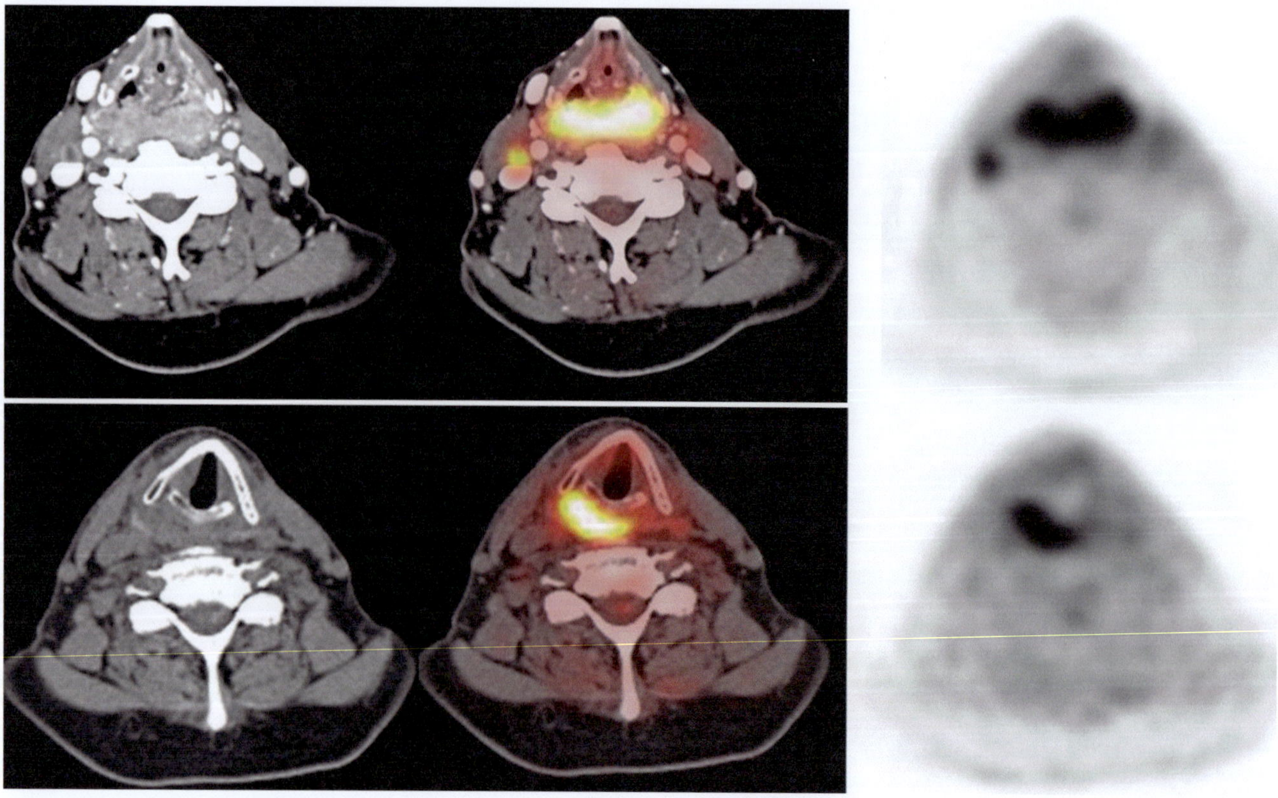

Fig. 4.12 PET/CT examinations before (*top*) and after chemoradiation (*bottom*) show major decrease of tumor volume and FDG uptake in the retrocricoid area and disappearance of the level III lymph node metastasis on the *right*

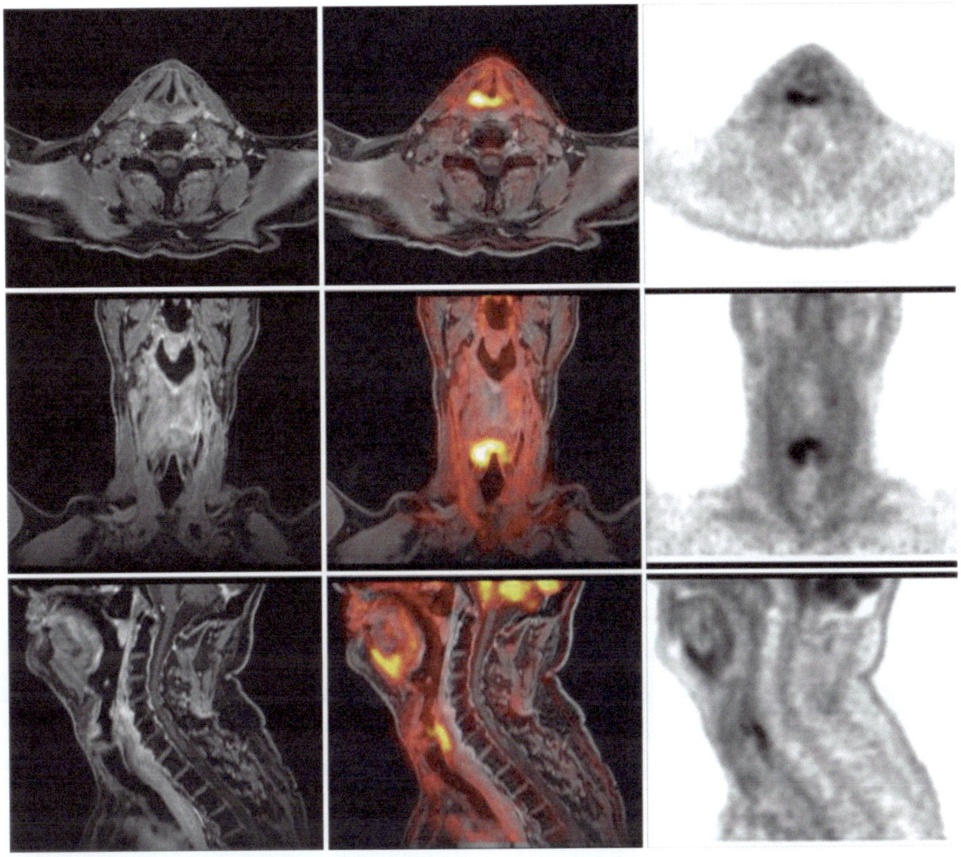

Fig. 4.13 Multi-planar reformatted PET/MRI images centered on the residual lesion allowing precise assessment of its cranio-caudal extent both on MRI and on fused PET/MRI images. The bilateral residual tumor spreads into the cervical esophagus. Note physiologic uptake of the sublingual glands on the sagittal reformatted images

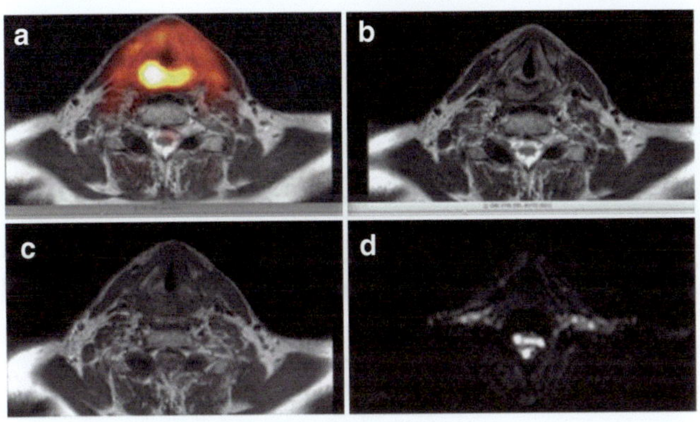

Fig. 4.14 Axial PET/MRI images at the level of the residual tumor: (**a**) Fused T2w TSE and PET (**b**) T2w TSE (**c**) T1w TSE (**d**) DWI. The tumor is easily seen on the first two images, however, it cannot be seen on the DWI image

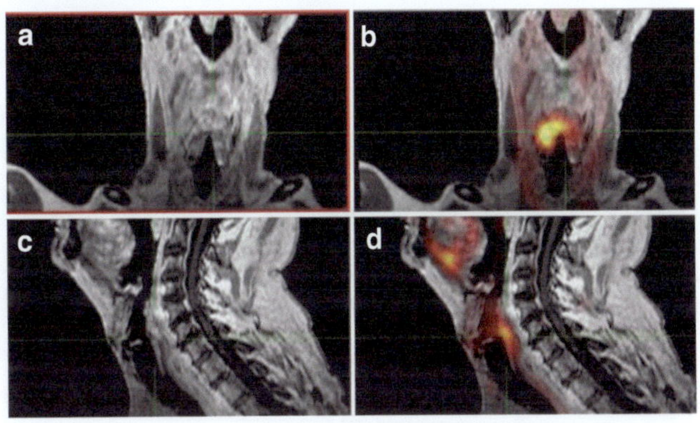

Fig. 4.15 Coronal and sagital PET/MRI images at the level of the residual tumor. Coronal T1w (**a**), sagittal T1w (**b**) and corresponding fused images (**c**, **d**). Same information as in Fig. 4.13. The T1w images are from the Dixon sequence

HNSCC of the Oropharynx with Lung Metastases

Clinical History

Fifty-five-year-old male with a history of radiotherapy for a T2N1M0 oropharyngeal HNSCC. Several years after initial treatment, the patient complained of odynophagia slowly increasing over a period of 1 year. Clinical examination revealed a base of the tongue tumor. Endoscopy revealed no other lesions.

Imaging Technique

Initial whole-body 18F-FDG PET/CT without contrast followed by Gd-enhanced PET/MRI that included whole body scan and axial T1w and T2w SE images, before and after intravenous administration of Gd.

Findings

PET/MRI shows a recurrent base of tongue tumor with a large area of ulceration best seen on the sagittal reconstructed images. There is involvement of a level VI lymph node on the right side, involvement of a pre-tracheal node and also multiple bilateral hypermetabolic nodules in the lungs suggesting metastatic lesions.

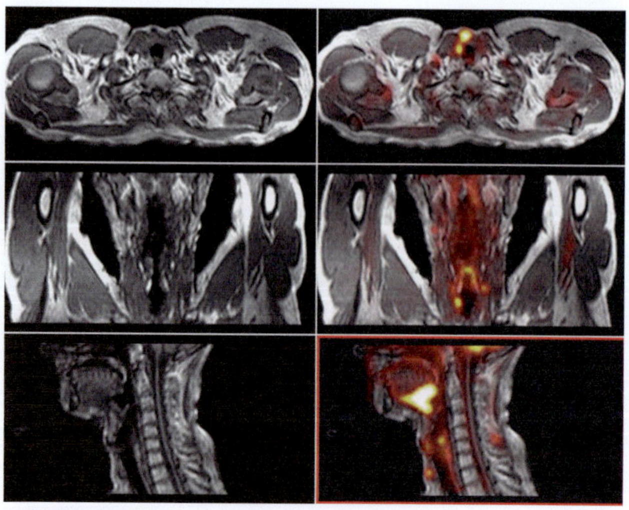

Fig. 4.16 2D multiplanar reformatted views of PET/MRI images of the base of the tongue tumor recurrence obtained from whole body low resolution T1W MRI used for localization of focal lesions on PET

> **Teaching Points**
>
> PET is primarily used for the work-up of distant metastases and to look for synchronous tumors, which may be seen in up to 20 % of patients with HNSCC.
>
> In recurrent tumors, the rate of synchronous second tumors and the probability of distant metastases is higher than in primary tumors.

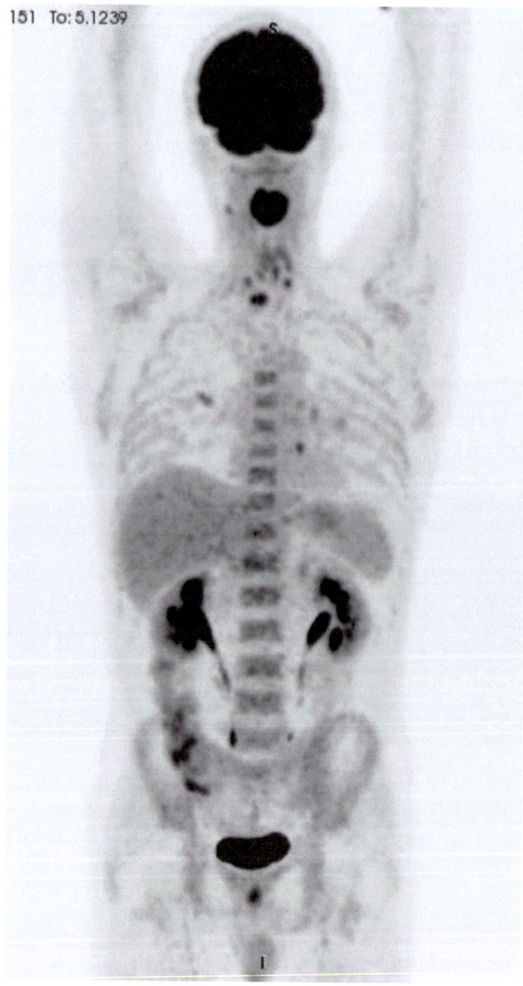

Fig. 4.17 Coronal MIP rendering of PET images showing the recurrent tumor and secondary focal lesions in the lungs

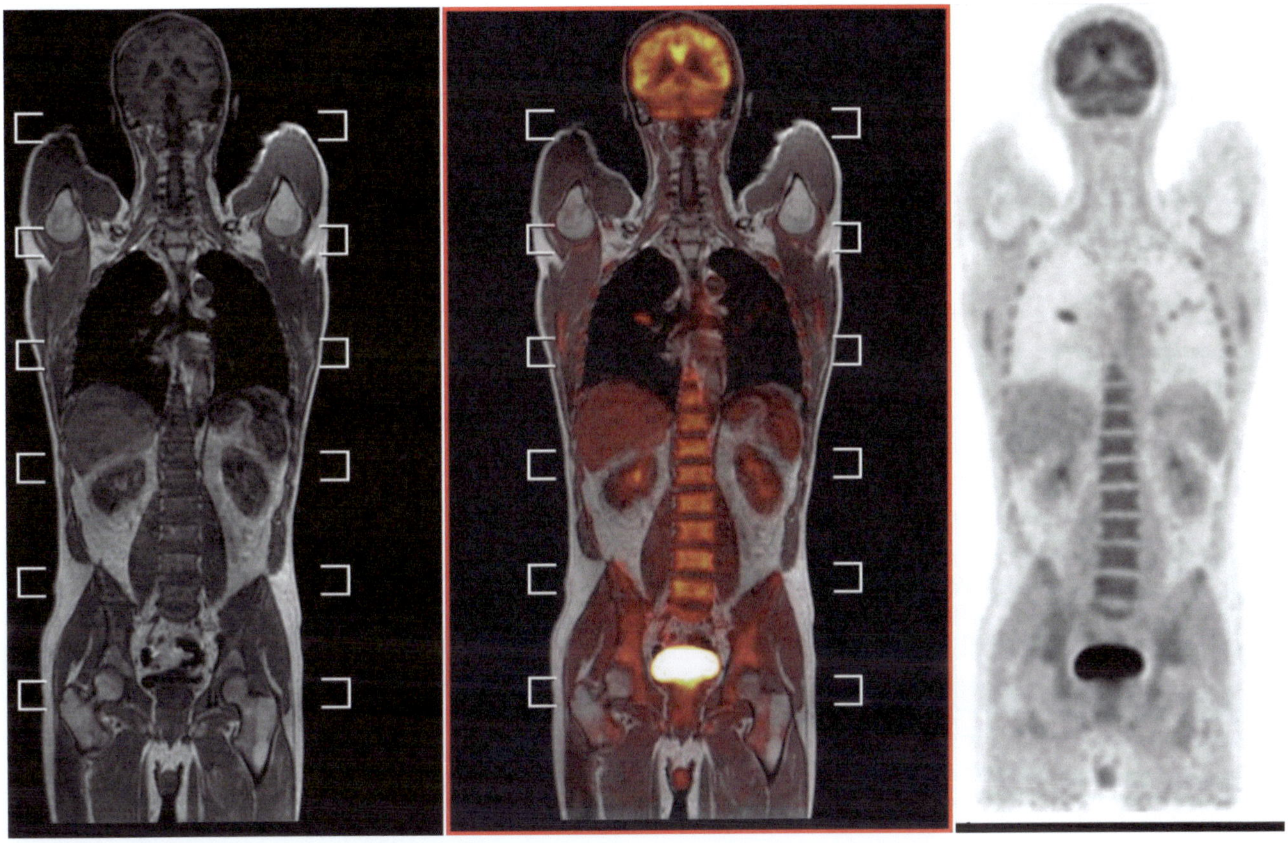

Fig. 4.18 Coronal views of whole body MRI (*left*), PET (*right*) and fusion of both (*middle*) showing lesions with focal FDG uptake in the lungs

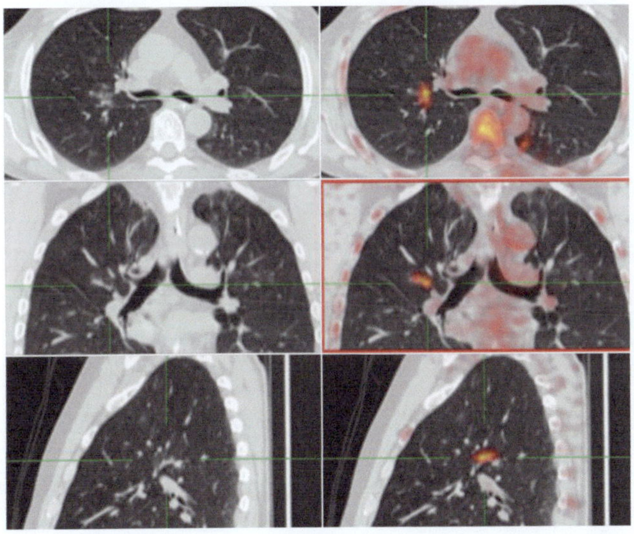

Fig. 4.19 Multiplanar reformatted PET/CT images in three orthogonal planes centered on the focal lesion of the right hilum

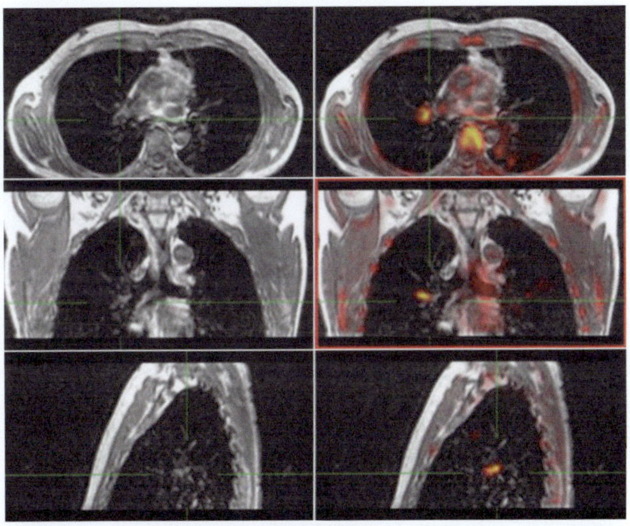

Fig. 4.20 Multiplanar reformatted PET/MRI images in three orthogonal planes centered on the focal lesion of the right hilum showing similar findings as on PET/CT. Biopsy confirmed lung metastases

SCCHN: Primary Staging

Clinical History

Forty-year-old HIV positive patient presenting with an ulcer at the floor the mouth on the left side and pain; biopsy revealed squamous cell carcinoma; patient is referred to PET/CT followed by PET/MR for primary staging.

Imaging Technique

Partial whole body PET/CT images acquired at 62 min after iv injection of 329 MBq 18F-FDG (7 bed positions a 2 min; with full diagnostic CT with i.v. contrast and dedicated head-and-neck study); PET/MR images acquired 92 min p.i., 52 kg.

Partial whole-body PET/MR: 4 beds × 4 min together with coronal T1w TSE and axial T2w haste fs. 1 bed (head-neck) a 15 min together with ax T1w ± Gd-DTPA, STIR ax and sag; T1w fatsat cor + Gd. Post CM axial T1w VIBE from chest to pelvis. Head/neck and TIM body coils.

Findings

The primary tumor on the left side of the floor of the mouth shows intense uptake of 18F-FDG and extends into the area of the left tonsil. The full extent and exact delineation of the tumor borders especially in the region of the left tonsil is better appreciated in the corresponding MR as compared to CT. Both CT and MR shows enlarged cervical lymph nodes on the left side. In PET, also smaller lymph nodes show intense tracer uptake, strongly suggesting lymph node metastases.

Teaching Points

For primary staging of squamous cell carcinoma of the head-and-neck area, MR is superior to CT for the delineation of primary tumors arising in the suprahyoid neck due to its excellent soft tissue contrast and can thus provide synergistic information together with 18F-FDG PET.

Concerning assessment of lymph nodes, PET can provide additional information in non-enlarged lymph nodes, suggesting malignancy despite of small size when the uptake is intense. On the other hand, the morphologic information of MR (or CT) is mandatory, because necrotic malignant lymph nodes can show only weak or moderate uptake, but can usually be defined as clearly malignant based on morphological criteria. This shows the synergistic value of morphological and biological imaging.

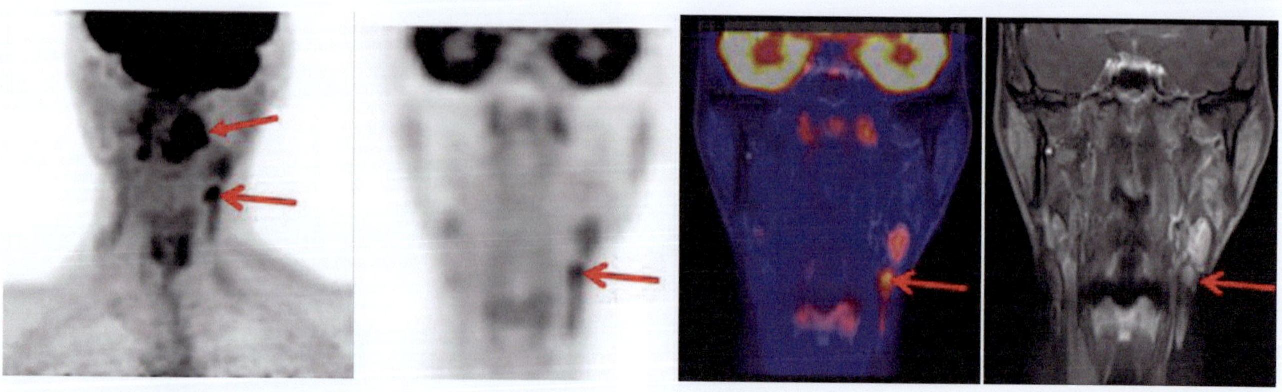

Fig. 4.21 PET/MR images from the head-and-neck area (*from left to right*): in the MIP of the PET you see the intense uptake in the primary tumor (*arrow*, *closed tip*) and several lymph nodes with variable uptake on the *left side*, the most intense one is marked with an *arrow* (*open tip*). The larger one directly above shows lesser uptake, but shows morphological criteria for malignancy, the small one marked with the *arrow* is unremarkable morphologically, however due to its intense uptake also has to be considered suspicious for malignancy

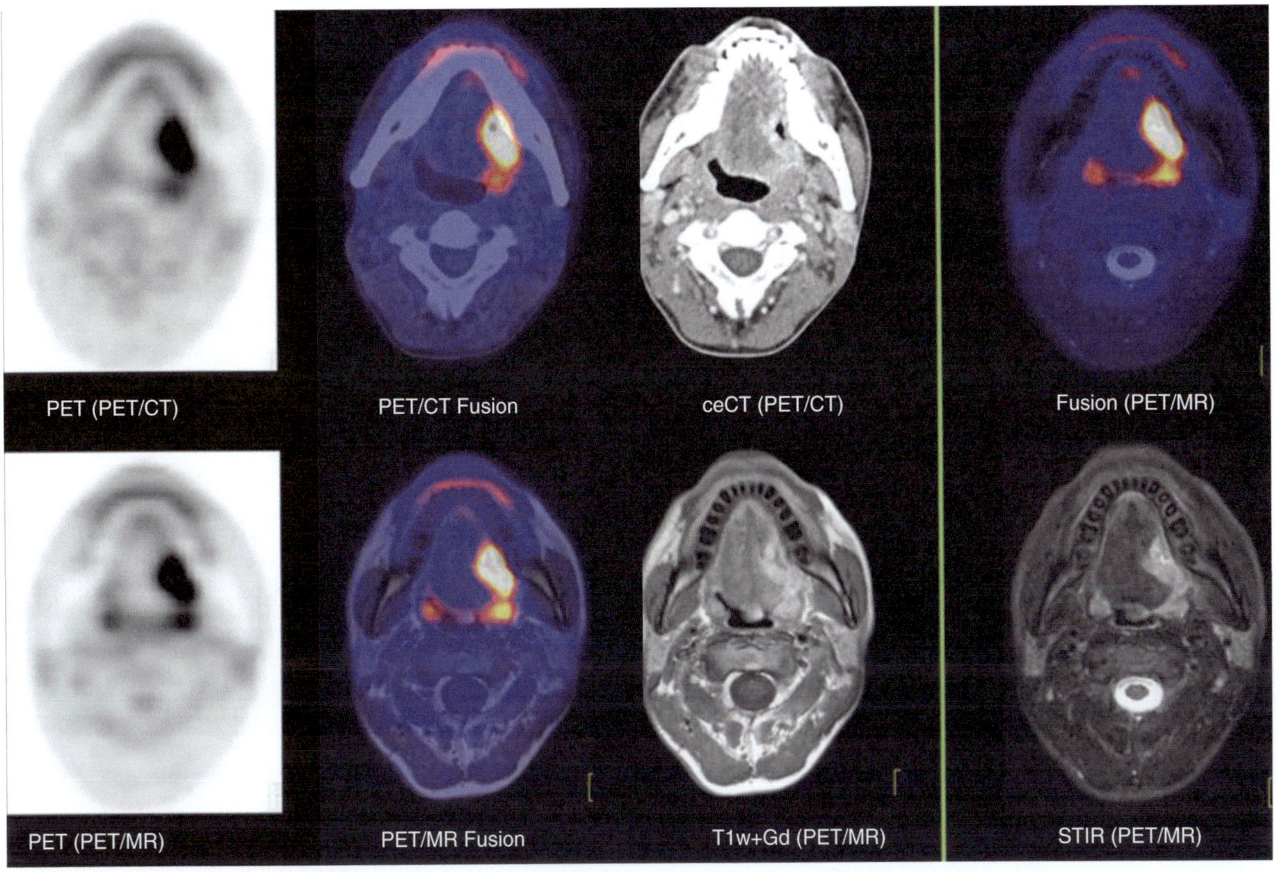

Fig. 4.22 Comparison PET/CT and PET/MR concerning the primary tumor (first 3 images *upper row* PET/CT, *lower row* PET/MR): the primary tumor shows intense 18F-FDG uptake, which can be clearly seen on both PET/CT and PET/MR. However the tumor borders and the extension of the tumor towards the left tonsillar area are better defined in the corresponding MR images as compared to CT. Note absence of mandibular invasion

SCCHN: Primary Staging, Dental Implants Artifacts

Clinical History

Fifty-three-year-old patient presenting with an ulcer at the right side of the tongue; biopsy revealed squamous cell carcinoma; patient is referred to PET/CT followed by PET/MR for primary staging.

Imaging Technique

Upper body PET/CT images acquired at 60 min after iv injection of 362 MBq 18F-FDG (6 bed positions a 2 min; with full diagnostic CT with i.v. contrast and dedicated head-and-neck study); PET/MR images acquired 94 min p.i., 64 kg.

Head and thoracic PET/MR: 4 beds × 4 min together with coronal T1w TSE and axial T2w haste fs. 1 bed (head-neck) a 15 min together with ax T1w ± Gd-DTPA, STIR ax and sag; T1w fatsat cor + Gd. Post CM axial T1w VIBE from chest to pelvis. Head/neck and TIM body coils.

Findings

The primary tumor involving the right anterior mobile tongue shows intense focal uptake of 18F-FDG both on PET from PET/CT and PET/MR. However due to extensive artefacts from dental implants adjacent to the tumor, the full extent and exact delineation of the tumor borders cannot be evaluated in the CT. However, in the MR from PET/MR, the exact tumor borders can be nicely seen, in particular involvement of the midline, undersurface of the right tongue and sublingual space. The tumor reaches the midline without crossing it. Both CT and MR show enlarged heterogeneous cervical lymph nodes on the right side in level 2, probably partially necrotic. In PET, weak to moderate tracer uptake is seen.

Teaching Points

In primary staging of SCCHN, delineation of the primary tumor in CT is often impaired by artefacts from adjacent dental implants. Depending on the imaging sequence, this can be less pronounced in MR.

However for lymph node staging, diagnostic CT with multiplanar reformations is at least equally good as MRI, especially in patients with low compliance due to the rather long examination times necessary for a comprehensive MR examination.

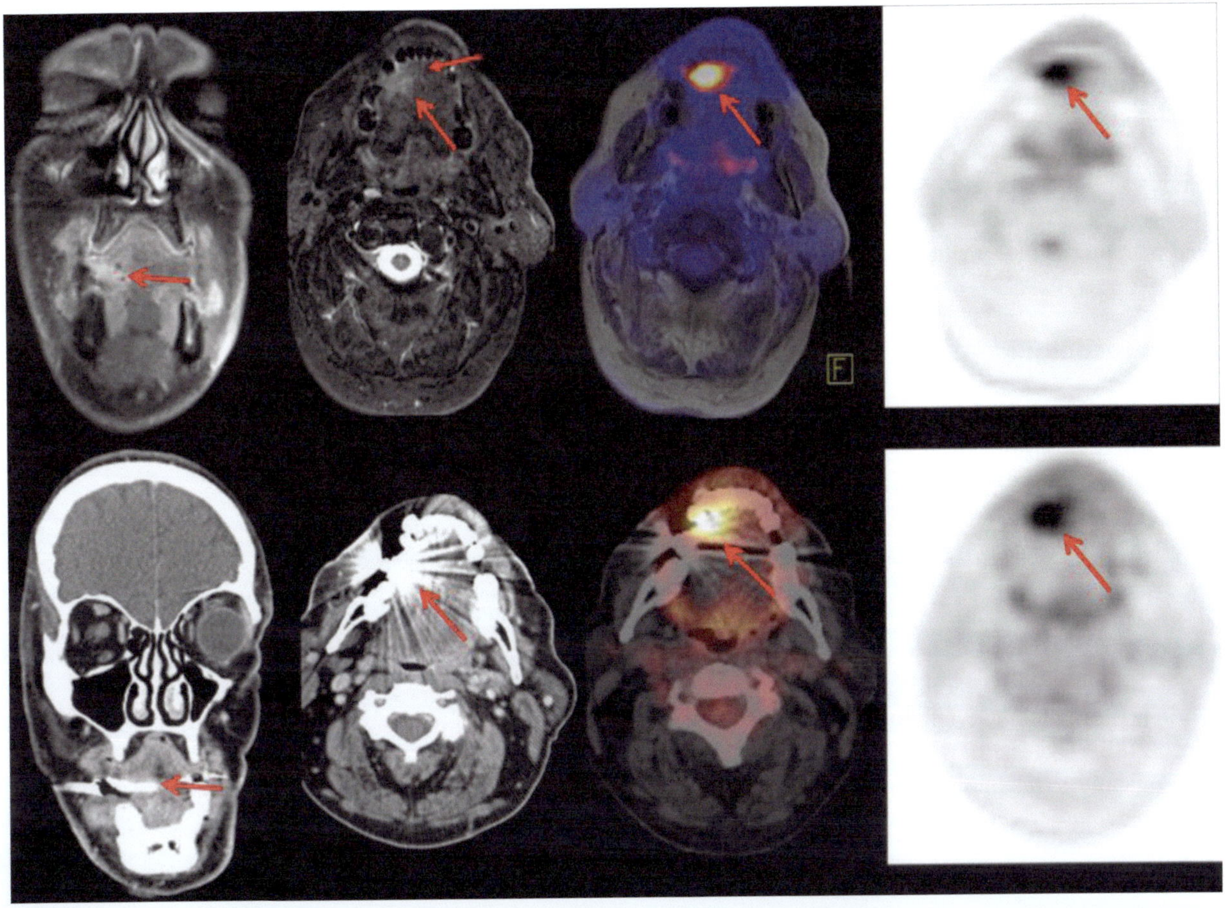

Fig. 4.23 PET/MR images (*upper row*) and PET/CT (*lower row*) from the head-and-neck area: the primary tumor (*arrow*, *open tip*) shows intense tracer uptake, but cannot be delineated on CT due to artefacts from adjacent dental implants. However in the MR from PET/MR, the tumor can be seen very well. The tumor borders reach but do not cross the midline (*arrow*, *closed tip*)

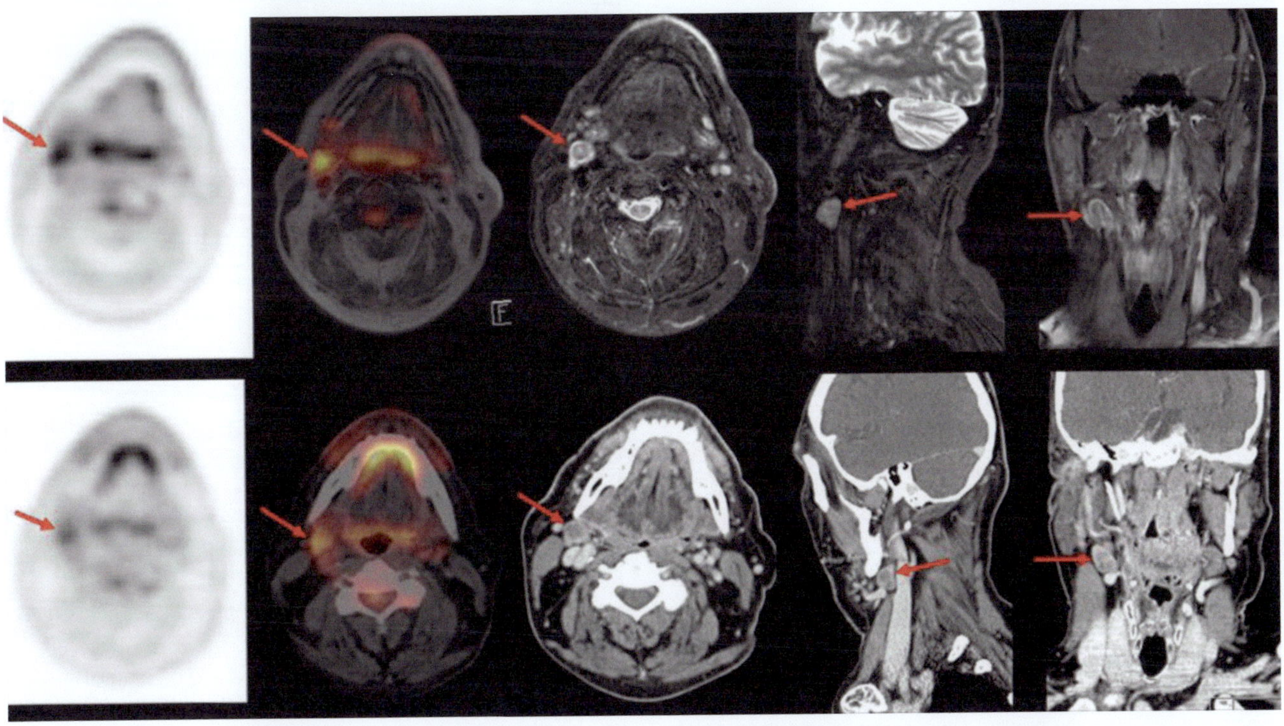

Fig. 4.24 Comparison of PET/CT and PET/MR concerning lymph node staging (*upper row* PET/MR, *lower row* PET/CT): the lymph node on the *right side* level 2 shows weak to moderate 18F-FDG uptake (*arrows*). However, both CT and MRI show substantial heterogeneity of the lymph node with a high signal on T2w images and peripheral rim enhancement on CT and MRI characteristic of central nodal necrosis. Thus the lymph node clearly has to be called metastatic. This also explains why the 18F-FDG uptake is not more intense. Here both PET/MR and PET/CT with diagnostic CT and multiplanar reformation perform equally well for lymph node assessment

SCCHN: Multiparametric Imaging

Clinical History

Seventy-six-year-old patient presenting with a bioptically proven squamous cell carcinoma of the left tonsil; patient is referred to PET/CT followed by PET/MR for primary staging and planning of radiochemotherapy.

Imaging Technique

Upper body PET/MR images acquired at 89 min after iv injection of 440 MBq 18F-FDG, 96 kg. 4 beds×4 min together with coronal T1w TSE and axial T2w haste fs. 1 bed (head-neck) a 15 min together with STIR ax and cor; DWI ax (b 50, 400, 800); Head/neck and TIM body coils.

Findings

The primary tumor in the left tonsil shows intense focal uptake of 18F-FDG in PET/MR. There are no enlarged or morphologically suspicious lymph nodes visible. However, in PET a moderate tracer uptake is seen in one small lymph node on the left side level 2. In the DWI images and the corresponding ADC map, we can see substantial restricted water movement in the primary tumor, which is better delineated from the surrounding tissue as compared to the STIR images alone. The area with low ADC values corresponds well to the area with intense 18F-FDG uptake. Note a small lymph node with the moderate tracer uptake shows low ADC values that is clearly delineated in the DWI images. The combination of low ADC values and tracer uptake suggest malignancy despite the small size.

Teaching Points

Combining functional information from MRI, like DWI or also DCE-MRI and MRS with the biological information from PET is feasible with high spatial precision with combined PET/MR.

In SCCHN, this combined information of DWI and biological information from PET might provide synergistic information on tumor biology, which in the future might be helpful for radiation therapy planning and/or classification of lymph nodes.

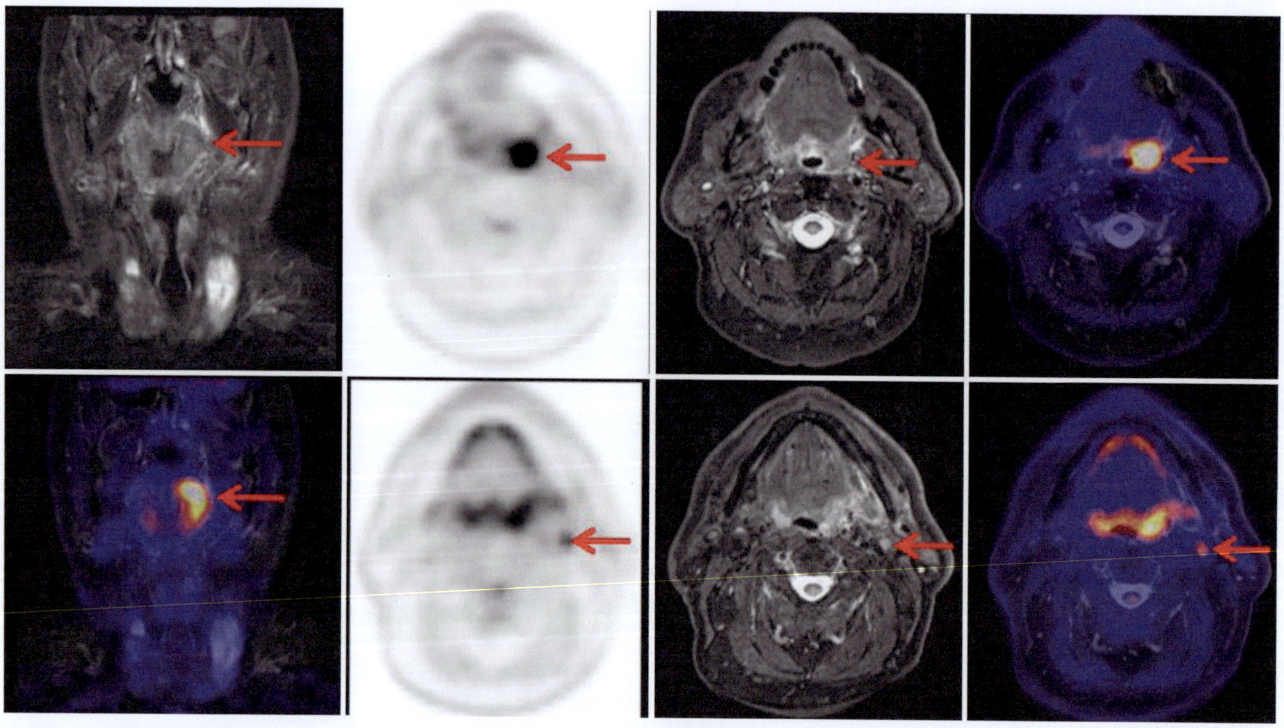

Fig. 4.25 PET/MR images from the head-and-neck area show the primary tumor (*upper row*, *arrows*) and lymph node on the *left side* level 2 (*lower row*, *arrows*): the primary tumor shows intense tracer uptake. The lymph node is small and shows only moderate tracer uptake, meaning that it could either be malignant or an unspecific benign reactive lymph node

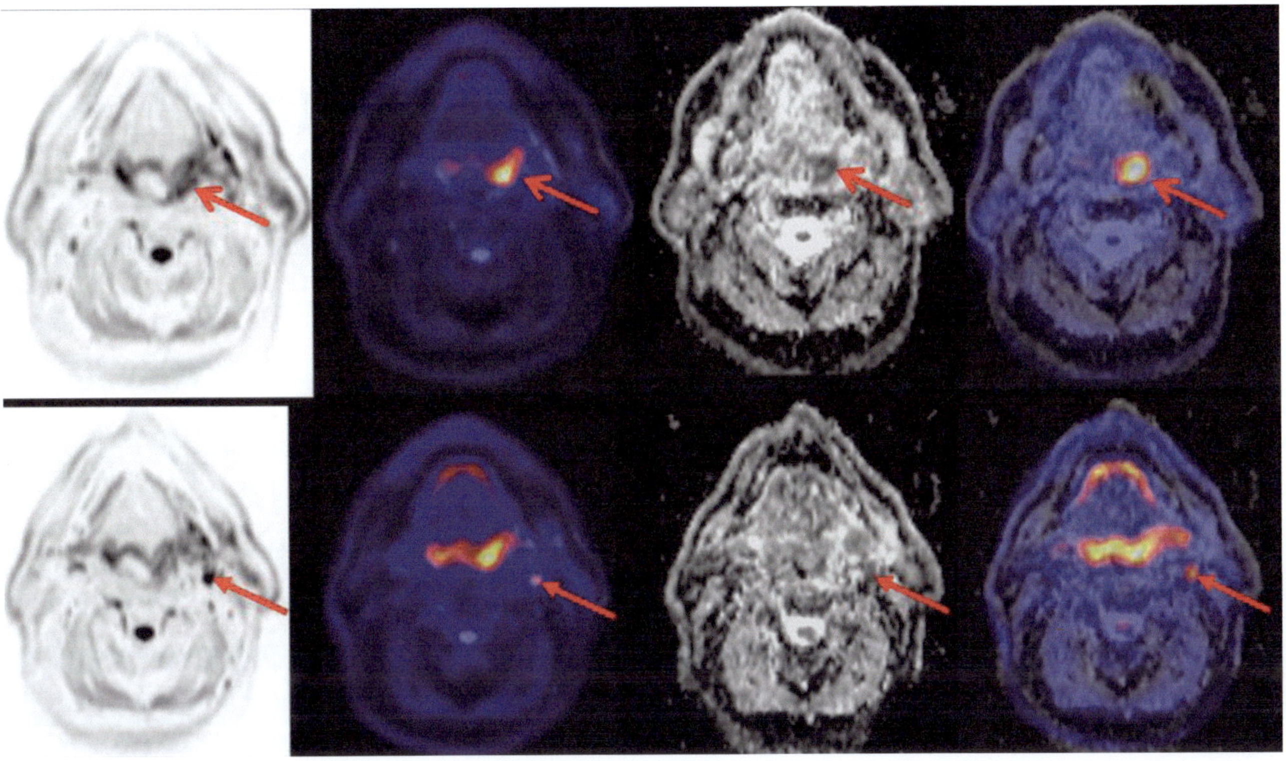

Fig. 4.26 Comparison of DWI and 18F-FDG PET in PET/MR for multiparametric imaging of tumor biology: primary tumor in the *upper row* (*arrow*, *open tips*), lymph node in the *lower row* (*arrow*, *closed tip*); *from left* to *right*: in the b 400 DWI images, the primary tumor and especially the small lymph node can be delineated very well, corresponding to the areas of tracer uptake in the DWI-PET fused images. On ADC maps we can also see the areas of restricted water movement with low ADC values corresponding to the areas of tracer uptake in the PET/ADC map fused images

Further Reading

Buchbender C, Heusner TA, Lauenstein TC, Bockisch A, Antoch G (2012) Oncologic PET/MRI, part 1: tumors of the brain, head and neck, chest, abdomen, and pelvis. J Nucl Med 53(6):928–938

Eiber M, Souvatzoglou M, Pickhard A et al (2012) Simulation of a MR-PET protocol for staging of head-and-neck cancer including Dixon MR for attenuation correction. Eur J Radiol 81(10): 2658–2665

Loeffelbein DJ, Souvatzoglou M, Wankerl V et al (2012) PET/MRI fusion in head-and-neck oncology: current status and implications for hybrid PET/MRI. J Oral Maxillofac Surg 70(2): 473–483

Nakamoto Y, Tamai K, Saga T et al (2009) Clinical value of image fusion from MR and PET in patients with head and neck cancer. Mol Imaging Biol 11(1):46–53

Platzek I, Beuthien-Baumann B, Schneider M et al (2013) PET/MRI in head and neck cancer: initial experience. Eur J Nucl Med Mol Imaging 40(1):6–11

Vargas MI, Becker M, Garibotto V et al (2013) Approaches for the optimization of MR protocols in clinical hybrid PET/MRI studies. MAGMA 26(1):57–69

Prostate Cancers

5

L. Allainmat, A. Baskin, T. De Perrot, M. Eiber,
M. Souvatzoglou, and J.-P. Vallée

Contents

L. Allainmat (✉) • A. Baskin
Department of Imaging, Division of Nuclear Medicine and Molecular Imaging, Geneva University Hospital, Geneva, Switzerland
e-mail: laurent.allainmat@hcuge.ch

T. De Perrot • J.-P. Vallée
Department of Imaging, Division of Radiology, Geneva University Hospital, Geneva, Switzerland

M. Eiber
Department of Radiology, Klinikum Rechts der Isar, Technische Universität München, Munich, Germany

M. Souvatzoglou
Department of Nuclear Medicine, Klinikum Rechts der Isar, Technische Universität München, Munich, Germany

Prostate Cancers

Prostate cancer is biologically and clinically a heterogeneous disease that makes imaging evaluation challenging because different stages of prostate cancer are managed with different treatment modalities.

The role of imaging in prostate cancer includes diagnosis, localization and characterization of the primary tumor, determination of extracapsular spread, guidance and evaluation of local therapy, staging of locoregional lymph nodes, detection of locally recurrent and metastatic disease in biochemical relapse, and planning of radiation treatment [1].

The most commonly used imaging modalities for diagnosing and staging prostate cancer are transrectal ultrasound, dedicated MRI and bone scintigraphy. New developments in radiotracers such as radiolabelled Choline and Acetate have brought a new scope of applications of PET in the diagnosis and follow-up of prostate cancers.

Prostate magnetic resonance imaging (MRI) plays an important role in the determination of tumor localization, characteristics, and extent [2]. Multiparametric MRI complementes T2W images with diffusion-weighted imaging, dynamic contrast-enhanced (DCE) imaging, and MR spectroscopy imaging (MRSI) to improve diagnostic accuracy. Multiparametric MRI still remains imperfect, with sensitivities and specificities ranging from 22–85 % to 50–99 % [3]. In particular morphologic lymph node assessment with MRI is limited.

PET has emerged as a promising imaging tool for prostate cancer. However, ^{18}F-FDG, has limited sensitivity for prostate cancer [4, 5] due to low glucose consumption in early prostate cancer [6, 7]. ^{18}F-choline and ^{11}C-Choline has shown promise in the detection of prostate cancer, especially in the setting of recurrent and metastatic disease [8–18].

Hybrid PET/MRI scanners introduced recently into clinical practice [19, 20] combine the advantages of both modalities with reduced ionizing radiation, shorter acquisition times and better diagnostic accuracy especially in recurrences and localized prostate cancers.

O. Ratib et al. (eds.), *Atlas of PET/MR Imaging in Oncology*,
DOI 10.1007/978-3-642-31292-2_5, © Springer-Verlag Berlin Heidelberg 2013

Prostate Focal Adenocarcinoma

Clinical History

Fifty-nine-year-old patient with a primary prostate adenocarcinoma discovered through clinical examination and further confirmed by biopsy (Gleason: 4+3).

Imaging Technique

PET: 10 min dynamic acquisition obtained immediately after injection of 240 MBq of F-18 Fluorocholine followed by whole body scan obtained 10 min after injection and a late acquisition centered on the prostate.

MRI: a complete diagnostic MRI study was acquired in the same session including a 2D T2 Fast SE (TR/TE 4,000/120 ms – slice thickness 3 mm – 432×386 for the axial acquisition – FOV 22 cm) with both an endorectal coil and an external 6 array coil, and after removal of the endorectal coil, a 3D T2 fast spin echo MR sequence (3D VISTA) (TR/TE 2,000/243 ms, matrix 392×448/×25, FOV 390 mm and slice thickness 1 mm), a diffusion SE EPI sequence (TR/TE 3,644/66 ms – slice thickness 3 mm – FOV 200 mm – matrix 88/×9, 4 b values 0, 500, 1,000, 1,500 s/mm^2).

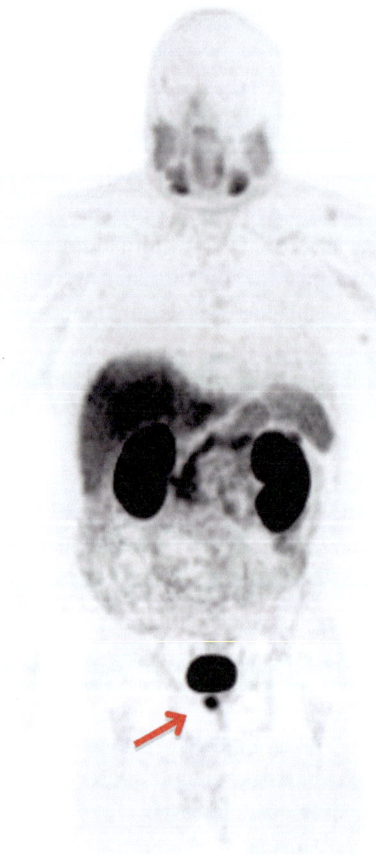

Fig. 5.1 3D MIP images of whole body PET showing focal uptake (*arrow*) in the prostate area but no other signs of dissemination or metastases

Findings

PET images show focal tracer uptake (SUV max 12.8) in the antero-apical area of the central zone predominantly on the right side matching the first lesion identified on MRI but not the second MRI lesion in the left peripheral zone.

MRI images showed two focal abnormalities: one in the right antero-apical area of the central zone with a hypointensity on the T2 images, and decreased diffusion (ADC at 800), and a second lesion in the left peripheral zone of the apex with decreased T2 signal and decreased diffusion (ADC at 900) adjacent to the central zone.

The histology performed after radical prostatectomy demonstrated an adenocarcinoma in the antero-apical area of the central zone and prostatic intraepithelial neoplasia in the left peripheral zone.

Teaching Points

Correlation between anatomical, functional and metabolic images: intra-epithelial neoplasia was a false positive on the T2 and diffusion MRI but not on the PET images.

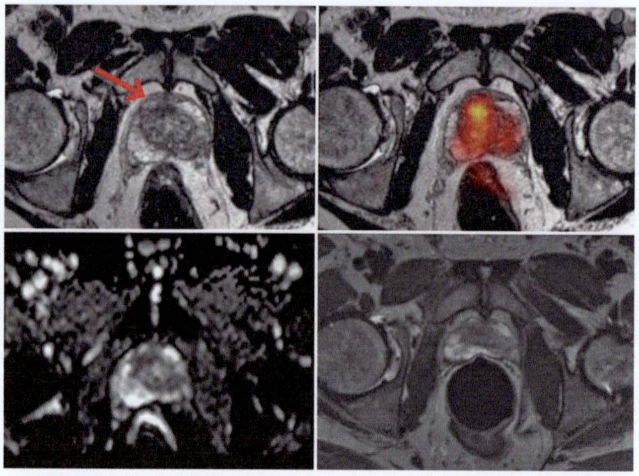

Fig. 5.2 Fused PET/MR images (*upper row*) showing the localization of a focal antero-apical lesion of decreased T2 MR signal (3D VISTA) (*red arrow*) and positive FDG uptake. *Lower row* shows additional diagnostic MR sequences with diffusion weighted images (DWI SSH) and a T2 TSE images obtained with endorectal coil. A prostatic intra-epithelial neoplasia in the left peripheral zone showed a decreased T2 and diffusion signal but no abnormality on the PET

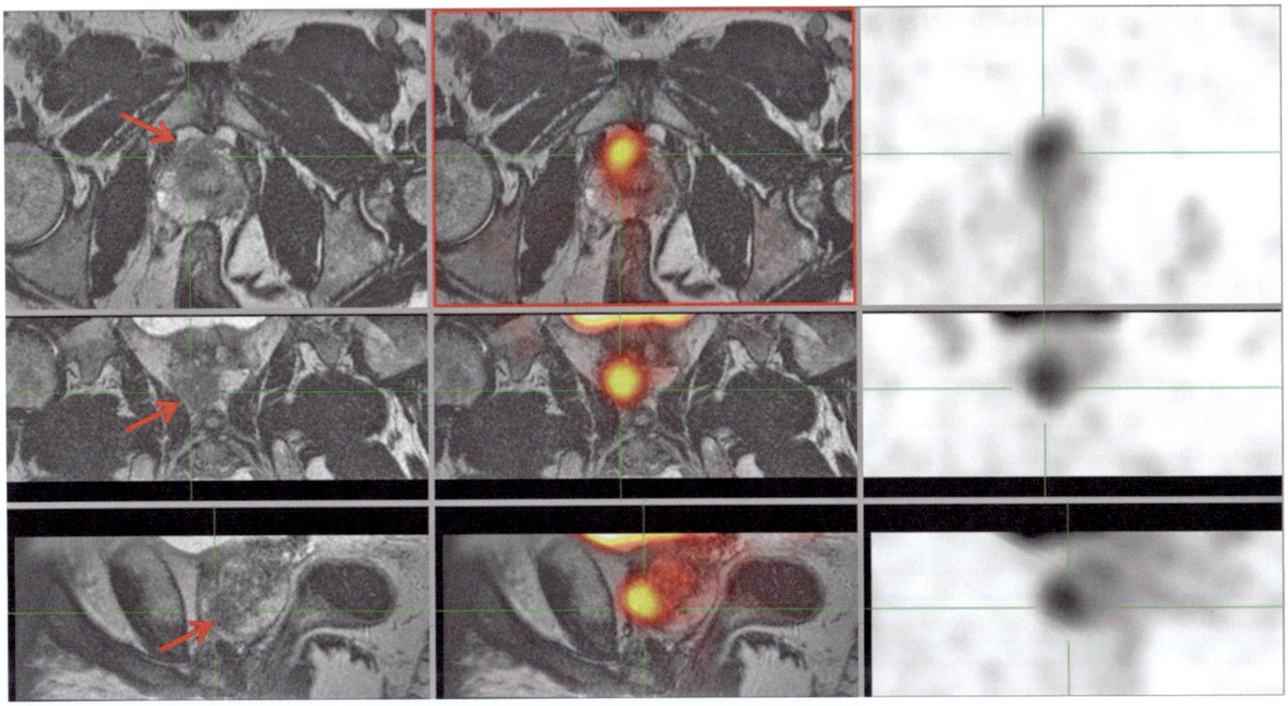

Fig. 5.3 Fused PET/MR images showing the localization (*red arrow*) of a focal antero-apical lesion of decreased T2 MR signal on a 3D VISTA and positive radiotracer uptake

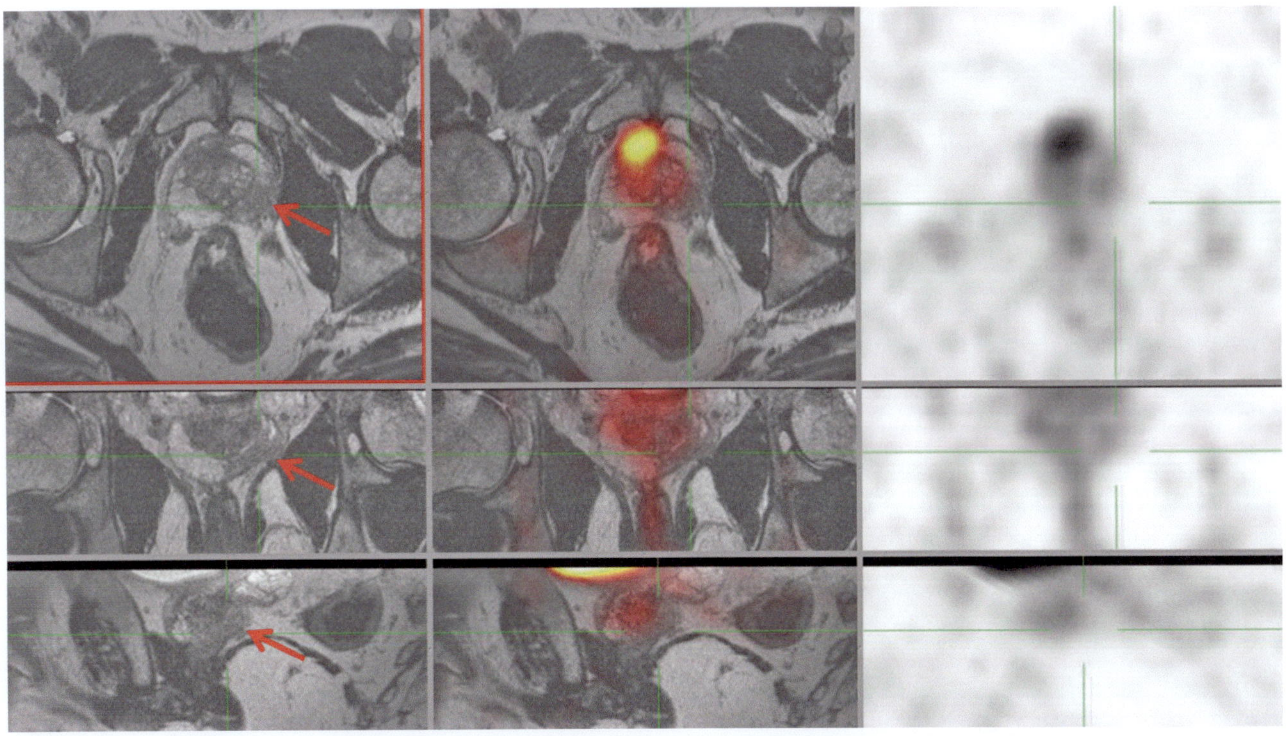

Fig. 5.4 Fused PET/MR images showing a lesion with decreased T2 MR signal (*red arrow*) on a 3D VISTA and no radiotracer uptake

Multifocal Prostate Cancer

Clinical History

Staging of a prostatic adenocarcinoma with a Gleason score 3+4.

Imaging Technique

PET: 10 min dynamic acquisition obtained immediately after injection of 317 MBq of F-18 Fluorocholine followed by whole body scan obtained 10 min after injection and a late acquisition centered on the prostate.

MRI: a complete diagnostic MRI study was acquired in the same session including a 2D T2 Fast SE (TR/TE 4,000/120 ms – slice thickness 3 mm – 432×386 for the axial acquisition – FOV 22 cm) with both an endorectal coil and an external 6 array coil, and after removal of the endorectal coil, a 3D T2 fast spin echo MR sequence (3D VISTA) (TR/TE 2,000/243 ms, matrix 392×448/×25, FOV 390 mm and slice thickness 1 mm), a diffusion SE EPI sequence (TR/TE 3,644/66 ms – slice thickness 3 mm – FOV 200 mm – matrix 88/×9, 4 b values 0, 500, 1,000, 1,500 s/mm^2) and a multiframe 3D T1 Fat Saturation gradient echo MR sequence (TR/TE 6.9 – 3.4 ms – matrix 192×189 – FOV 210 mm – slice thickness 3 mm) during 5 min after Gd-chelate injection.

Findings

The left peripheral zone at 4 o'clock in the base of the prostate showed a high tracer uptake (SUV max=4) as well as reduced T2 signal and apparent diffusion coefficient ADC and an increase wash-in on the perfusion MRI after Gd injection. In the right peripheral zone at 7 o'clock, there was also an area of T2, diffusion and perfusion abnormalities on MRI but only a weak tracer uptake on the PET images (SUV max=2.3). Note also a moderate hypermetabolism in the central zone associated with an hyperperfusion and a mild restriction of the apparent coefficient of diffusion but no T2 abnormality in the right central zone.

Histology confirmed an adenocarcinoma in both the left and right peripheral zone.

Teaching Points

A low tracer uptake of a lesion does not exclude a prostatic cancer. The normal central gland can show moderate tracer uptake by comparison to the peripheral zone.

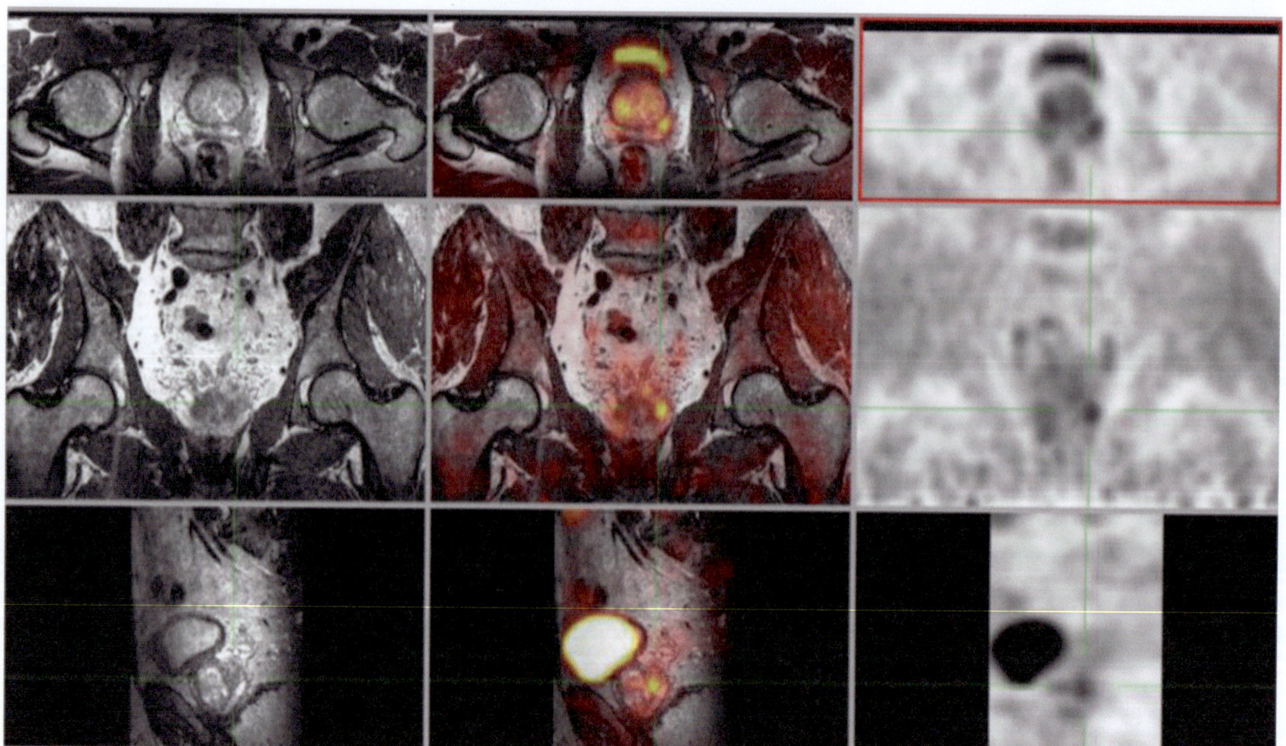

Fig. 5.5 Fused PET/MR images showing the localization of a left peripheral zone at the base of decreased T2 MR signal on a 3D VISTA and positive radiotracer uptake. Note the absence of abnormal lymph nodes

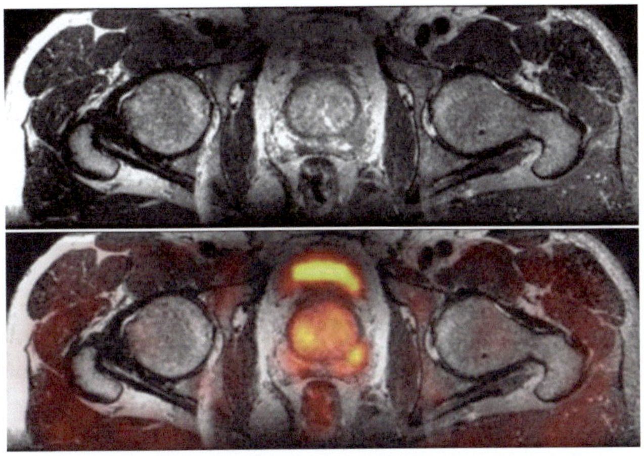

Fig. 5.6 T2 weighted 3D VISTA axial MRI images (*upper row*) and after fusion with PET (*lower row*) showing tracer uptake in the left peripheral zone at 4 o'clock as well as a T2 hyposignal. At 7 o'clock there is also a weak tracer uptake a as well as a T2 hypointensity

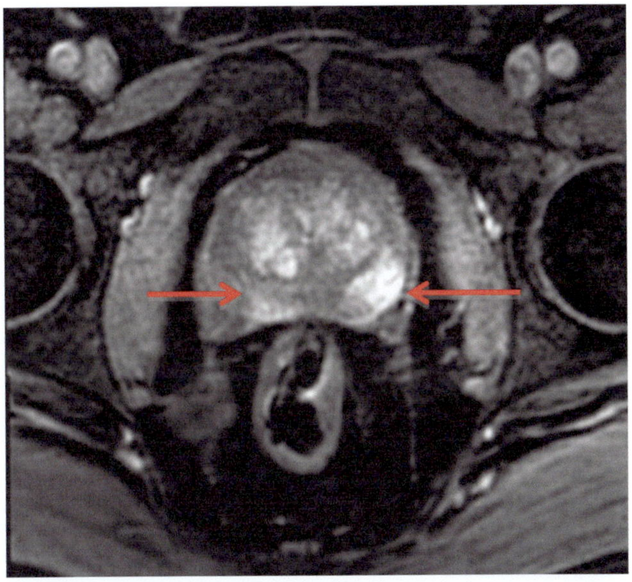

Fig. 5.8 Perfusion MRI with 3D fast GRE after Gd injection demonstrates foci of hyperperfusion in the right central zone and in the peripheral zone at 4 o'clock and 7 o'clock (*arrows*)

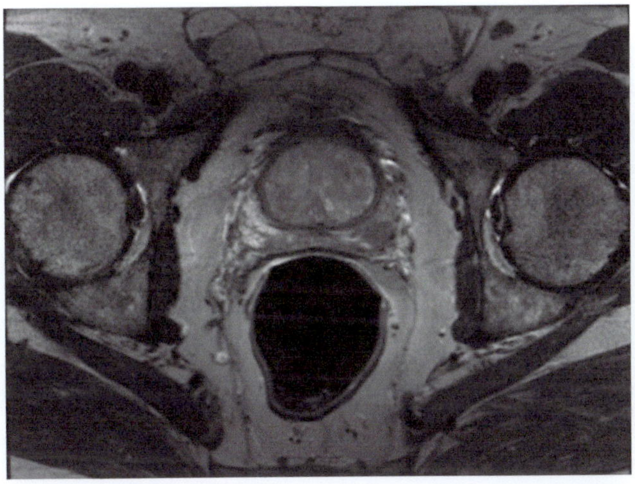

Fig. 5.7 Hypointense T2 signal at 4 o'clock and at 7 o'clock in the peripheral zone of the prostate with a T2 FSE MR sequence and an endorectal coil

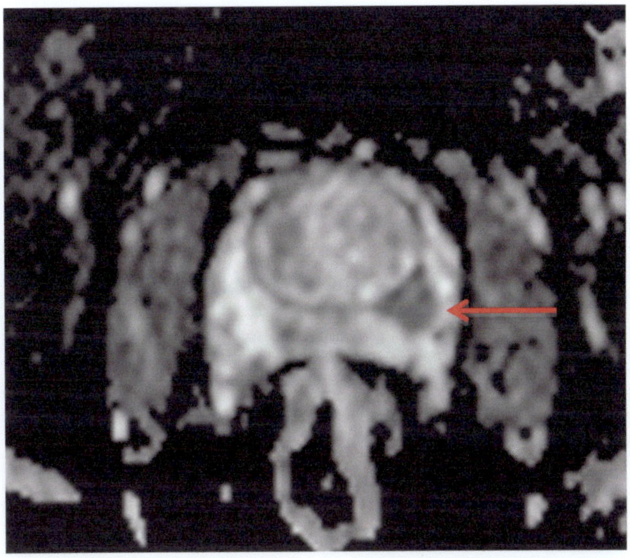

Fig. 5.9 The diffusion MRI shows an area of strong restriction of the apparent diffusion coefficient in the left peripheral zone at 4 o'clock (*arrow*)

Prostate Cancer with Invasion of Regional Lymph Nodes

Clinical History

Staging of a prostatic adenocarcinoma with a Gleason score of 4+4 discovered by an increased PSA serum level (14.7 ng/ml).

Imaging Technique

PET: 10 min dynamic acquisition obtained immediately after injection of 240.3 MBq of F-18 Fluorocholine followed by whole body scan obtained 10 min after injection and a late acquisition centered on the prostate.

MRI: a complete diagnostic MRI study was acquired in the same session including a 2D T2 Fast SE (TR/TE 4,000/120 ms – slice thickness 3 mm – 432×386 for the axial acquisition – FOV 22 cm) with both an endorectal coil and an external 6 array coil, and after removal of the endorectal coil, a 3D T2 fast spin echo MR sequence (3D VISTA) (TR/TE 2,000/243 ms, matrix 392×448/×25, FOV 390 mm and slice thickness 1 mm), a diffusion SE EPI sequence (TR/TE 3,644/66 ms – slice thickness 3 mm – FOV 200 mm – matrix 88/×9, 4 b values 0, 500, 1,000, 1,500 s/mm^2) and a multi-frame 3D T1 Fat Saturation gradient echo MR sequence (TR/TE 6.9 – 3.4 ms – matrix 192×189 – FOV 210 mm – slice thickness 3 mm during 5 min after Gd-chelate injection.

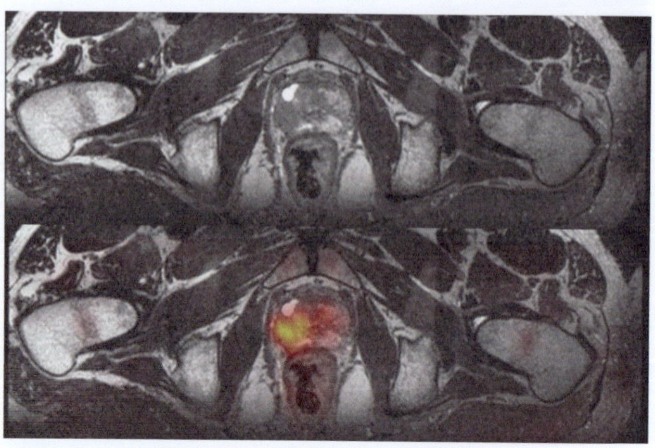

Fig. 5.10 T2 3D vista with (*bottom*) and without (*top*) fusion with the PET data. The adenocarcinoma in the right peripheral zone is hypointense in T2 and hypermetabolic on the PET

Findings

Large lesion in the right peripheral zone from 7 to 9 o'clock extending from the base to the apex with an hypointensity on the T2 MR sequences, a restriction of the apparent diffusion coefficient (ADC) and an hypervascularisation as well as an increased radiotracer uptake (SUV max=6.8) associated to a loss of the adjacent capsule reflecting an extracapsular dissemination. In the right anterior part of the prostate, a retention cyst is also seen that is hyperintense on T2, with a high ADC and no metabolism on the PET images. In addition, both MRI and PET (SUV max=10.4) show an abnormal right iliac lymph node. PET also detected a bone metastasis on the roof of the left acetabulum (SUV max=4.0) that was difficult to diagnose on the T2 Fast SE MR sequences optimized for the prostate but not for bone analysis.

Teaching Points

Good correlation between MRI and PET for the detection of the adenocarcinoma.

Extracapsular dissemination is best diagnosed by T2 2D FSE with the endorectal coil.

PET is a very efficient tool for the detection of bone metastasis due to the limited bone marrow contrast of MR sequences used for the prostate evaluation.

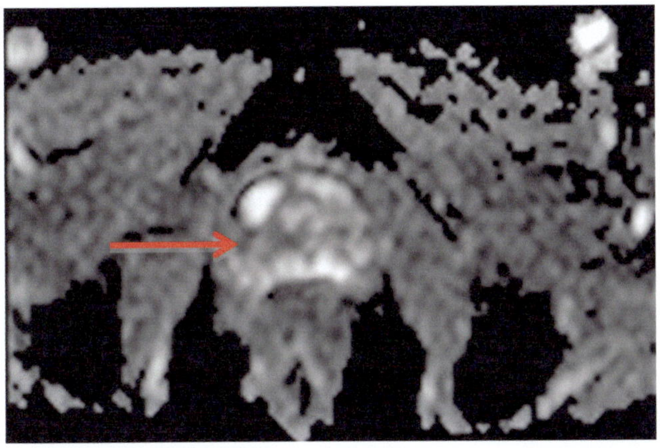

Fig. 5.11 Diffusion weighted image. An area of restriction of the apparent coefficient of diffusion (ADC) is present in the right peripheral zone between 7 and 9 o'clock (*arrow*). Note the presence of retention cyst located anterior to this zone with a high ADC

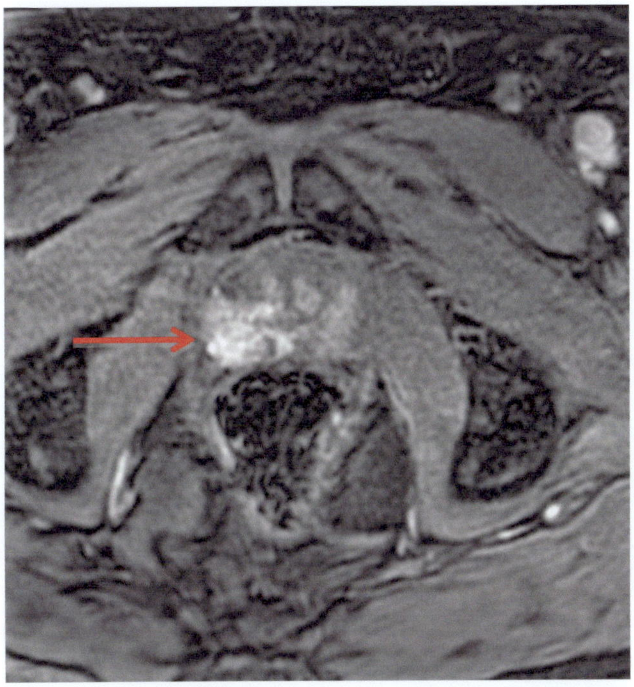

Fig. 5.12 Dynamic thrive image sequence; the adenocarcinoma in the right peripheral zone (*arrow*) is hypervascularized on the perfusion MRI obtained after Gd injection

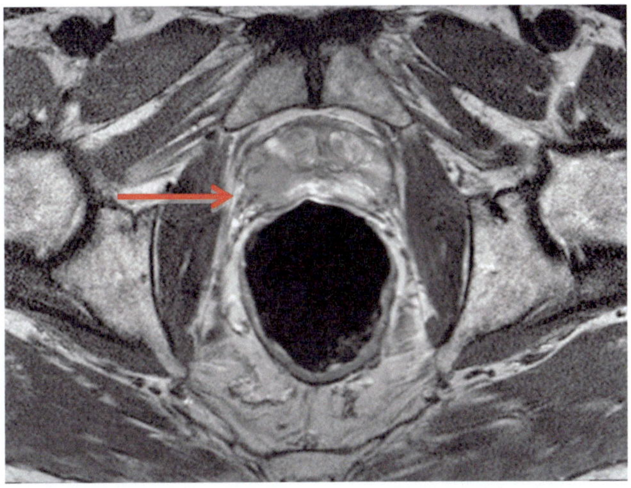

Fig. 5.13 The 2D T2 FSE MR sequence acquired with an endorectal coil shows a hypointense area (*red arrow*) in the right peripheral zone with a loss of the prostatic capsule in front of the right neurovascular bundle corresponding to an extracapsular extension of the tumor

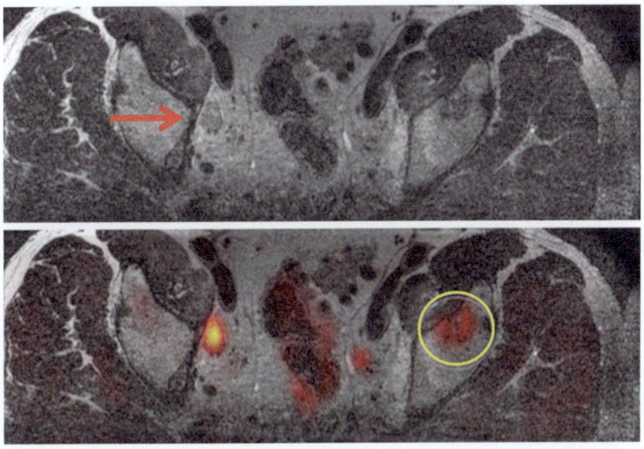

Fig. 5.14 Fused PET/MR images showing a right iliac adenopathy on the 3D VISTA with an abnormal radiotracer uptake (*red arrow*). There is also an abnormal radiotracer uptake on the roof of the left acetabulum corresponding to a bone metastasis that is barely visible on the fast SE 3D VISTA MR sequence (*yellow circle*)

Prostate Cancer with Capsular Invasion

Clinical History

Staging of extension of primary prostate cancer in a 72 year old patient with a primary prostate adenocarcinoma discovered through clinical examination. Gleason (3+4). PSA at 13 μg/l.

Imaging Technique

PET: 10 min dynamic acquisition obtained immediately after injection of 240 MBq of F-18 Fluorocholine followed by whole body scan obtained 10 min after injection and a late acquisition centered on the prostate.

MRI: a complete diagnostic MRI study was acquired in the same session including a 2D T2 Fast SE (TR/TE 4,000/120 ms – slice thickness 3 mm – 432×386 for the axial acquisition – FOV 22 cm) with both an endorectal coil and an external 6 array coil, and after removal of the endorectal coil, a 3D T2 fast spin echo MR sequence (3D VISTA) (TR/TE 2,000/243 ms, matrix 392×448/×25, FOV 390 mm and slice thickness 1 mm), a diffusion SE EPI sequence (TR/TE 3,644/66 ms – slice thickness 3 mm – FOV 200 mm – matrix 88/×9, 4 b values 0, 500, 1,000, 1,500 s/mm^2) and a multi-frame 3D T1 Fat Saturation gradient echo MR sequence (TR/TE 6.9 – 3.4 ms – matrix 192×189 – FOV 210 mm – slice thickness 3 mm) during 5 min after Gd-chelate injection.

Findings

PET images show focal hypermetabolic nodule (SUV max of 3) at the lower right quadrant (8 o'clock) measuring approximately 6 mm in diameter and depicted with hyposignal on T2 weighted images and hypervascular irregular shape extending beyond the external capsule.

A second lesion measuring 2.5 × 0.4 cm with hypointense signal on T2 images and focal hypermetabolism (SUVmax = 2.6) is identified in the left apical area with extension beyond the external capsule.

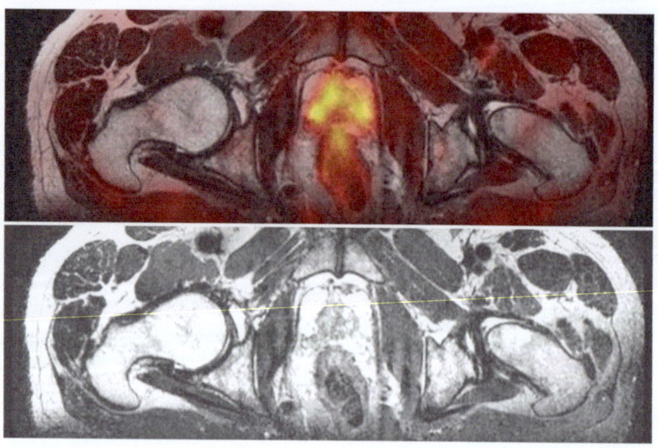

Fig. 5.15 T2-PET MR (3D VISTA) fusion image showing two hypointense and hypermetabolic lesions in the right and left lobes, with heterogeneous pattern of the prostate capsule in contact with the tumor

Teaching Points

This case illustrates the added value of MRI for the assessment of capsular invasion of tumoral tissue that can hardly be detected by PET images.

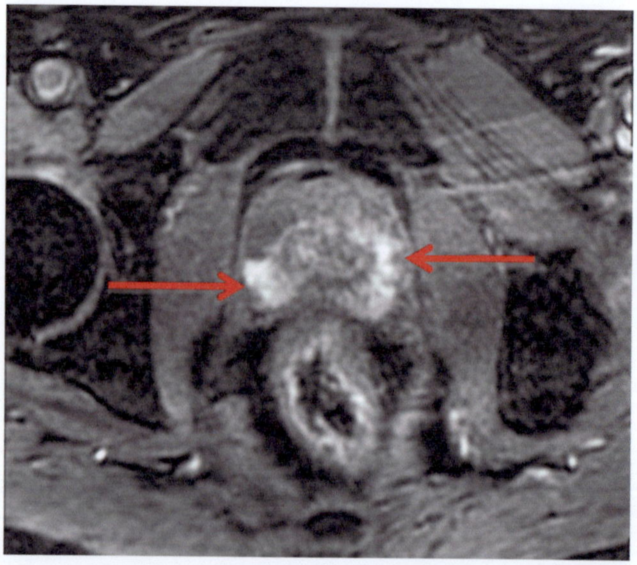

Fig. 5.16 Perfusion weighted images (WIP DYN THRIVE NEW SENSE) showing the hypervascular nature of the lesions on both sides (*arrows*)

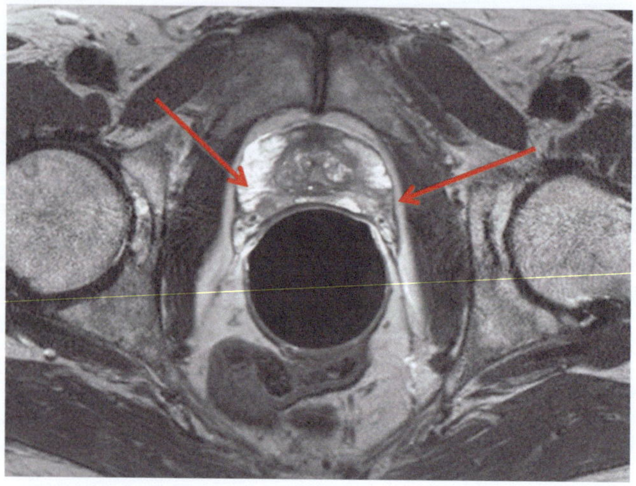

Fig. 5.17 T2 TSE images obtained with rectal coil showing two hypointense lesions (*arrows*) more visible in this sequence

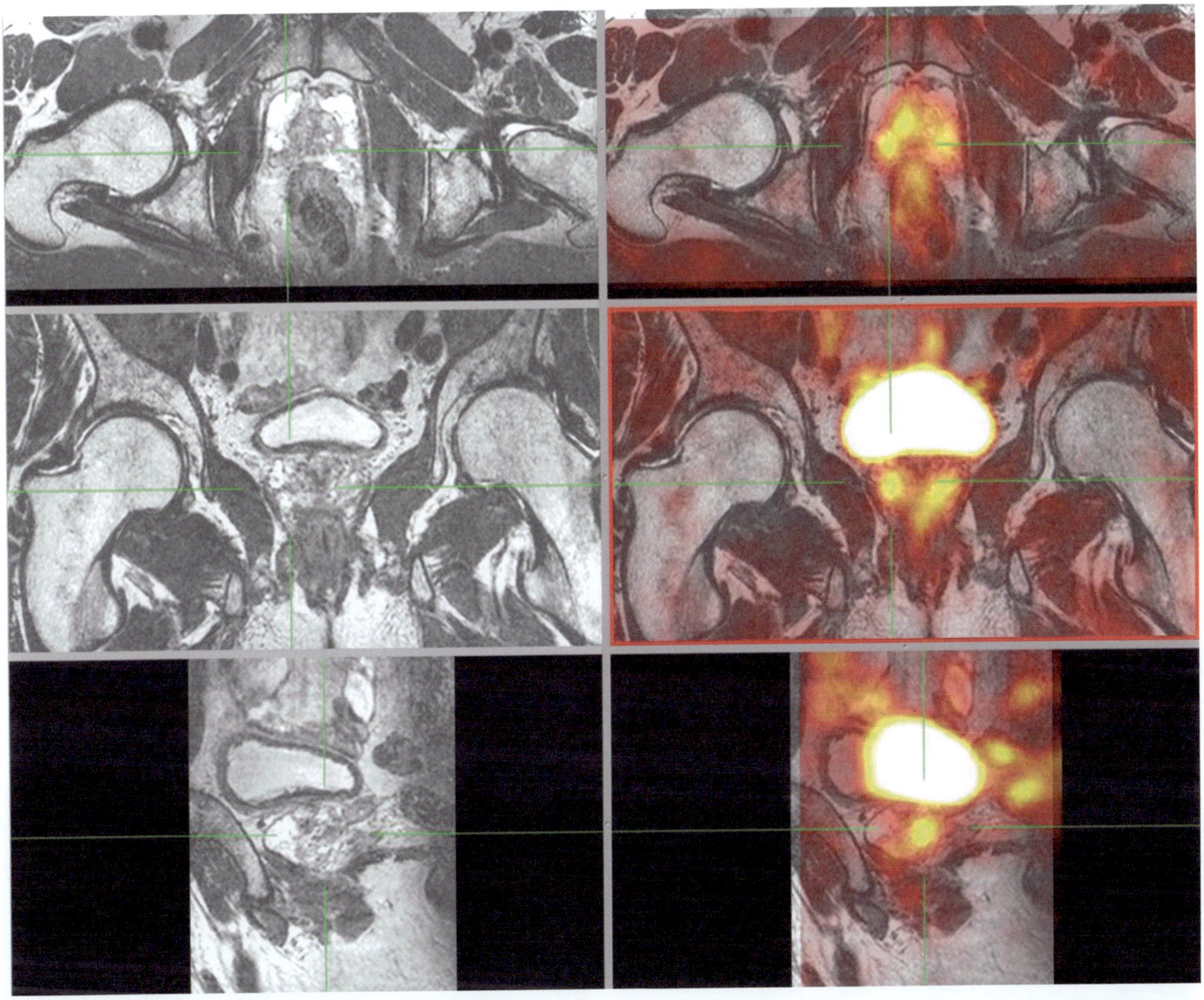

Fig. 5.18 3D VISTA, multiplanar image fusion centered on the most hypermetabolic lesion, showing two lesions on the right and left with heterogeneous appearance of the prostate capsule in contact with the tumor

Prostate Cancer with Lymph Node Extension

Clinical History

Staging of a prostatic adenocarcinoma with a Gleason score of 5+4 and a PSA level at 13.7 µg/l.

Imaging Technique

PET: 10 min dynamic acquisition obtained immediately after injection of 240 MBq of F-18 Fluorocholine followed by whole body scan obtained 10 min after injection and a late acquisition centered on the prostate.

MRI: a complete diagnostic MRI study was acquired in the same session including a 2D T2 Fast SE (TR/TE 4,000/120 ms – slice thickness 3 mm – 432×386 for the axial acquisition – FOV 22 cm) with both an endorectal coil and an external 6 array coil, and after removal of the endorectal coil, a 3D T2 fast spin echo MR sequence (3D VISTA) (TR/TE 2,000/243 ms, matrix 392×448/×25, FOV 390 mm and slice thickness 1 mm), a diffusion SE EPI sequence (TR/TE 3,644/66 ms – slice thickness 3 mm – FOV 200 mm – matrix 88/×9, 4 b values 0, 500, 1,000, 1,500 s/mm^2) and a multi-frame 3D T1 Fat Saturation gradient echo MR sequence (TR/TE 6.9 – 3.4 ms – matrix 192×189 – FOV 210 mm – slice thickness 3 mm during 5 min after Gd-chelate injection.

Findings

Large prostatic tumor invading all the right peripheral zone with some extension on the left side with a strong hypointensity on T2 images, an hypervascularization on perfusion MRI as well as a strong restriction of the apparent diffusion coefficient (ADC). On the PET images, this lesion has a strong uptake of the radiotracer (SUV max=9.3). In front of the right neurovascular bundle, there is a loss of the capsule reflecting extracapsular dissemination. In addition, three lymph nodes of the right iliac chain demonstrated a strong uptake of the radiotracer corresponding to metastasic adenopathies (max SUVmax from 4.6 to 8.1). On the MRI, two of these abnormal lymph nodes were infracentimetric (6 and 5 mm) and were erroneously classified as benign lymph nodes.

Teaching Points

This case demonstrates strong correlation between MRI and PET for the tumor localization.

Advantage of MRI for identification of the transgression of the prostatic capsule.

Advantage of PET for lymph node staging.

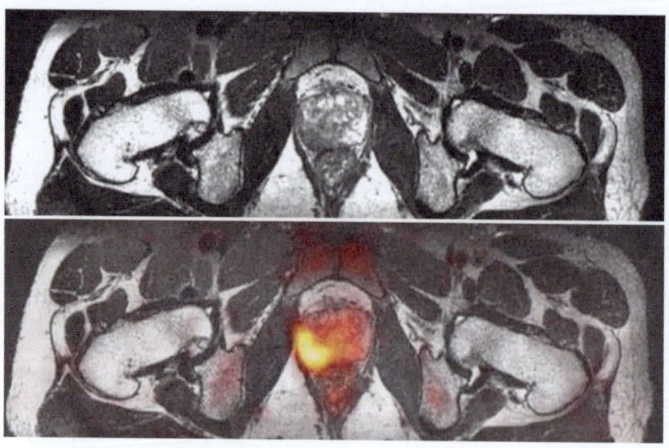

Fig. 5.19 T2 weighted MR image and PET/MR fusion showing the hypointense lesion on the right

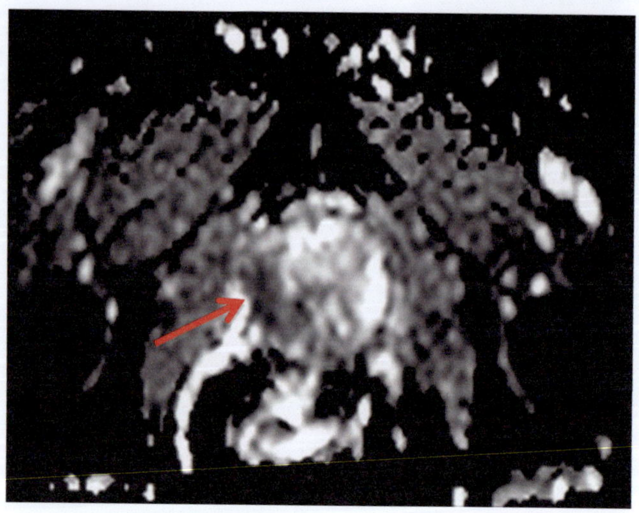

Fig. 5.20 The apparent diffusion coefficient (ADC) map demonstrates a significant reduction of the ADC in the right peripheral zone (*arrow*) with some extension on the left side. This reflects an increased cellular density specific of prostatic tumor

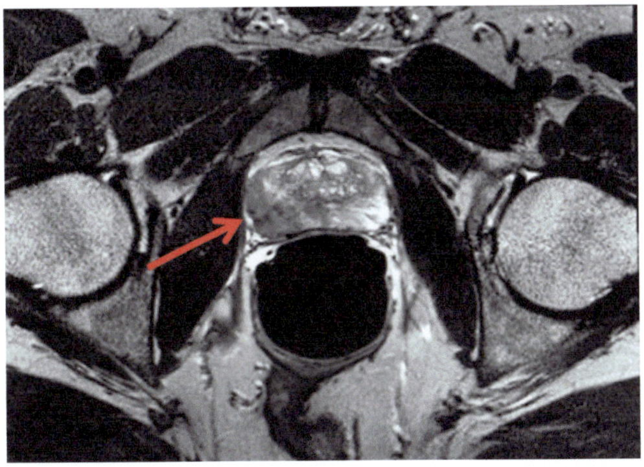

Fig. 5.21 Large prostatic tumor invading the entire right peripheral zone (*arrow*) with some extension on the left side with a strong hypointensity on T2 images with endorectal coil. On the right size there is a bulging of the capsule associated to some capsule loss reflecting an extra-capsular dissemination

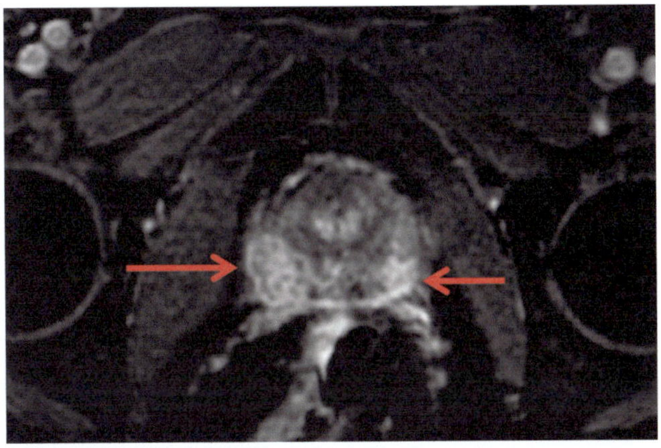

Fig. 5.22 Perfusion MRI after Gd injection. The right peripheral zone and to some extend also on the left peripheral zone (*arrows*) demonstrate a hypervascularization in the area of T2 hypointensity corresponding to the adenocarcinoma

Fig. 5.23 Fused PET/MR images showing the localization of the prostatic tumor in the right peripheral zone on T2 3D VISTA as well as positive radiotracer uptake in three abnormal lymph nodes. Note that two of these abnormal lymph nodes measure less than a centimeter in diameter and there would have been classified as benign lymph node

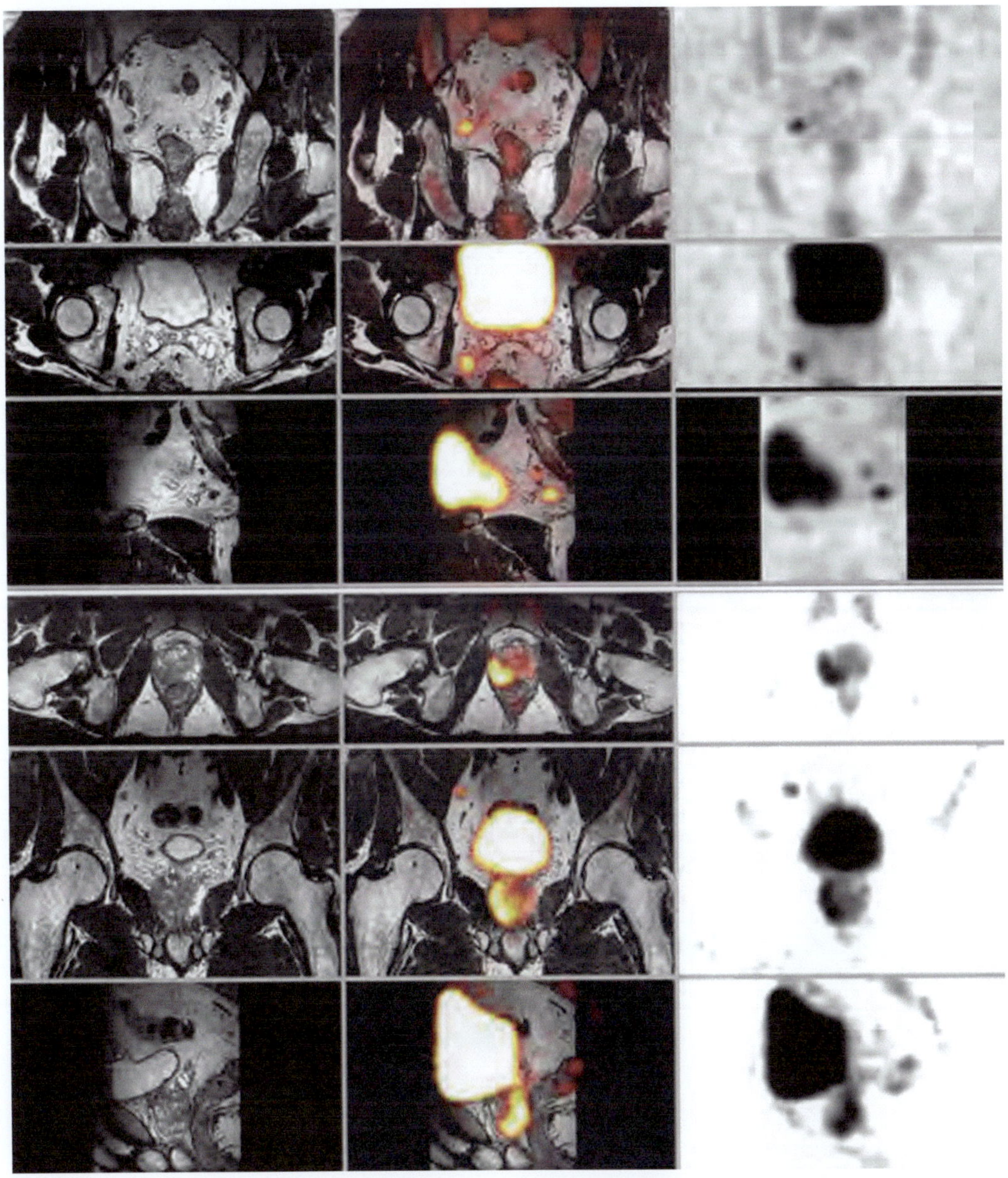

Multiple Bone Metastases of Prostate Cancer

Clinical History

Sixty-seven-year-old patient with prostate adeno-carcinoma, Gleason score 5+5 and PSA at 5.98 μg/l.

Imaging Technique

PET: 10 min dynamic acquisition obtained immediately after injection of 240 MBq of F-18 Fluorocholine followed by whole body scan obtained 10 min after injection and a late acquisition centered on the prostate.

MRI: a complete diagnostic MRI study was acquired in the same session including a 2D T2 Fast SE (TR/TE 4,000/120 ms – slice thickness 3 mm – 432×386 for the axial acquisition – FOV 22 cm) with both an endorectal coil and an external 6 array coil, and after removal of the endorectal coil, a 3D T2 fast spin echo MR sequence (3D VISTA) (TR/TE 2,000/243 ms, matrix 392×448/×25, FOV 390 mm and slice thickness 1 mm) and a diffusion SE EPI sequence (TR/TE 3,644/66 ms – slice thickness 3 mm – FOV 200 mm – matrix 88/Å~ 9, 4 b values 0, 500, 1,000, 1,500 s/mm^2).

Findings

Hypermetabolic prostate tumor covering entire left lobe from apex to base and also spreading to the right lobe. Extracapsular invasion is consistent with local invasion covering left neurovascular bundle.

PET images showing a hypermetabolic lymph node below the iliac bifurcation with SUV 3.1 and a millimetric hypermetabolic left ilio-obturator lymph with SUV max. 2.1.

Multifocal hypermetabolic bone lesions at the right iliac (SUV max. 3.5), at the left iliac wing (SUV max. 3.7) at the left sacroiliac joint, at the ilio-pubic branch right (SUV max. 7.3), the right ischio-pubic branch (SUV 6.3) and at left ischial tuberosity (SUV max. 5.5) are present.

> **Teaching Points**
>
> PET/MRI imaging allows a comprehensive staging of remote metastasis by combining the two modalities in a single examination.

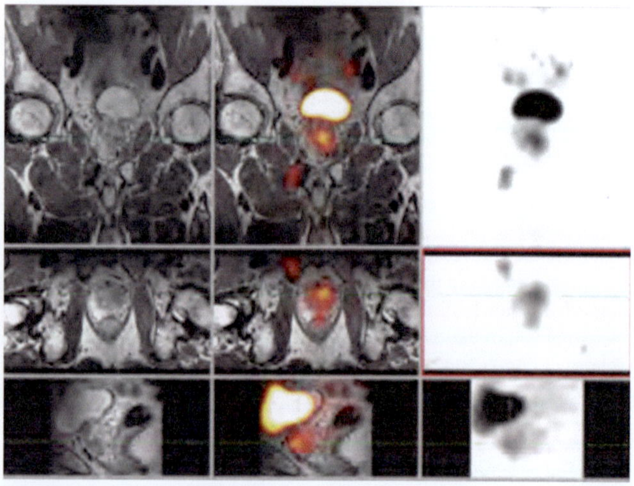

Fig. 5.24 The large hypermetabolic tumor in two lobes of the prostate also visible in T2 MR images

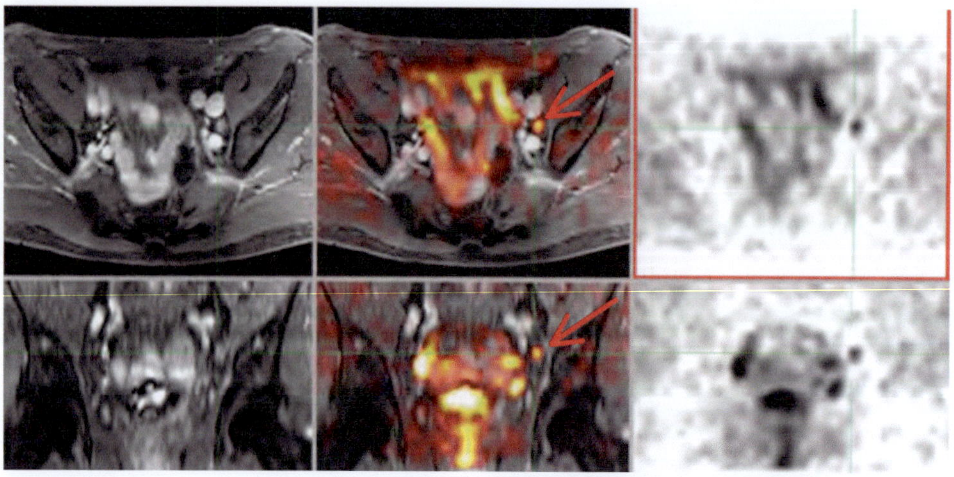

Fig. 5.25 eThrive MR image showing the iliac lymph node below the bifurcation with SUV max. of 2.1 (*arrows*)

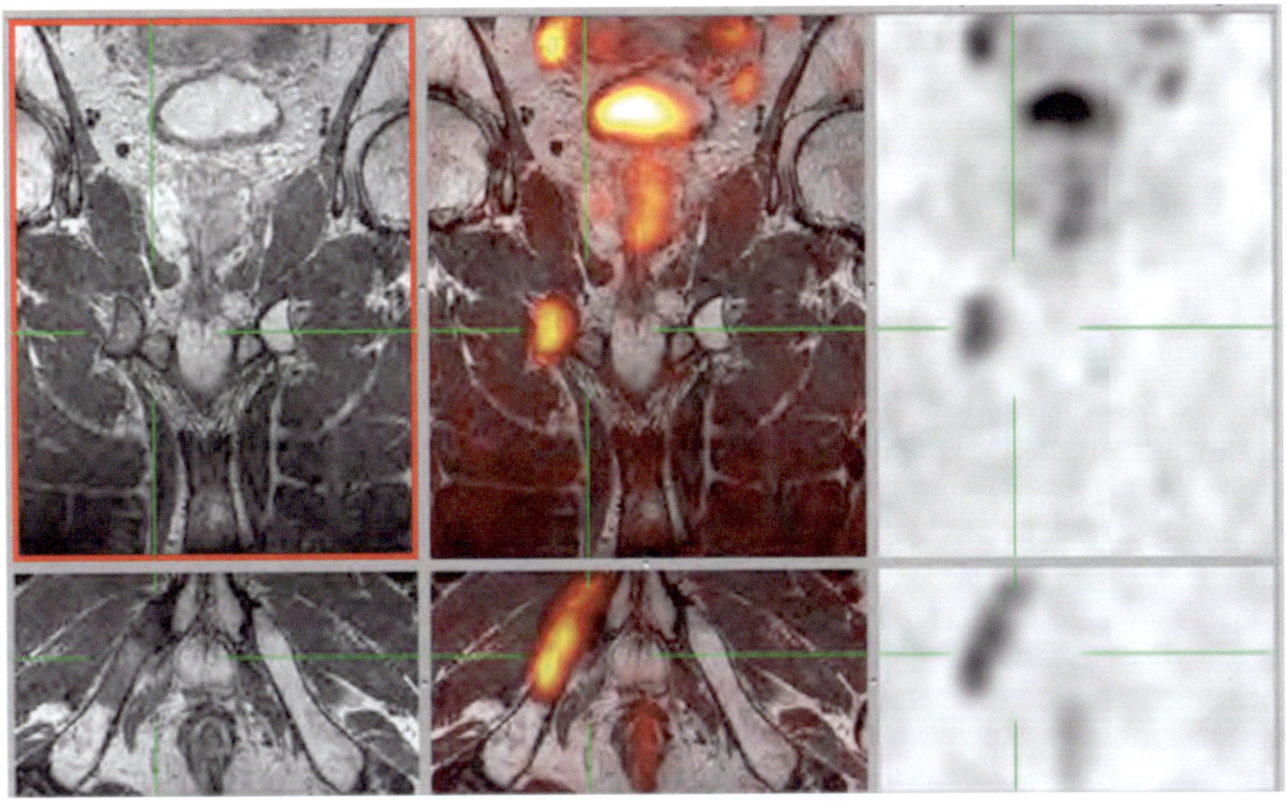

Fig. 5.26 Coronal (*top*) and axial (*bottom*) PET/MR images of the pelvis showing the metastatic bone lesions of the right iliac branch also clearly visible on T2 weighted 3D VISTA MR images

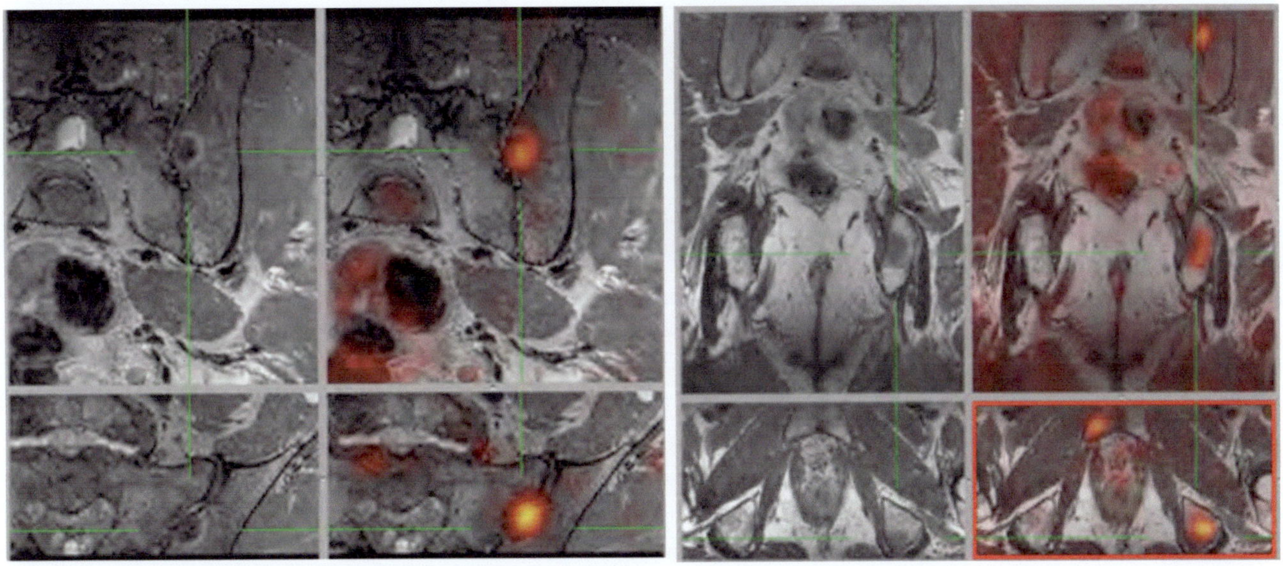

Fig. 5.27 Coronal (*top*) and axial (*bottom*) PET/MR images of the pelvis showing multiple bone metastases of the left pelvic and iliac bones also visible on T2 weighted 3D VISTA MR images

Primary Prostate Cancer with Extraprostatic Extension

Clinical History

Sixty-five-year-old patient presents with an initial PSA-value of 11.2 ng/ml. Endorectal biopsy confirmed prostate cancer (cT3a, Gleason 4+5=9).

Imaging Technique

Whole body PET/MR images acquired 37 min after iv injection 811 MBq ^{11}C-Choline, 77 kg.

3 beds × 4 min together with coronal T1w TSE and axial T2w haste fs. 1 bed (pelvis) a 15 min together with ax T2 TSE, ax T1 TSE, ax DWI, ax T1w TWIST CM dynamic. Post gadolinium axial T1w VIBE from chest to pelvis. Head/neck and two body coils.

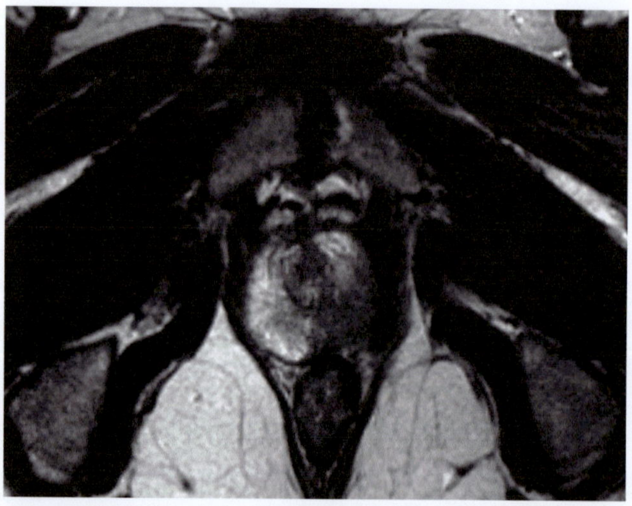

Fig. 5.28 Axial T2w TSE of prostatic apex shows a relative hypointense signal in the peripheral zone of the *left side* highly suspicious for prostate cancer. The missing delineation of the capsule (compared to the *right side*) raises the suspicion of extracapsular extension

Findings

T2w TSE sequences are very sensitive in the detection of prostate cancer in the peripheral zone which normally shows a hyperintense signal. Missing delineation of the prostatic capsule is suspicious for extracapsular extension.

Teaching Points

The superb anatomical delineation of the prostate fossa in MRI allows local staging of prostate cancer. This is a clear advantage of PET/MR compared to PET/CT.

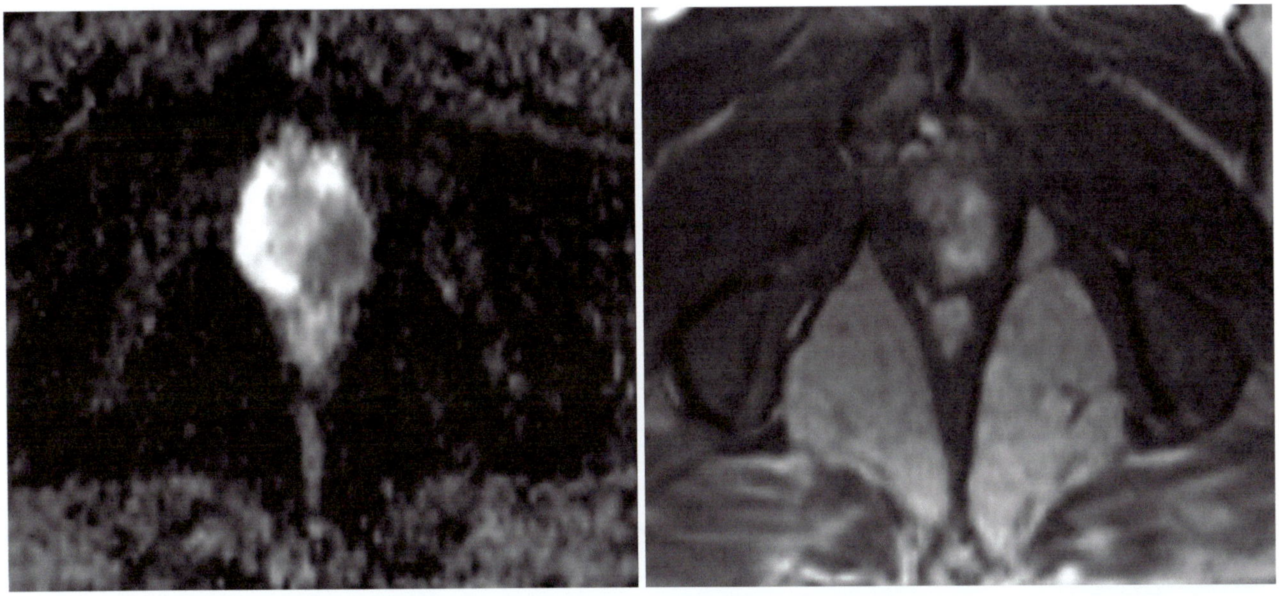

Fig. 5.29 Axial diffusion weighted imaging (DWI) demonstrate a highly restricted diffusion (low ADC-value) in the left peripheral zone (*left*). An intense and early enhancement of the corresponding region can be found in the arterial phase of the dynamic contrast enhanced MRI sequence (*right*). Both findings support the uspicion of prostate cancer from the T2w TSE sequence

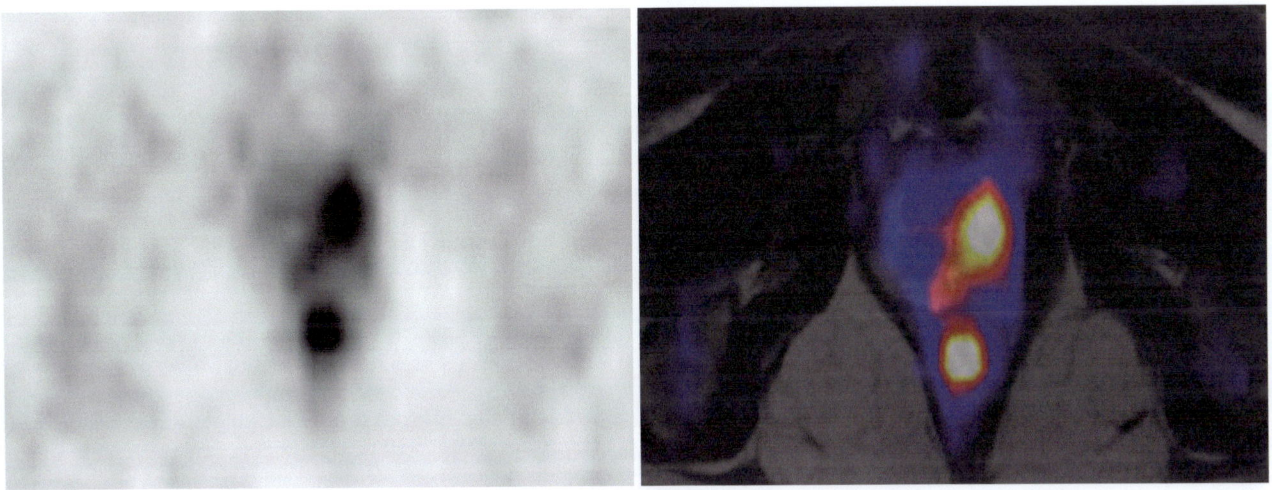

Fig. 5.30 A high focal uptake in ^{11}C-Choline PET (*left*) is located exactly in the area of the abnormalities presented by MRI shown in the fused PET/T2w TSE image (*right*)

Prostate Cancer in the Central Zone

Clinical History

Seventy-three-year-old patient with a PSA-value of 34 ng/ml suspicious for prostate cancer. No prior endorectal biopsy has been performed.

Imaging Technique

Whole body PET/MR images acquired 32 min after iv injection 809 MBq ^{11}C-Choline, 71 kg.

3 beds × 4 min together with coronal T1w TSE and axial T2w haste fs. 1 bed (pelvis) a 15 min together with ax T2 TSE, ax T1 TSE, ax DWI, ax T1w TWIST CM dynamic. Post CM axial T1w VIBE from chest to pelvis. Head/neck and two body coils.

Findings

T2w sequences show superb anatomical details of the prostate with a hypointense region in the anterior part on the left side. With morphological sequences alone in MRI no definite differentiation between prostate cancer and benign prostatic hyperplasia (BPH) can be made. Functional imaging with diffusion-weighted imaging (DWI) and ^{11}C-Choline PET confirm the presence of prostate cancer in the anterior portion of the gland.

Teaching Points

Detection of prostate cancer in the central zone is often unambiguous with morphological MR sequences. However DWI and ^{11}C-Choline PET can help in the differentiation between BPH and prostate cancer.

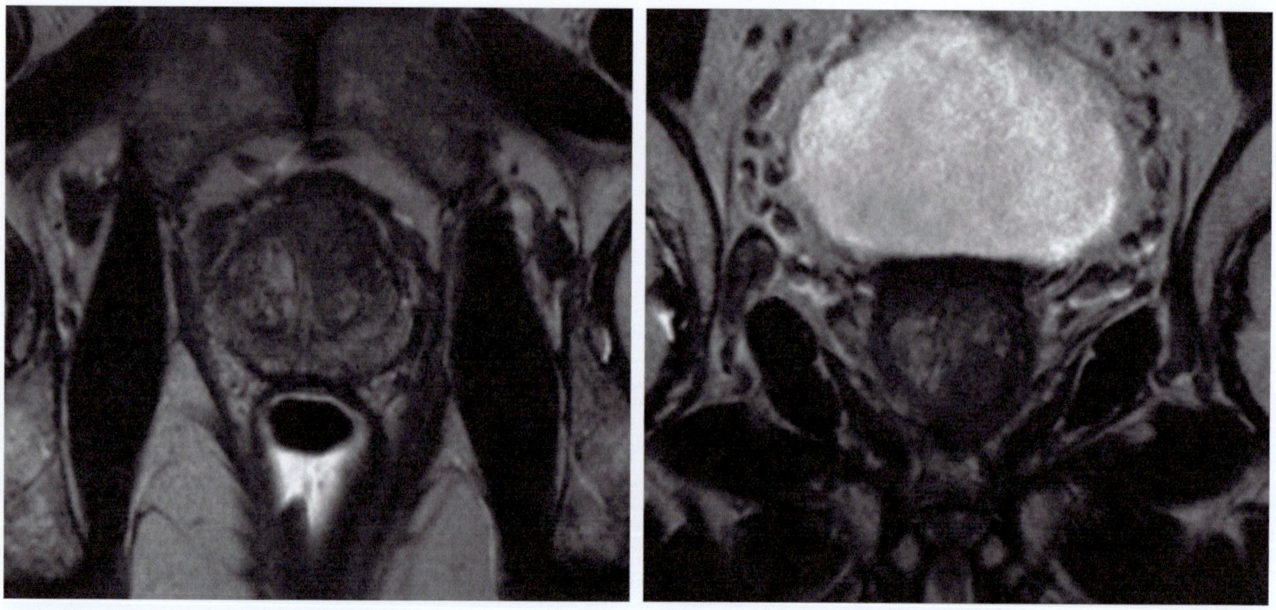

Fig. 5.31 Morphological T2w TSE sequences in the axial and the coronal plane demonstrate superb anatomical details of the prostate fossa. A hypointense region in the anterior part of the left side is suspicious for prostate cancer. However benign prostatic hyperplasia can have similar appearance on MRI

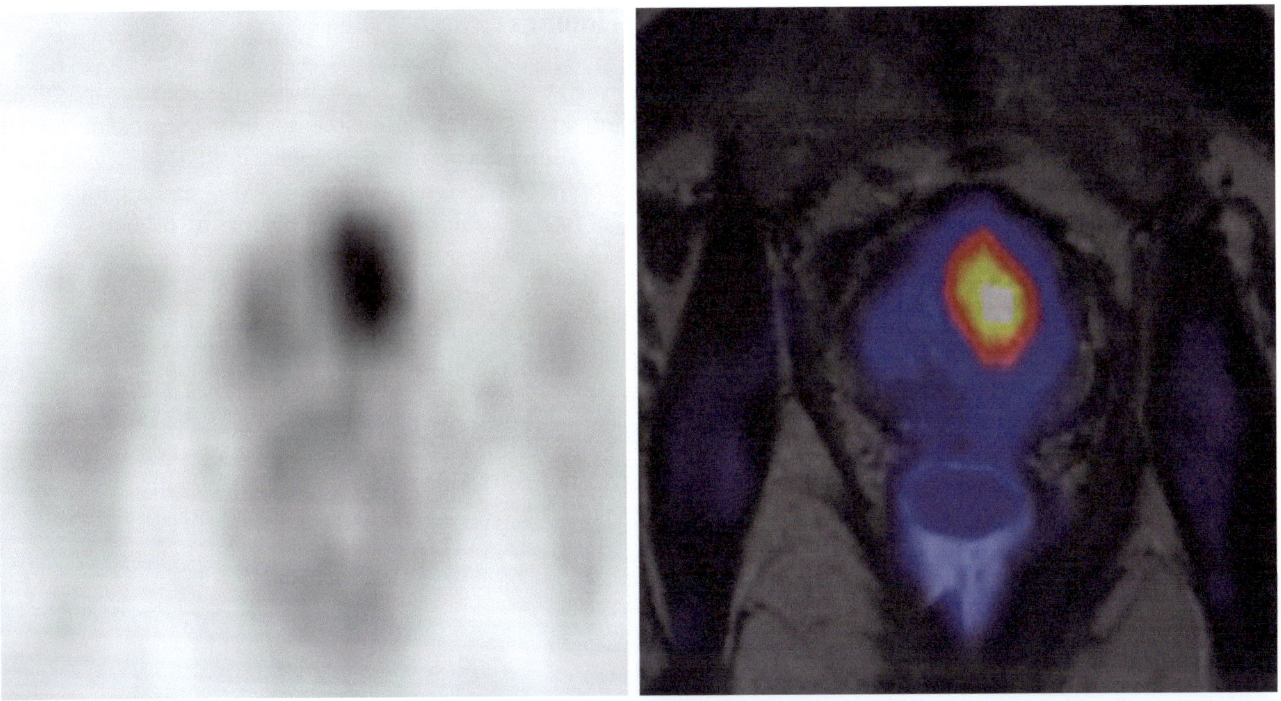

Fig. 5.32 ^{11}C-Choline PET shows an intense focal uptake in the left anterior part of the prostate highly suspicious for prostate cancer

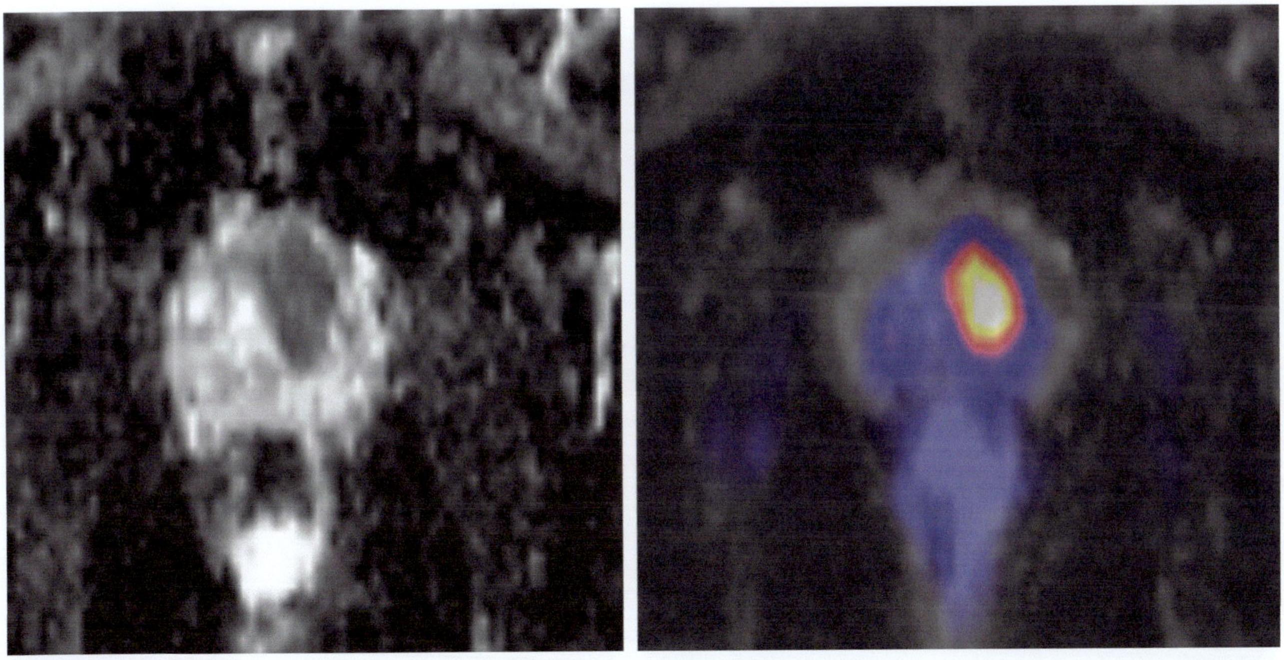

Fig. 5.33 The parametric ADC (apparent diffusion coefficient) map derived from diffusion-weighted imaging sequences shows an area of highly restricted diffusion (low ADC-value) in the left anterior part of the prostate. In the central zone this can be more specific for prostate cancer than hypointensity in T2w sequences. Fusion with ^{11}C-Choline PET demonstrates a good concordance between the findings in PET and DWI

Multiparametric Imaging in Primary Prostate Cancer

Clinical History

Fifty-nine-year-old patient with slowly rising PSA-value over 5 years and a history of negative biopsy 3 years ago. The current PSA-value is 11.3 ng/ml.

Imaging Technique

Whole body PET/MR images acquired 66 min after iv injection 750 MBq ^{11}C-Choline, 58 kg.

3 beds × 4 min together with coronal T1w TSE and axial T2w haste fs. 1 bed (pelvis) a 15 min together with ax T2 TSE, ax T1 TSE, ax DWI, ax T1w TWIST CM dynamic. Post CM axial T1w VIBE from chest to pelvis. Head/neck and two body coils.

Findings

A T2w-hypointense lesion in the peripheral zone of the left side is highly suspicious for primary prostate cancer. In addition focal increased uptake in PET, restricted diffusion in DWI, high wash-in DCE-MRI and a pathological choline peak in MRS are indicative of primary prostate cancer.

Teaching Points

Multiparametric PET/MR imaging of primary prostate cancer can further increase tumor detection and possibly guide biopsy especially in patients with prior negative histopathology.

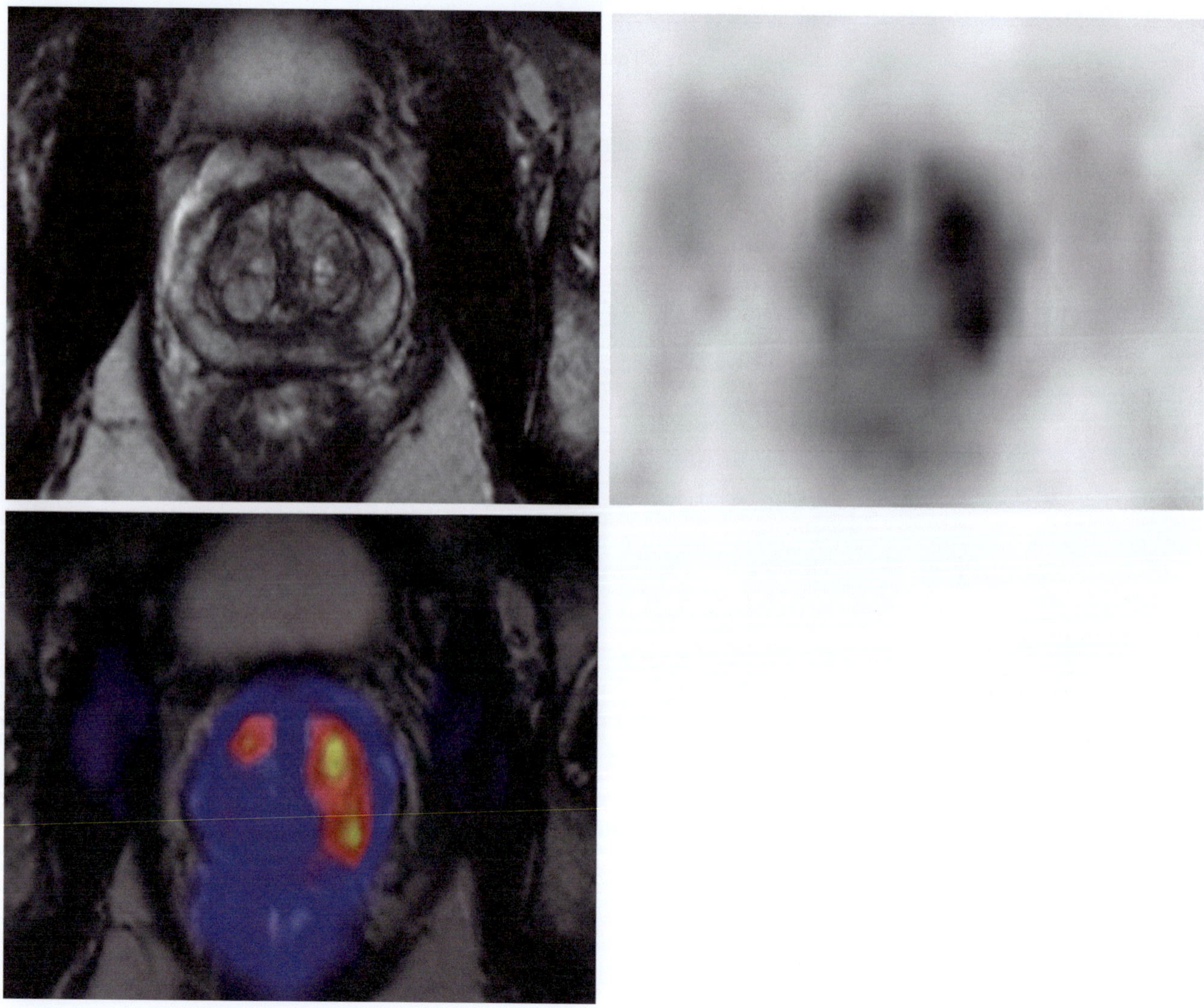

Fig. 5.34 The axial T2w TSE sequence shows a hypointense lesion in the peripheral zone on the left side which is highly suspicious for primary prostate cancer (*left top*). Diffuse partially focal uptake is demonstrated in the central zone with a focus of high uptake in the left peripheral zone (*right top*). Fused PET/T2w image documents a good correlation of the abnormal findings in the left peripheral zone (*bottom*)

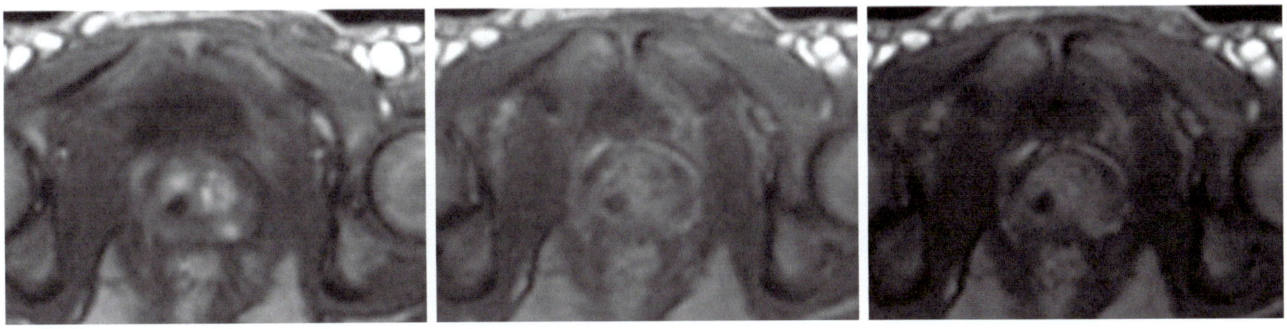

Fig. 5.35 Dynamic contrast enhancement (DCE) MRI of the prostate gland. Arterial phase (*left*) shows an early enhancement in the left peripheral zone suspicious for primary prostate cancer and a diffuse inhomogeneous enhancement in the central zone typical for BPH. In the later phases (*center* and *right*) an inhomogeneous enhancement is found in the whole prostate nearly completely obscuring the lesion in the peripheral zone

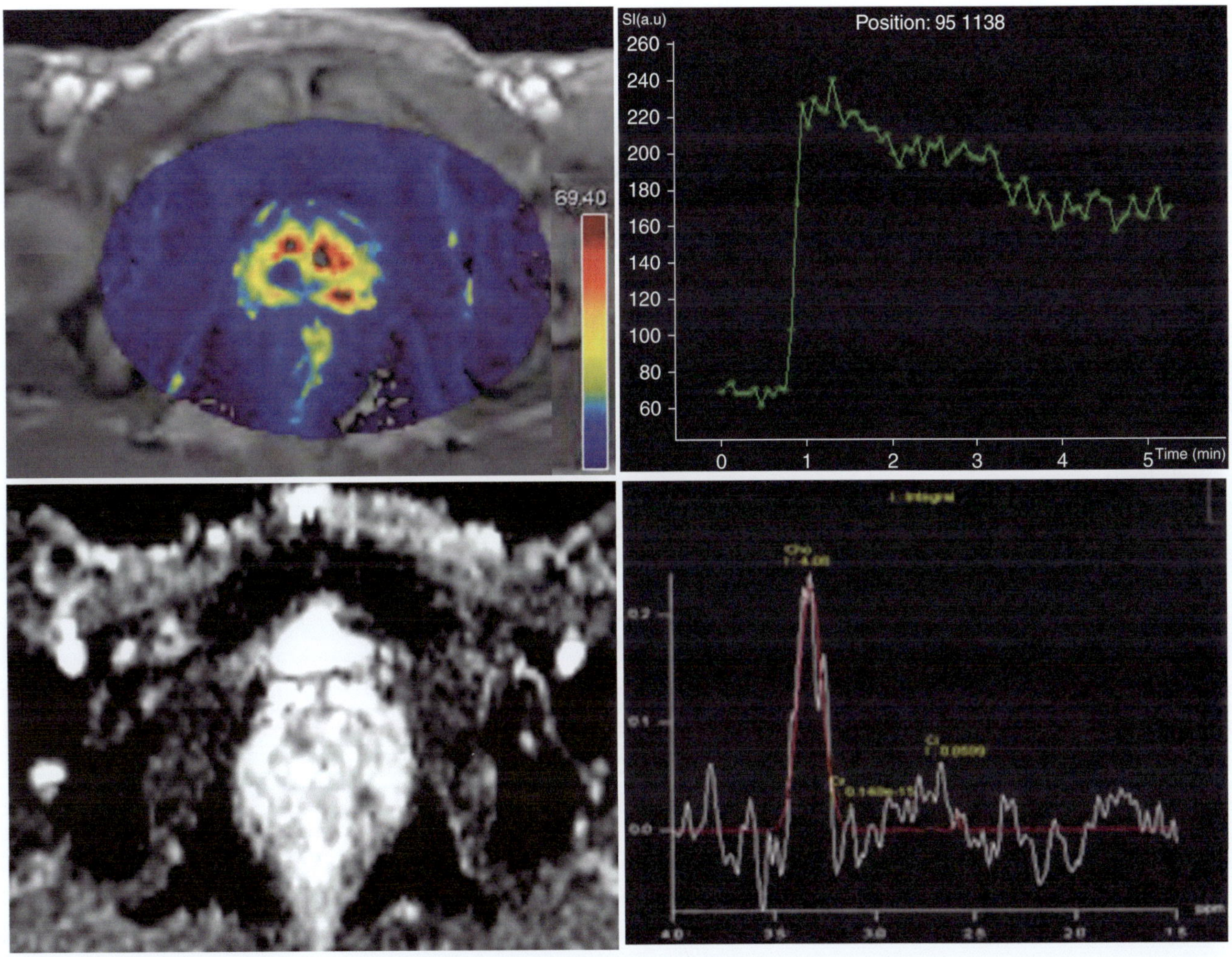

Fig. 5.36 Parametric map of the DCE-images show an increased AUC (area under the *curve*) in the left peripheral zone (*left top*). ROI analysis demonstrates an early wash-in as well as an wash-out typical for a malignant lesion (*top right*). Restricted diffusion with a low ADC-value can be found in this region in DWI-MRI (*bottom left*). MR-spectroscopy reveals a high peak of choline

Recurrence After Brachytherapy

Clinical History

Seventy-two-year-old patient presenting with rising PSA (10.6 ng/ml) 2 years after brachytherapy.

Imaging Technique

Whole body PET/MR images acquired 46 min after iv injection 883 MBq ^{11}C-Choline, 86 kg.

4 beds × 4 min together with coronal T1w TSE and axial T2w haste fs. 1 bed (pelvis) a 15 min together with ax T2 TSE, ax DWI, ax T1w TWIST CM dynamic. Post CM axial T1w VIBE from chest to pelvis. Head/neck and two body coils.

Findings

A high focal uptake of ^{11}C-Choline in PET strongly indicates local recurrence. MRI is impaired due to metal artifacts from the implanted seeds. However it demonstrates a relative sparing of the seeds in the zone with the recurrent tumor.

Teaching Points

The metallic seeds from Brachytherapy create susceptibility artifacts in MRI. In these cases information from PET can become crucial for detection of local recurrence.

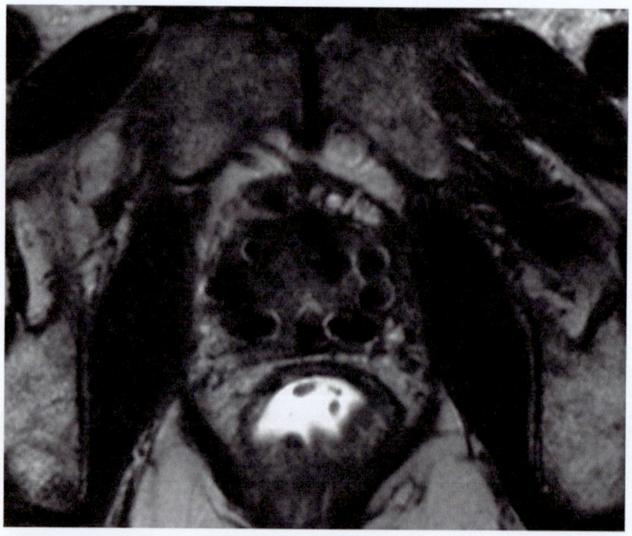

Fig. 5.37 Usually in MRI of the prostate gland a T2w sequence with small field-of-views serves for anatomical delineation of the prostate gland and enables detection of prostate cancer especially in the peripheral zone. Hence after Brachytherapy image quality is impaired

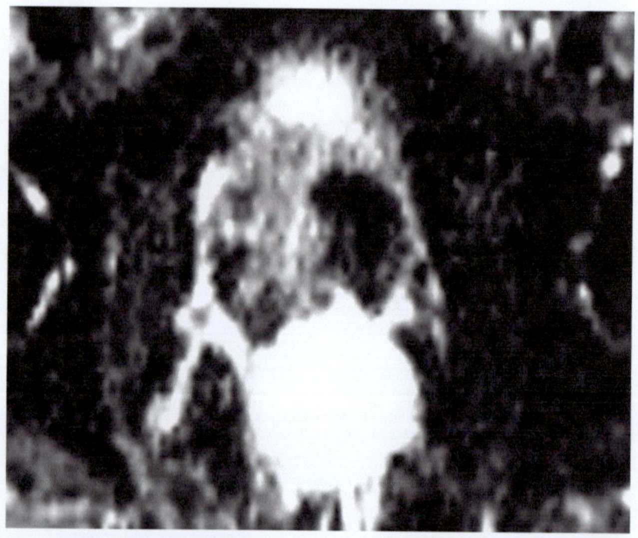

Fig. 5.38 Modern imaging techniques like DWI (diffusion weighted imaging) enable higher detection rates of recurrent local prostate cancer. However the use is hampered by implanted metal

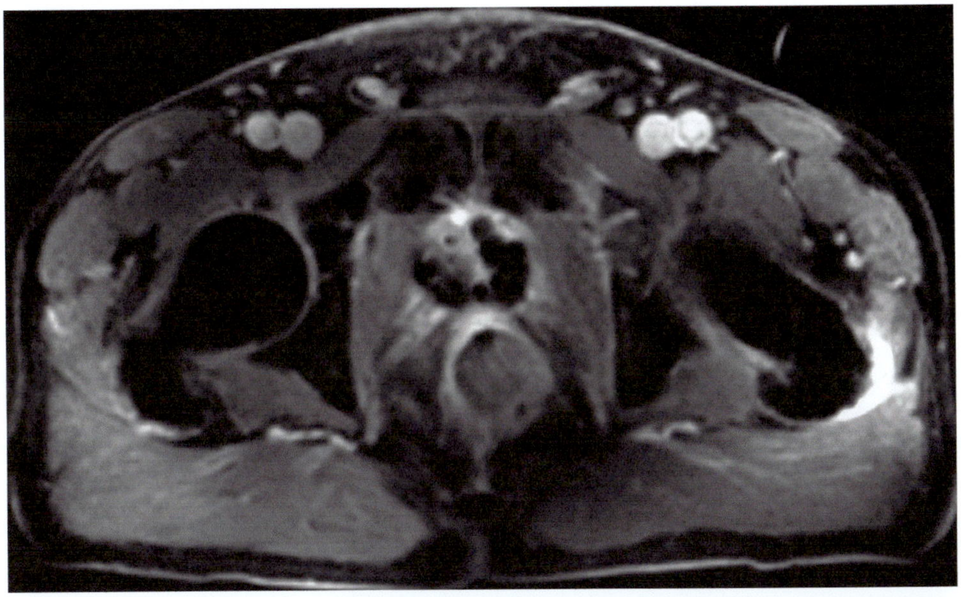

Fig. 5.39 In the T1w VIBE GRE-sequence intense susceptibility artifacts demonstrate the location of the seeds with a relative sparing of the right anterior part of the prostate

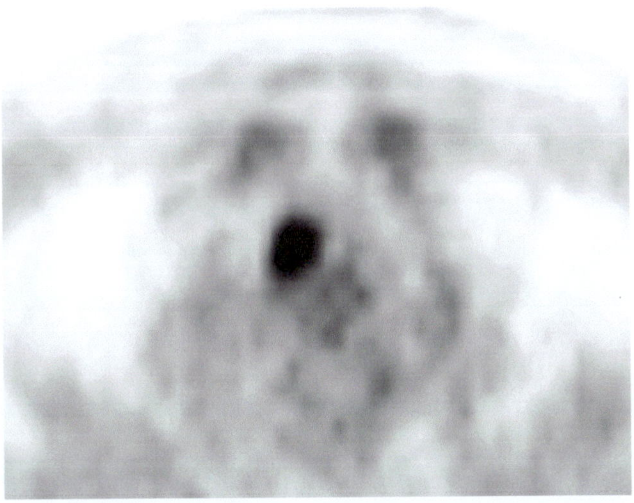

Fig. 5.40 High focal uptake of ^{11}C-Choline in PET indicates local recurrence/remaining tumor

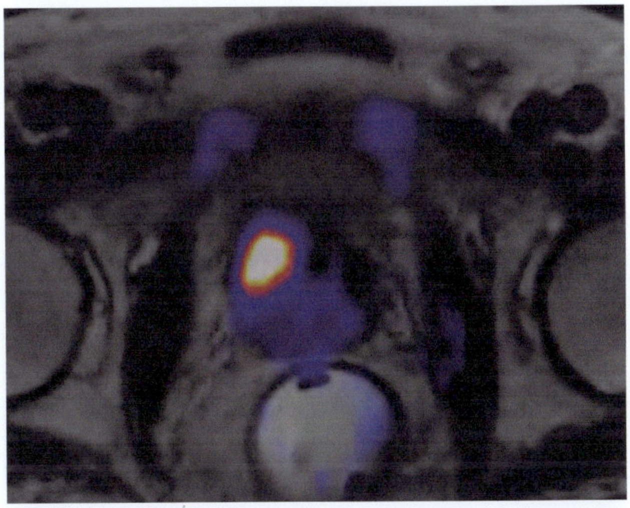

Fig. 5.41 Fusion from PET and T2w demonstrates the exact anatomical location of the local recurrence

Lymph Node Metastasis from Recurrent Prostate Cancer

Clinical History

Seventy-one-year-old patient presenting with rising PSA (34.5 ng/ml) 3 years after radiation therapy of the prostate.

Imaging Technique

Whole body PET/MR images acquired 56 min after iv injection 770 MBq ^{11}C-Choline, 74 kg.

4 beds × 4 min together with coronal T1w TSE and axial T2w haste fs. 1 bed (pelvis) a 15 min together with ax T2 TSE, ax DWI, ax T1w TWIST CM dynamic. Post CM axial T1w VIBE from chest to pelvis. Head/neck and two body coils.

Findings

A pararectal lymph node which is slightly enlarged and rounded appears suspicious in morphological imaging. Highly restricted diffusion and high uptake of ^{11}C-Cholin confirm the malignant nature.

Teaching Points

This case demonstrates the additional value of multiparametric PET/MR compared to PET/CT. Besides the functional information from PET, PET/MR can also provide molecular information from MRI – in this case the restricted diffusion in a malignant lymph node in prostate cancer.

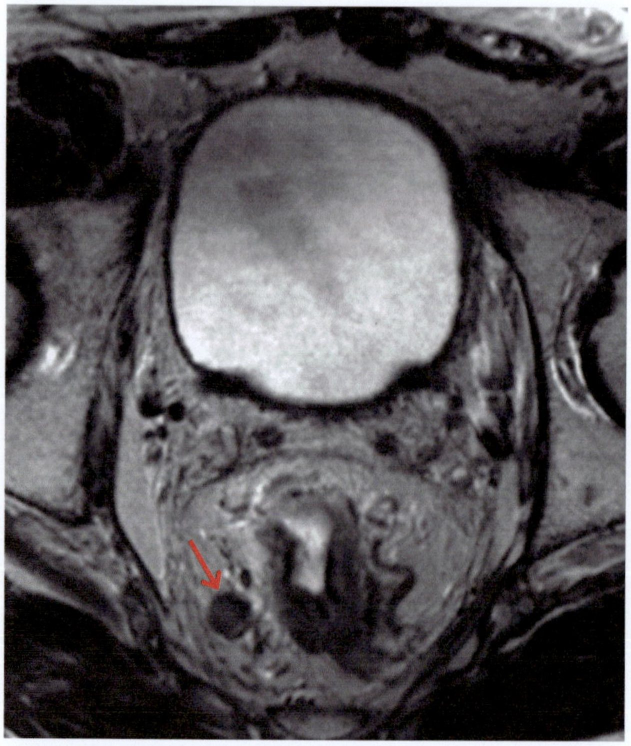

Fig. 5.42 Anatomical T2w TSE demonstrate an enlarged lymph node in the mesorectal fascia which is an untypical location for a lymph node metastases in prostate cancer (*arrow*)

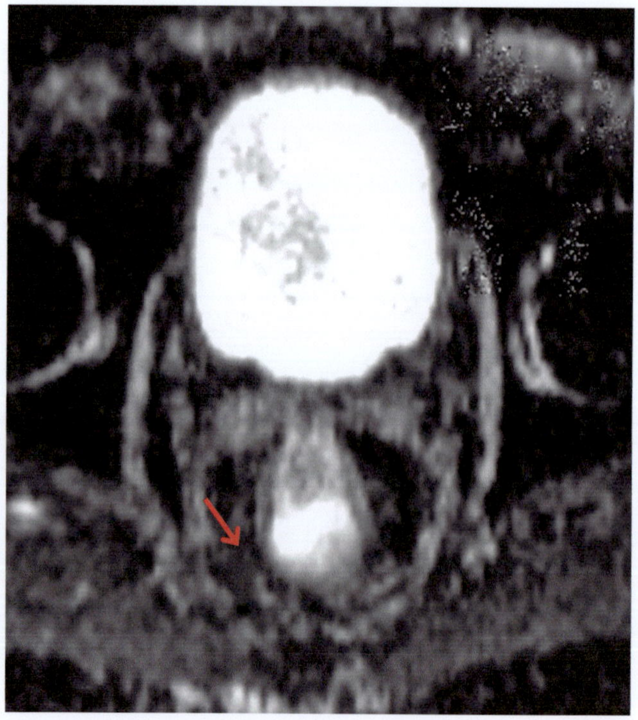

Fig. 5.43 The ADC (apparent diffusion coefficient) – map of DWI shows highly restricted diffusion in the suspicious lymph node (*arrow*)

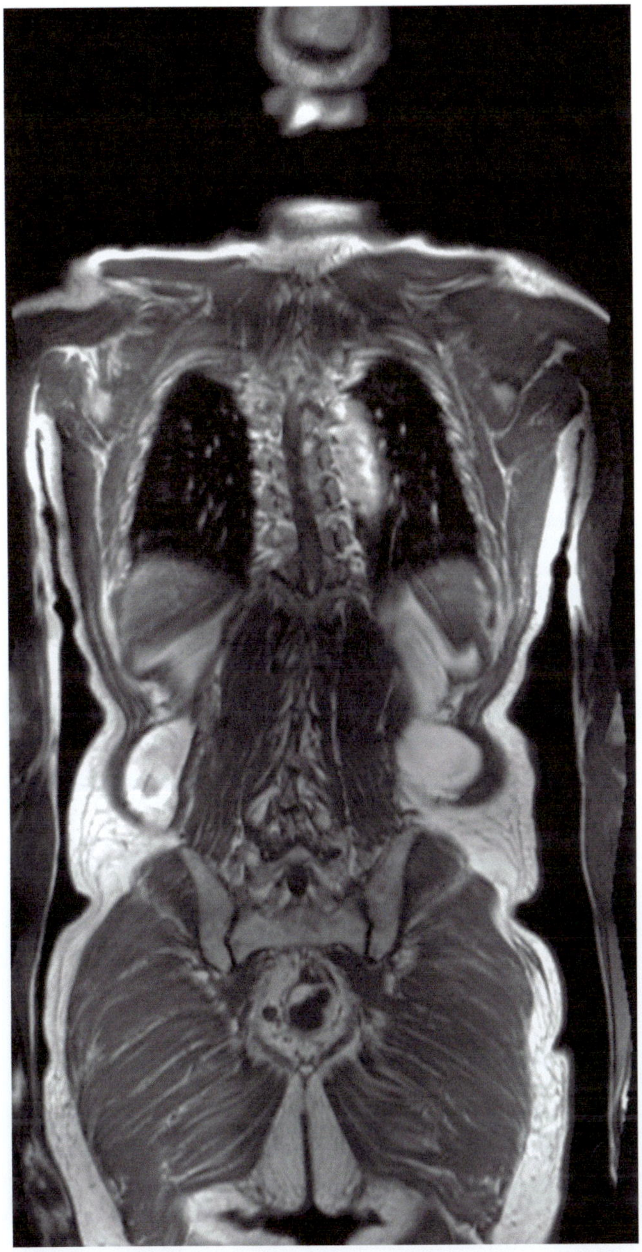

Fig. 5.44 Coronal T1w TSE demonstrates the whole field-of-view from PET/MR and also outlines the lymph node in the mesorectal fat

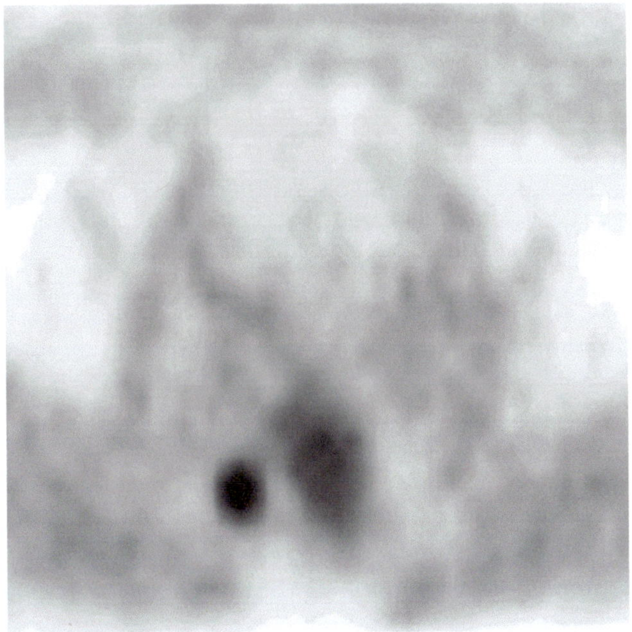

Fig. 5.45 High uptake of ^{11}C-Choline in a morphologically enlarged lymph node can be regarded as diagnostic for a metastases in the case of PSA-recurrent prostate cancer

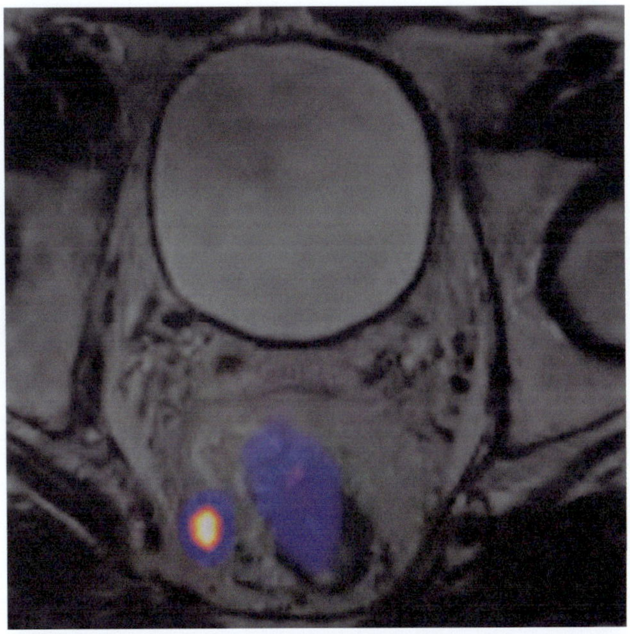

Fig. 5.46 Fusion of PET and T2w TSE shows a perfect anatomical coregistration of the focal increased uptake in PET and the suspicious lymph node

Bone Metastases in Prostate Cancer After Radiotherapy

Clinical History

Eighty-five-year-old patient status post radical prostatectomy 8 years ago. He presents with rising PSA (25.9 ng/ml) despite radiation of multiple bone metastases in the last 2 years.

Imaging Technique

Whole body PET/MR images acquired 53 min after iv injection 850 MBq ^{11}C-Choline, 70 kg.

4 beds × 4 min together with coronal T1w TSE and axial T2w haste fs. 1 bed (pelvis) a 15 min together with ax T2 TSE, ax DWI, ax T1w TWIST CM dynamic. Post CM axial T1w VIBE from chest to pelvis. Head/neck and two body coils.

Findings

In this patient with prior radiotherapy T1w SE sequences show the conversion to fatty bone marrow in the whole spine. Additional T1w hypointense areas with high uptake of ^{11}C-Choline indicate new/residual bone metastases which now could be treated with focused radiation therapy.

Teaching Points

MRI with T1w SE sequences is superior to CT in outlining the anatomical extent of bone metastases. Therefore it can serve for a more exact planning of radiation therapy especially in patient who underwent prior radiotherapy.

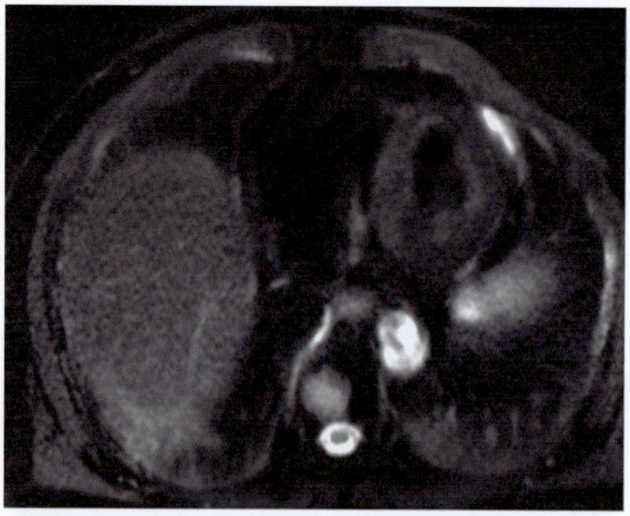

Fig. 5.47 The axial T2w fs sequence shows a round hyperintense area in the thoracic spine. T2w hyperintensity of a bone metastasis usually indicates viable tumor tissue compared to T2w hypointensity which is a sign of prior effective treatment (esp. by radiation therapy)

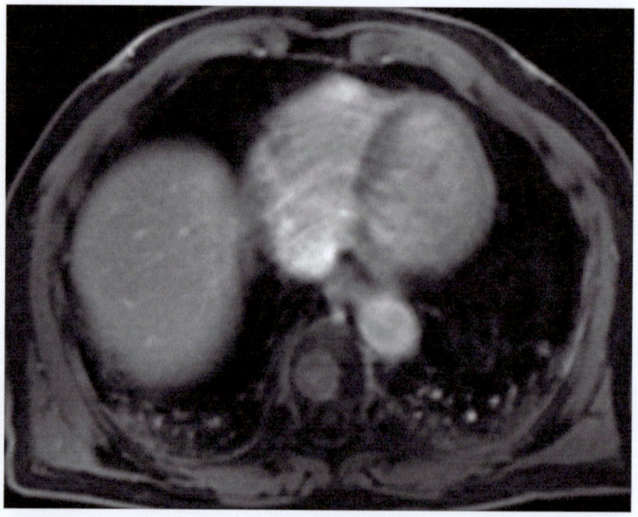

Fig. 5.48 Axial post contrast VIBE sequence with fat saturation shows a moderate contrast enhancement of the lesion

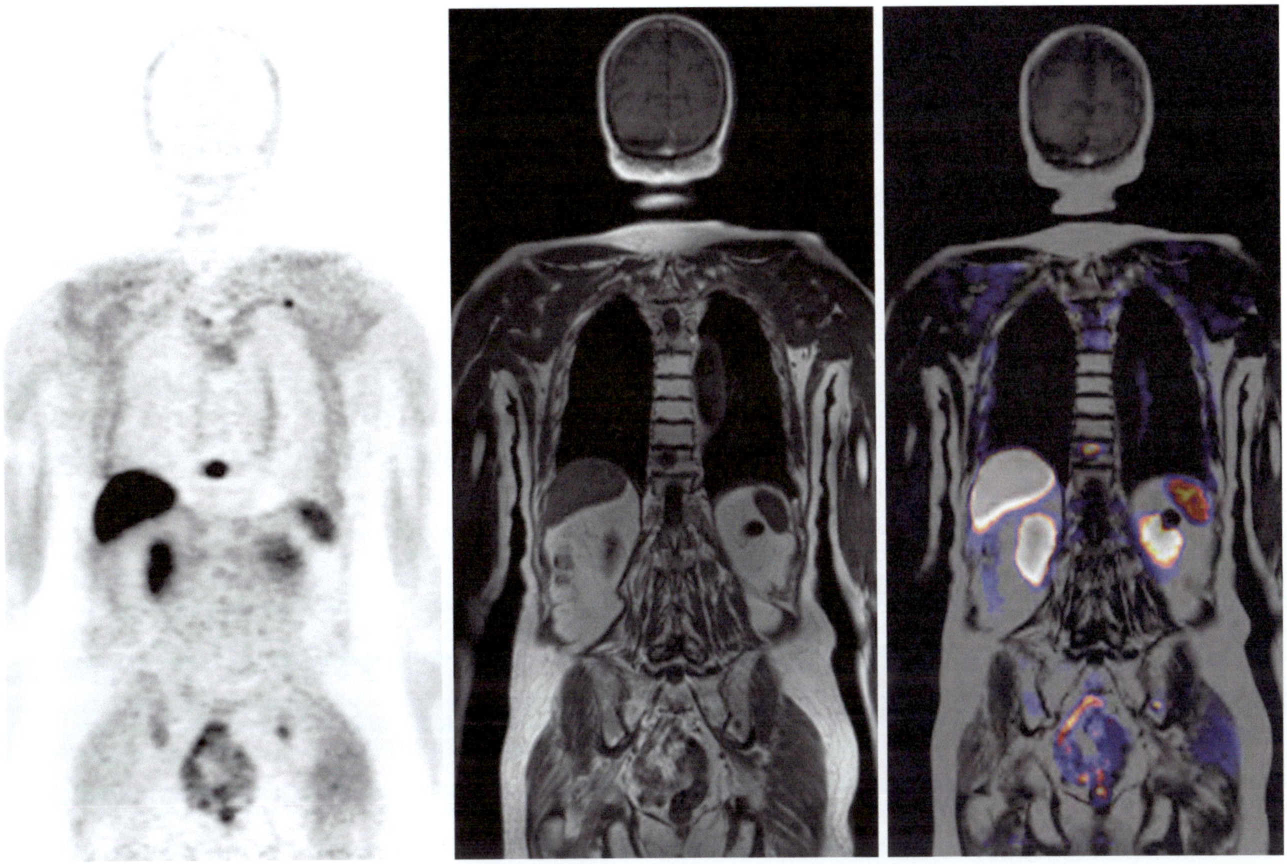

Fig. 5.49 Coronal images show the extent of bone metastases in this patient. PET demonstrates the highest uptake of ^{11}C-Choline in a lesion of the lower thoracic spine. Other lesions are located in the left pelvis and the ribs (*left*). T1w TSE show fatty conversion of the bone marrow indicating prior radiation therapy and hypointense lesions corresponding with the high uptake in PET (*middle*). Fused T1w TSE and PET demonstrate good correlation between the uptake in PET and the hypointense lesions in MRI

Discrimination of Viable and Effectively Treated Bone Metastases

Clinical History

Sixty-year-old patient after with increasing PSA over 2 years (21.5 ng/ml) after radical prostatectomy and prior radiation of the right pelvis due to a single bone metastases.

Imaging Technique

Whole body PET/MR images acquired 42 min after iv injection 764 MBq ^{11}C-Choline, 75 kg.

3 beds × 4 min together with coronal T1w TSE and axial T2w haste fs. 1 bed (pelvis) a 15 min together with ax T2 TSE, ax DWI, ax T1w TWIST CM dynamic. Post CM axial T1w VIBE from chest to pelvis. Head/neck and two body coils.

Findings

The patients presents with a treated bone metastasis in the right pelvis which shows no uptake of 11_C-Cholin and only faint contrast enhancement. In contrast, a new bone metastasis in the sternum has a high uptake in PET as well as an intense contrast enhancement in MRI.

Teaching Points

In contrast to CT, MRI can give additional information about the viability of bone metastases in prostate cancer complementing the information provided by PET.

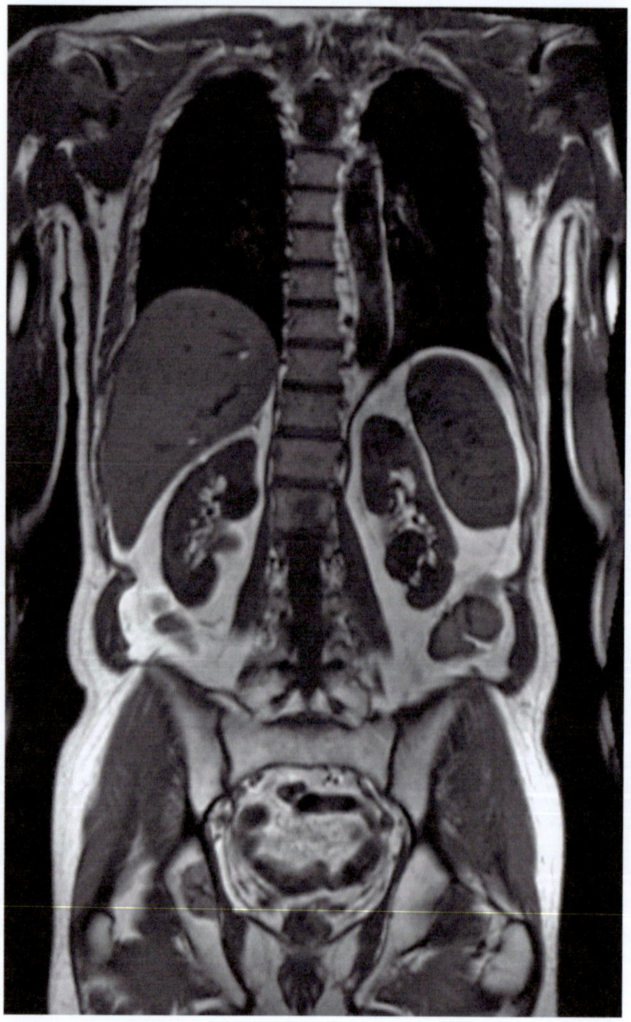

Fig. 5.50 Coronal T1w TSE shows a hypointense lesion in the right pelvis. T1w alone does not allow to discriminate between active or effectively treated bone lesions

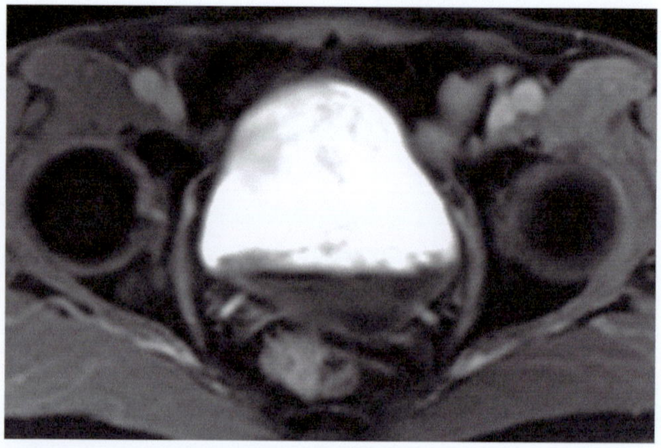

Fig. 5.51 Axial T1w VIBE fs after contrast media show only faint enhancement of a bone lesion in the right pelvis suggesting effective treatment

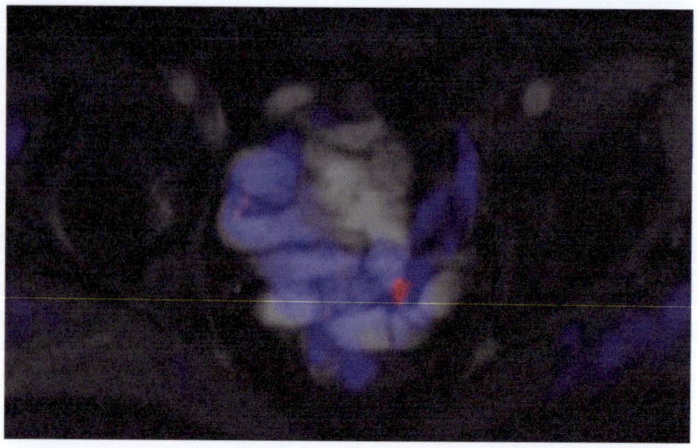

Fig. 5.52 In axial PET/MR no uptake is noted in the region of the right pelvis

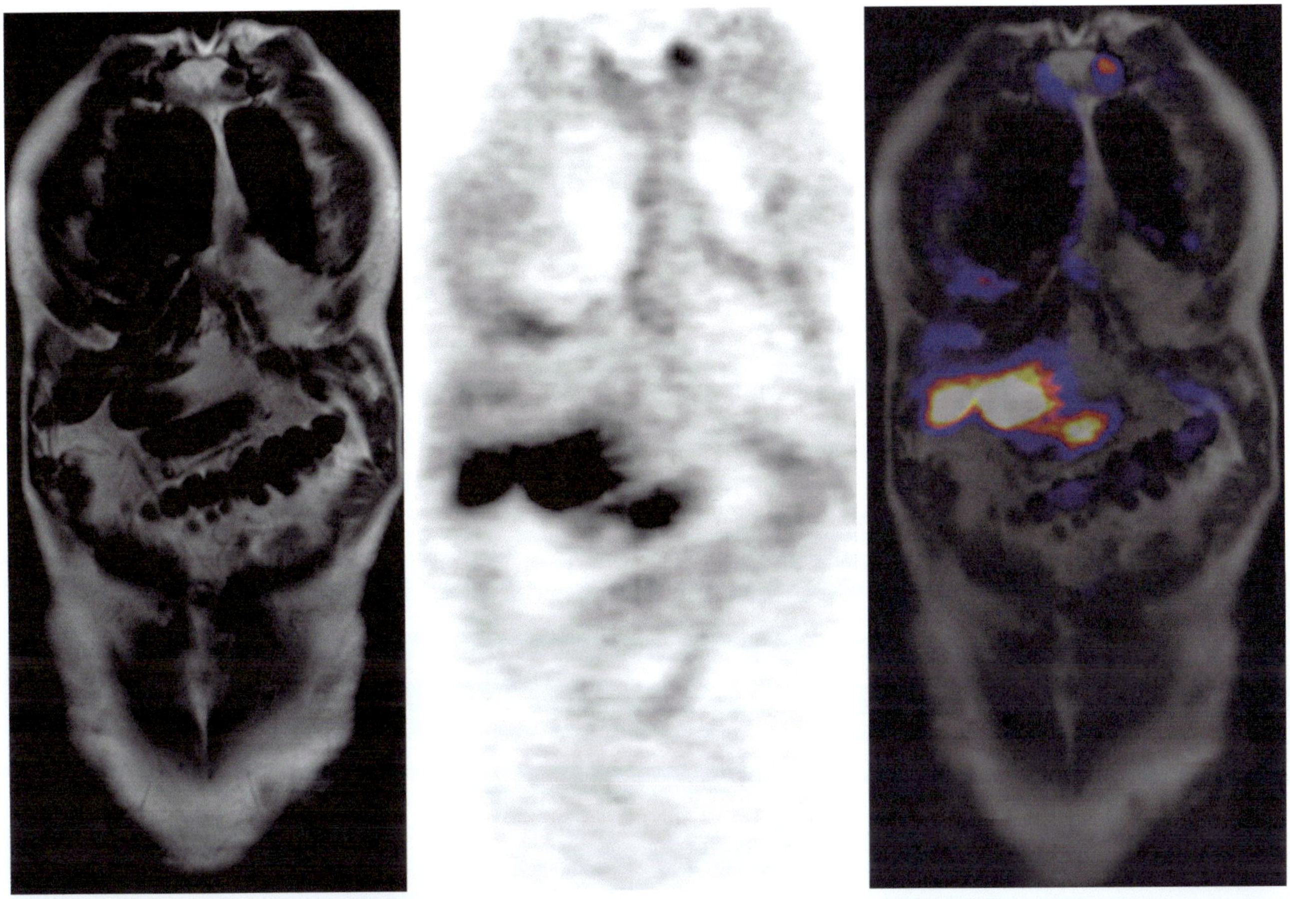

Fig. 5.53 Coronal PET and T1w TSE show a lesion in the proximal sternum with T1w hypointensity in MRI and high Choline metabolism in PET

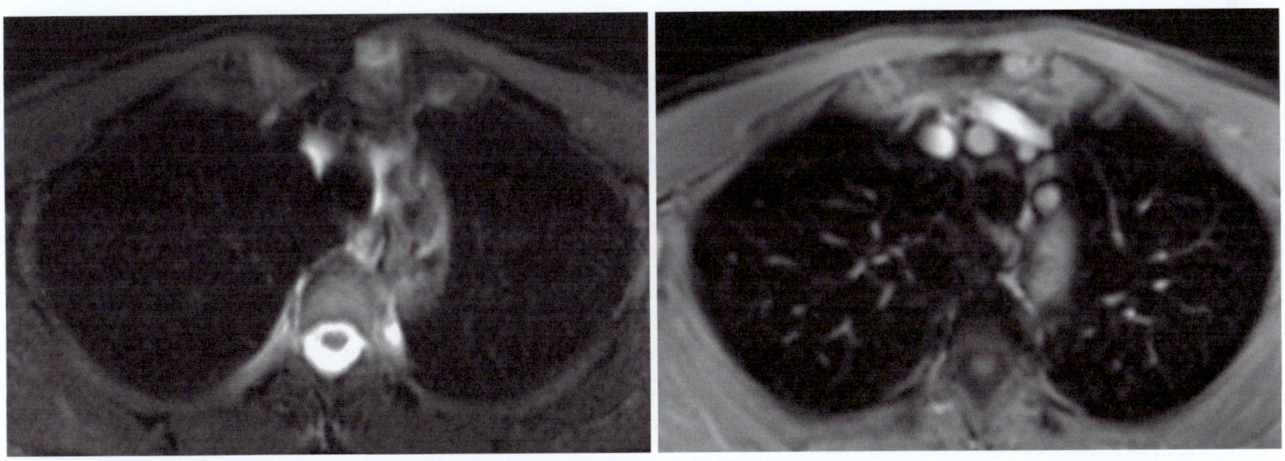

Fig. 5.54 Axial T2w HASTE fs shows relative hyperintensity of the lesion in the sternum (*left*). In addition T1w VIBE fs after contrast media demonstrates an intense enhancement (*right*). Both findings are indicating a viable bone metastases

Local Recurrence After Radical Prostatectomy

Clinical History

Seventy-one-year-old patient presenting with a slow increase of PSA-value from 0.07 ng/ml (nadir) after radical prostatectomy 5 years ago to a current value of 0.31 ng/ml.

Imaging Technique

Whole body PET/MR images acquired 43 min after iv injection 798 MBq ^{11}C-Choline, 102 kg.

3 beds × 4 min together with coronal T1w TSE and axial T2w haste fs. 1 bed (pelvis) a 15 min together with ax T2 TSE, ax DWI, ax T1w TWIST CM dynamic. Post CM axial T1w VIBE from chest to pelvis. Head/neck and two body coils.

Findings

PET demonstrates a moderate uptake of ^{11}C-Choline in the area of the former prostate gland. Dynamic contrast enhanced MRI shows an arterial hypervascularisation in the corresponding region.

> **Teaching Points**
>
> Especially in cases with low PSA-value PET and MRI can provide complimentary information. Hereby accumulating evidence for a possible local recurrence increases the certainty in reporting these findings.

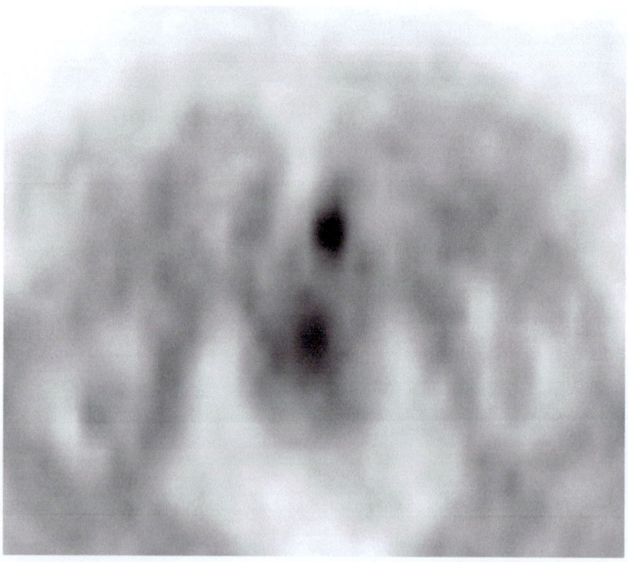

Fig. 5.55 Moderate uptake of ^{11}C-Choline in the pelvis is suspicious for local recurrence

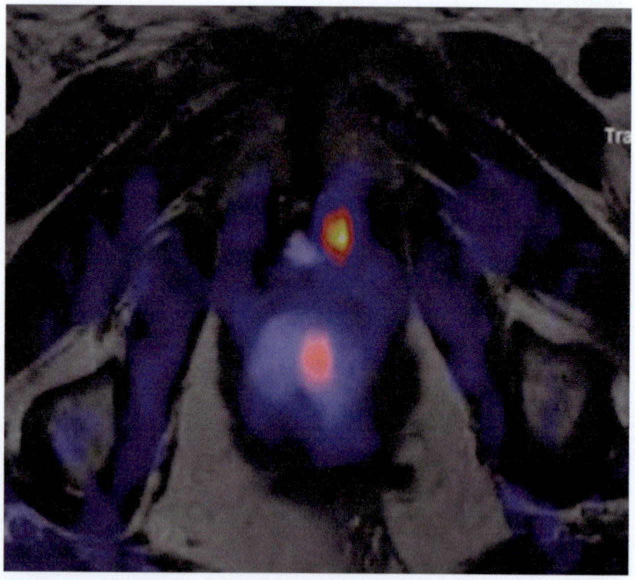

Fig. 5.56 Axial fused imagines show that the uptake in PET is located at the base of the bladder in the region of the former prostate gland

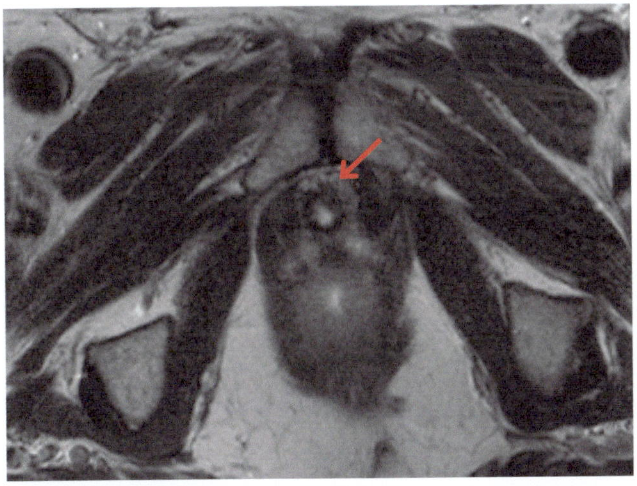

Fig. 5.57 High resolution T2w provides superb anatomical resolution with high soft tissue contrast in the pelvis. A slight asymmetry is found at the base of the bladder (*arrow*)

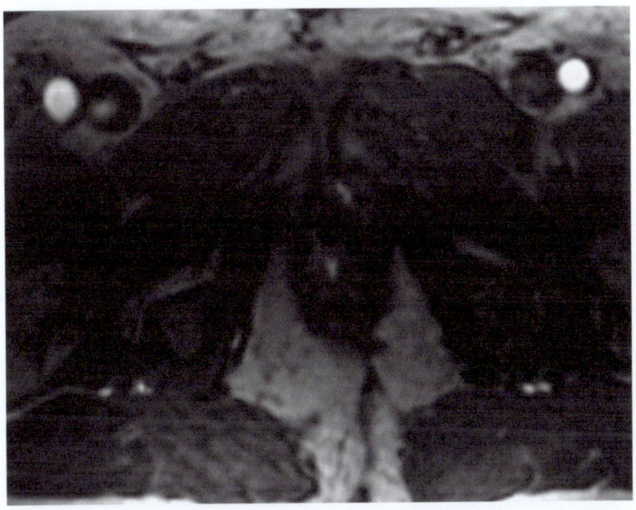

Fig. 5.58 Axial dynamic contrast enhanced T1 TWIST show a hypervascularized region at the base of the bladder corresponding with the uptake in PET

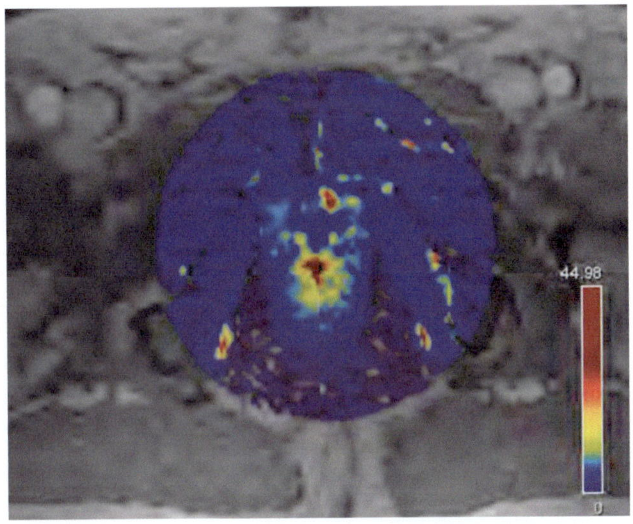

Fig. 5.59 A parametric map illustrating the influx of contrast media in the first 60s (iAUC60) demonstrates this finding more clearly

References

1. Boyle P, Ferlay J (2005) Cancer incidence and mortality in Europe 2004. Ann Oncol 16(3):481–488
2. Carrol CL, Sommer FG, McNeal JE, Stamey TA (1987) The abnormal prostate; MR imaging at 1.5 T with histopathologic correlation. Radiology 163:521–525
3. Turkbey B, Albert PS, Kurdziel K, Choyke PL (2009) Imaging localized prostate cancer: current approaches and new developments. AJR Am J Roentgenol 192:1471–1480
4. Liu IJ, Zafar MB, Lai YH, Segall GM, Terris MK (2001) Fluorodeoxyglucose positron emission tomography studies in diagnosis and staging of clinically organ-confined prostate cancer. Urology 57:108–111
5. Hofer C, Laubenbacher C, Block T, Breul J, Hartung R, Schwaiger M (1999) Fluorine-18-fluorodeoxyglucose positron emission tomography is useless for the detection of local recurrence after radical prostatectomy. Eur Urol 36:31–35
6. Takahashi N, Inoue T, Lee J, Yamaguchi T, Shizukuishi K (2007) The roles of PET and PET/CT in the diagnosis and management of prostate cancer. Oncology 72:226–233
7. Schöder H, Larson SM (2004) Positron emission tomography for prostate, bladder, and renal cancer. Semin Nucl Med 34:274–292
8. Scher B, Seitz M, Albinger W et al (2007) Value of ^{11}C-choline PET and PET/CT in patients with suspected prostate cancer. Eur J Nucl Med Mol Imaging 34:45–53
9. Picchio M, Crivellaro C, Giovacchini G, Gianolli L, Messa C (2009) PET/CT for treatment planning in prostate cancer. Q J Nucl Med Mol Imaging 53:245–268
10. Picchio M, Briganti A, Fanti S et al (2011) The role of choline positron emission tomography/computed tomography in the management of patients with prostate-specific antigen progression after radical treatment of prostate cancer. Eur Urol 59:51–60
11. Castellucci P, Fuccio C, Rubello D et al (2011) Is there a role for ^{11}C-choline PET/CT in the early detection of metastatic disease in surgically treated prostate cancer patients with a mild PSA increase <1.5 ng/ml? Eur J Nucl Med Mol Imaging 38:55–63
12. Jadvar H, Gurbuz A, Li X et al (2008) Choline autoradiography of human prostate cancer xenograft: effect of castration. Mol Imaging 7:147–152
13. Kotzerke J, Prang J, Neumaier B et al (2000) Experience with carbon-11 choline positron emission tomography in prostate carcinoma. Eur J Nucl Med 27:1415–1419
14. De Jong IJ, Pruim J, Elsinga PH et al (2003) 11C-choline positron emission tomography for the evaluation after treatment of localized prostate cancer. Eur Urol 44:38–38
15. Reske SN (2008) [11C]choline uptake with PET/CT for the initial diagnosis of prostate cancer: relation to PSA levels, tumor stage and anti-androgenic therapy. Eur J Nucl Med Mol Imaging 35: 1740–1741
16. Reske SN, Blumstein NM, Glatting G (2008) [11C]choline PET/CT imaging in occult local relapse of prostate cancer after radical prostatectomy. Eur J Nucl Med Mol Imaging 35:9–17
17. Hara T, Bansal A, DeGrado TR (2006) Effect of hypoxia on the uptake of [methyl-3H] choline, [1-14C]acetate and [18F]FDG in cultured prostate cancer cells. Nucl Med Biol 33:977–984
18. Breeuwsma AJ, Pruim J, Jongen MM et al (2005) In vivo uptake of [11C]choline does not correlate with cell proliferation in human prostate cancer. Eur J Nucl Med Mol Imaging 32:668–673
19. Pichler BJ, Judenhofer MS, Pfannenberg C. Multimodal imaging approaches: PET/CT and PET/MRI. Handb Exp Pharmacol 2008: 109–132.
20. Boss A, Bisdas S, Kolb A et al (2010) Hybrid PET/MRI of intracranial masses: initial experiences and comparison to PET/CT. J Nucl Med 51:1198–1205

Breast Cancers

6

C. Tabouret-Viaud, A. Baskin, A.J. Beer, M. Eiber, C. Gerngross, and P. Loubeyre

Contents

C. Tabouret-Viaud (✉) • A. Baskin
Department of Imaging, Division of Nuclear Medicine and Molecular Imaging, Geneva University Hospital, Rue Gabrielle Perret Gentil 4, 1211 Geneva 4, Switzerland
e-mail: claire.tabouretviaud@hcuge.ch

A.J. Beer • C. Gerngross
Department of Nuclear Medicine, Klinikum Rechts der Isar, Technische Universität München, Munich, Germany

M. Eiber
Department of Radiology, Klinikum Rechts der Isar, Technische Universität München, Munich, Germany

P. Loubeyre
Department of Imaging, Division of Radiology, Geneva University Hospital, Rue Gabrielle Perret Gentil 4, 1211 Geneva 4, Switzerland

Breast Cancers

Breast cancer is the leading cancer and the second leading cause of mortality in women in most European countries, North America, and Australia. In Europe, 1 out of every 10–15 women will develop breast cancer in her lifetime, and the risk is even higher in the United States, where it is 1 out of every 8 women.

MRI plays an important role in the characterization of breast lesions for patients with suspected breast cancer [1, 2], and may change the surgical approach at least for young women or women with dense breast or in cases of high risk of multifocal/multicentric lesions [3]. However, MRI's positive predictive value and specificity vary over a wide range [4]. 18F-FDG whole body PET/CT on the contrary is highly specific [4], and stages not only axillary and internal mammary nodes but also the whole body for unexpected sites of disease. Its utility as a staging procedure in primary stage II and III breast cancer has now been proven [5], as well as for inflammatory breast cancers at diagnosis [6, 7]. PET/CT is also useful for detecting recurrence in breast cancer patients, for restaging [8], and for treatment response assessment [9–11]. Therefore, ^{18}F-FDG PET/CT has become more widely adopted in selected categories of patients, where PET is complementary to breast MRI resulting in both modalities to be part of patient clinical workup.

On those patients, the emergence of hybrid PET/MR scanners offers the advantage of combining both studies in a single session, reducing radiation dose of CT and allowing more accurate localization of lesion detection. Optimized whole-body PET/MR protocols, can also be acquired if necessary in addition to dedicated breast MRI using specific breast coils compatible with PET, allowing full diagnostic quality of both modalities. This could become the modality of choice in those indications, reducing the effective dose of radiation compared to PET/CT, and decreasing the total time of the examination in a single session instead of two separate exams [12].

O. Ratib et al. (eds.), *Atlas of PET/MR Imaging in Oncology*,
DOI 10.1007/978-3-642-31292-2_6, © Springer-Verlag Berlin Heidelberg 2013

Invasive Ductal Carcinoma (IDC)

Clinical History

Forty-one-year-old patient with cT2 N1a invasive ductal carcinoma, G2, of the junction of the inferior quadrants of the left breast. PET/MR was performed for staging.

Imaging Technique

Whole-body PET acquired 60 min after injection of 371 MBq of 18F-FDG, 57 kg/168 cm patient, with 3.7 mmol/L of fasting glycemia. Whole body atMR (T1 weighted), supine position.

T2 TSE axial, 3D e-thrive native, arterial and veinous post-gadolinium, and breast PET in a SENSE breast-coil, prone position.

Findings

Breast MR showed a 50 mm maximal diameter tumor of the junction of the left inferior quadrants, and a suspicious retroareolar linear enhancement. PET imaging showed a 25 mm diameter hypermetabolic suspicious area of the junction of the left inferior quadrants. No ipsilateral axillary lymph node involvement was noted. Pathological examination of left mastectomy found a 95×45×20 mm invasive ductal carcinoma of the central area of the breast. Sentinel lymph node biopsy was negative.

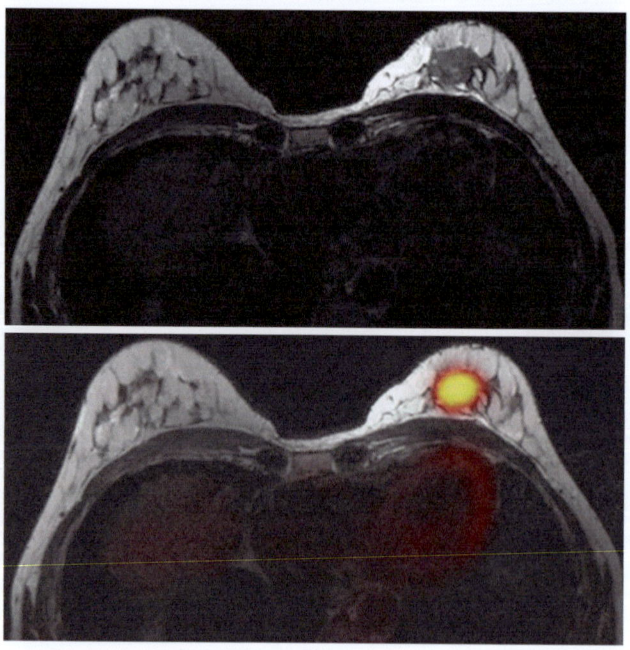

Fig. 6.1 T2 TSE axial MRI sequence acquired using dedicated breast coil (*top*), fused with PET acquired in the same PET-compatible coil (*bottom*), showing the left breast hypermetabolic lesion

> **Teaching Points**
>
> MRI is more effective than PET to assess tumor extent when the tumor infiltration is along the linear galactophoric channels both techniques may underestimate the tumor extension in these cases.

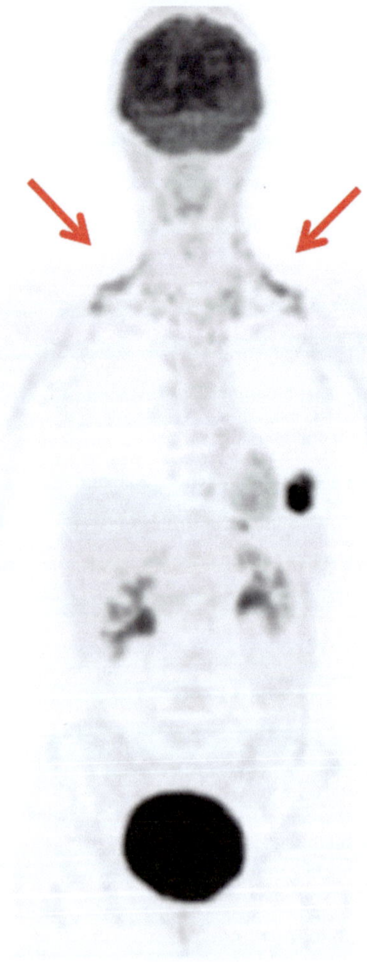

Fig. 6.2 Coronal MIP from whole-body PET showing cervical and supra-clavicular brown fat tracer uptake (*arrows*) for this young patient, and the breast tumor without evident distant extension

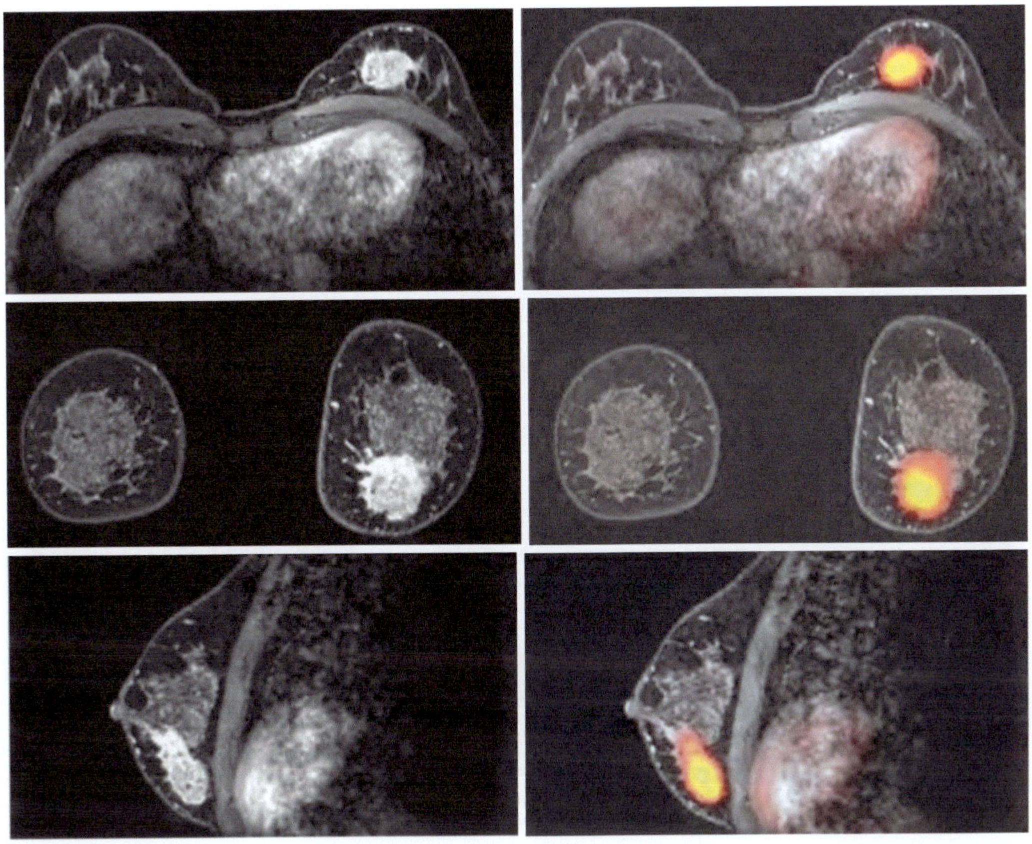

Fig. 6.3 E-thrive arterial MRI sequence in the three orthogonal planes, showing the hypermetabolism and the contrast enhancement of the single left breast lesion

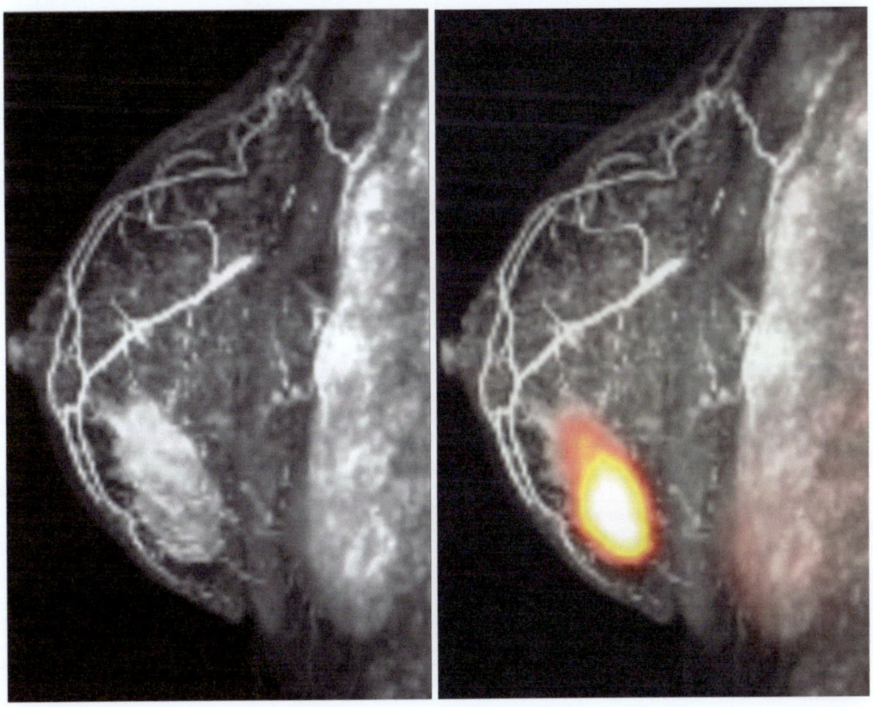

Fig. 6.4 3D volume rendering of an e-thrive arterial phase MRI sequence in a sagittal view, showing the hypermetabolism and the contrast enhancement of the single left breast lesion

Recurrence of Axillary Lymph Node

Clinical History

Sixty-four-year-old patient with history of left lumpectomy and axillary lymph node dissection 14 years ago for invasive lobular carcinoma (ILC) and tumorectomy of a right invasive ductal carcinoma with radiotherapy and chemotherapy 8 years ago. Patient presented with a clinically suspicious 2-cm single left axillary nodule.

Imaging Technique

Whole-body PET acquired 60 min after injection of 382 MBq of 18F-FDG, 70 kg patient, with 5 mmol/L of fasting glycemia. Whole body atMR (T1 weighted), supine position.

T2 TSE axial, 3D e-thrive native, arterial and venous post-gadolinium, and breast PET in a SENSE breast-coil, prone position.

Findings

PET/MR showed a 3-cm single tumoral lesion of the lower limit of the left axillary region. Subsequent pathological examination of axillary tumorectomy showed a single 28-mm G2 invasive ductal carcinoma.

Teaching Points

In this case, both MRI and PET gave the same information: they confirmed the presence of a suspicious left axillary nodule. PET provided no evidence for other metastatic lesions which is important for the surgeon. This patient already had extensive left axillary dissection and performing additional exploratory surgery can be risky and difficult. Radiotherapy of the region is indicated in the absence of axillary invasion either clinically and / or on imaging.

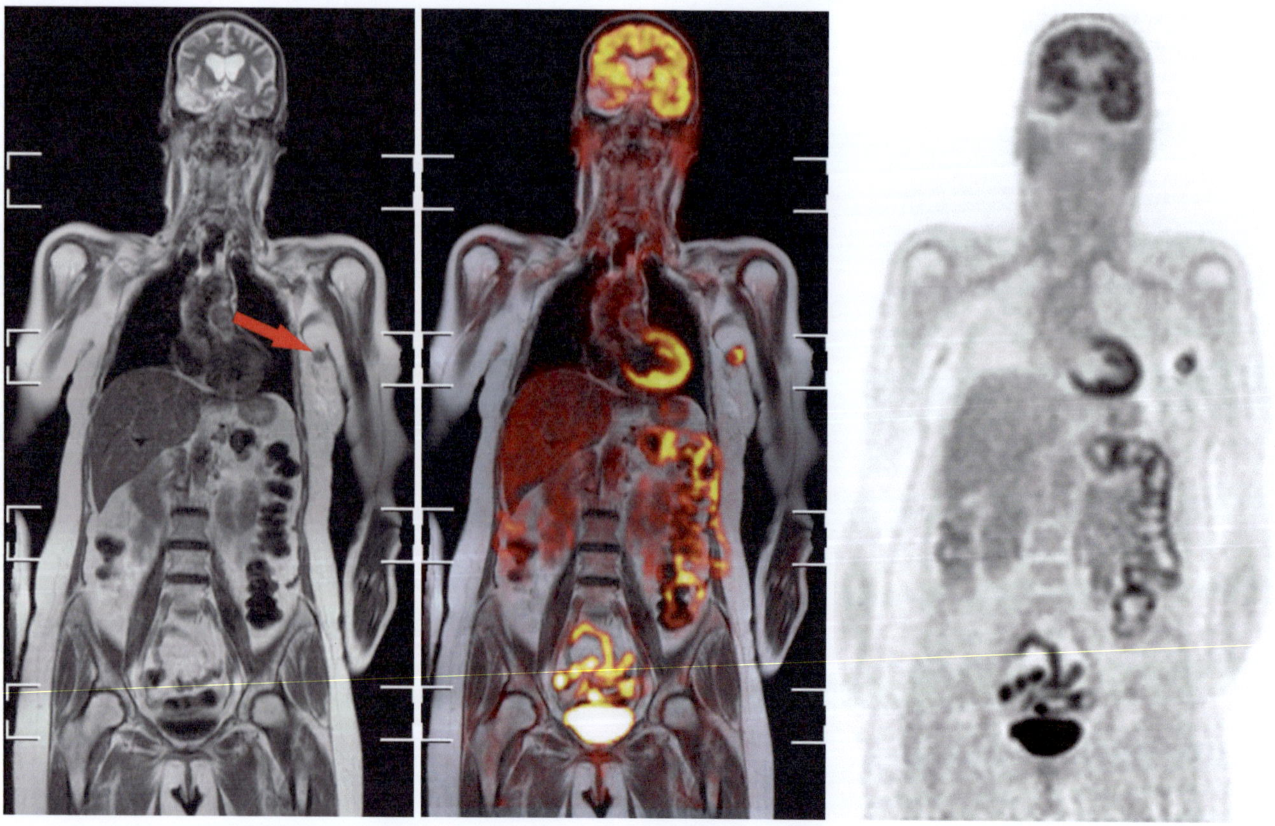

Fig. 6.5 Whole-body T2W MRI sequence fused with PET, and FDG-PET alone, *from the left to the right*, showing the main lesion in the left axillary region (*arrow*)

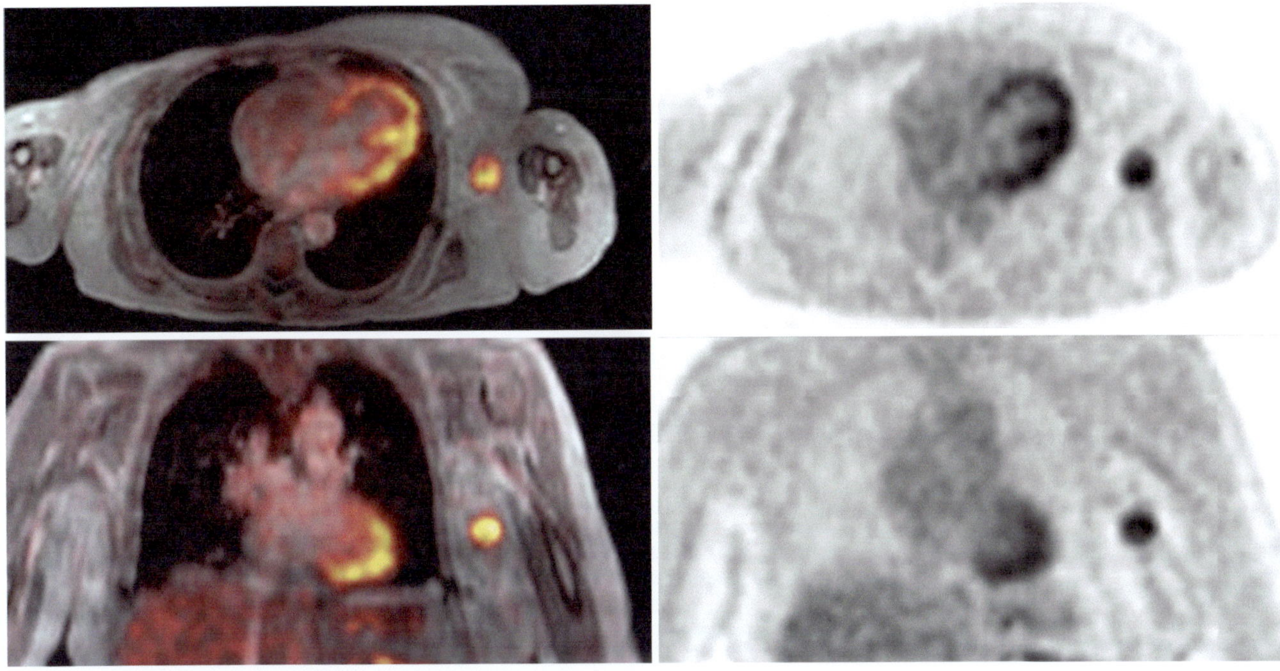

Fig. 6.6 Axial (*top*) and coronal (*bottom*) views of fused PET/MR (*left*) and PET (*right*) images centered over the left axillary region showing a single lesion with no evidence of additional axillary lymph node invasion

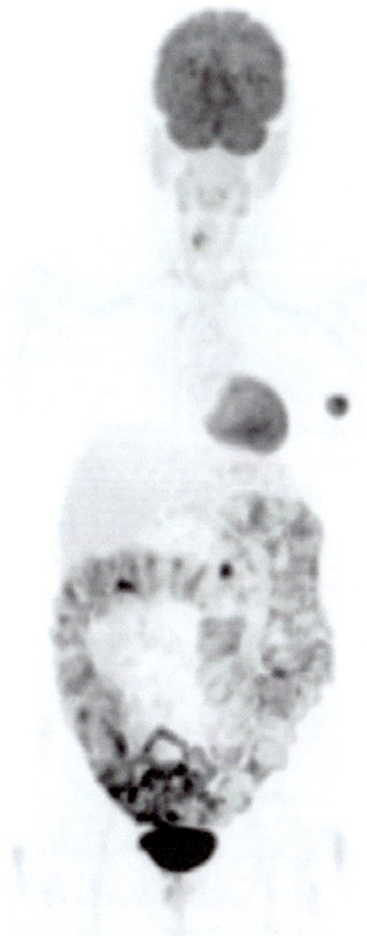

Fig. 6.7 Whole body MIP image showing the single left axillary region with no evidence of other dissemination or lymph node involvement

Breast Cancer with Lymph Nodes Invasion

Clinical History

Forty-one-year-old patient with invasive ductal carcinoma (IDC) cT4b N3b G2 of the right breast. PET/MR was performed for staging before neoadjuvant chemotherapy.

Imaging Technique

Whole-body PET acquired 60 min after injection of 375 MBq of 18F-FDG, 74 kg/177 cm patient, with 4.1 mmol/L of fasting glycemia. Whole body atMR (T1 weighted), supine position.

T2 TSE axial, T2W TSE STIR, 3D e-thrive native, arterial and venous post-gadolinium, and breast PET in a SENSE breast-coil, prone position.

Findings

PET/MR showed a right breast multifocal/multicentric carcinoma, with highly suspicious right axillary and internal mammary lymph nodes. Note a post-biopsy collection of the right inner superior quadrant. Post chemotherapy pathological examination of right mastectomy and axillary lymph node dissection showed a residual lymphangitic carcinomatosis and ductal carcinoma in-situ (DCIS) of 13-cm maximal diameter.

Teaching Points

Internal mammarian lymph node involvement is more difficult to assess on MRI compared to PET, but this information is important to adjust the radiation field of the thoracic radiotherapy after mastectomy in this case.

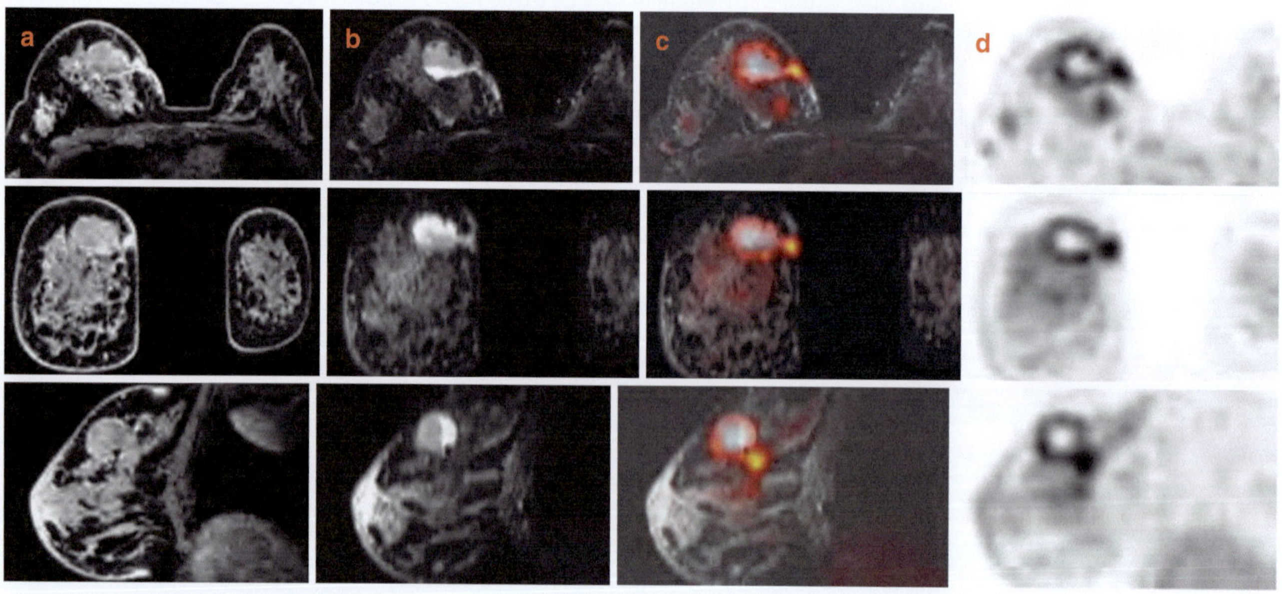

Fig. 6.8 Three orthogonal plane images showing the right breast lesion, *from left to right*: (**a**) T1 dynamic e-thrive MRI sequence; (**b**) T2 TSE STIR MRI sequence; (**c**) Fusion of PET and MRI; and (**d**) PET images

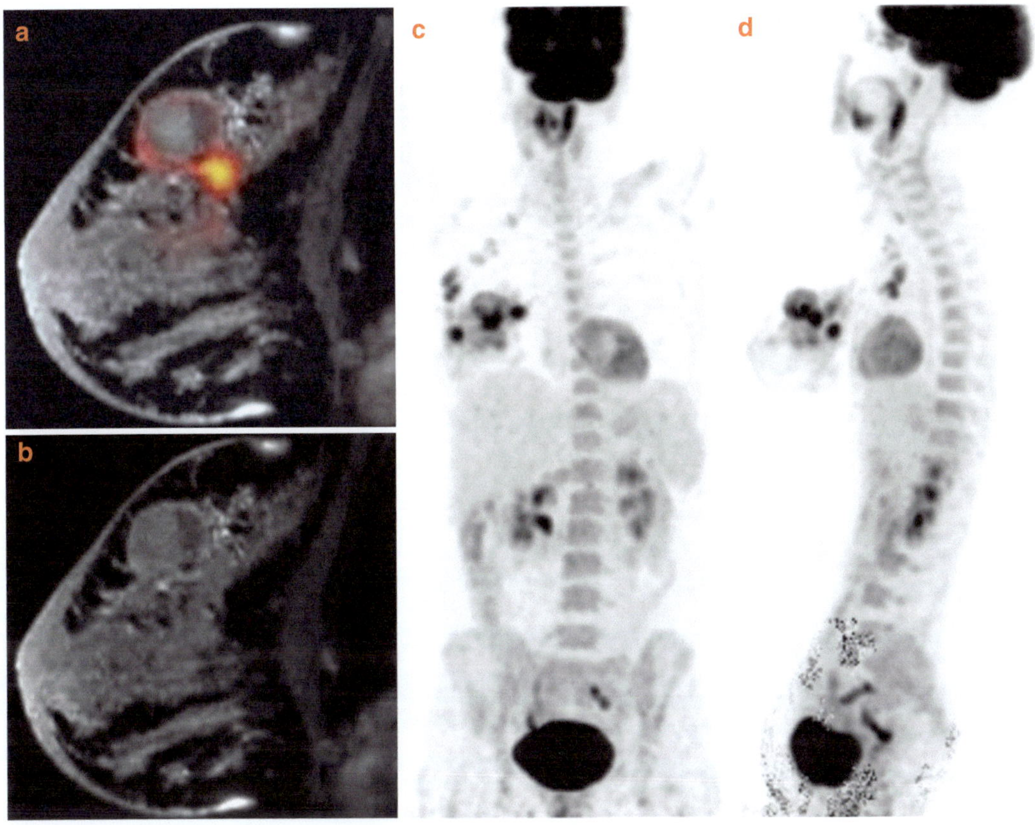

Fig. 6.9 Dynamic e-thrive MRI sequence fused with PET (**a**) and dynamic e-thrive MRI sequence alone (**b**) showing the tumor lesion and a fluid/air cavity. Coronal (**c**) and sagittal (**d**) whole body MIP images of PET showing the multifocal tumor of the left breast and the extension along the axillary and mammary lymph nodes

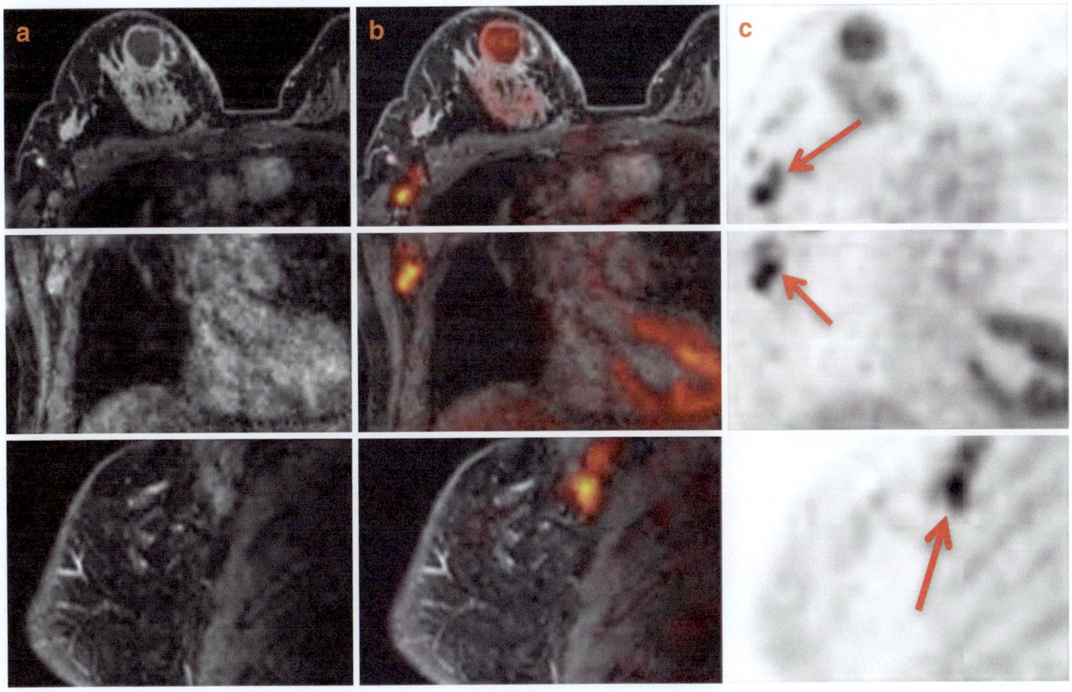

Fig. 6.10 Three orthogonal plane images showing the axillary lymph nodes with high FDG uptake (*arrows*), *from left to right*: (**a**) T1 dynamic e-thrive sense MRI sequence; (**b**) PET/MR with same MRI sequence; and (**c**) PET images

Invasive Ductal Carcinoma (IDC)

Clinical History

Forty-two-year-old patient with a G3 cT3 N1a invasive ductal carcinoma (IDC) of the junction of the superior quadrants of the left breast. PET/MR was performed for staging.

Imaging Technique

Whole-body PET acquired 60 min after injection of 380 MBq of 18F-FDG, 62 kg patient, with 5.1 mmol/L of fasting glycemia. Whole body atMR (T1 weighted), supine position.

T2 TSE axial, 3D e-thrive native, arterial and venous post-gadolinium, and breast PET in a SENSE breast-coil, prone position.

Findings

Whole body and breast PET/MR showed multifocal/bicentric tumoral involvement of the superior quadrants of the left breast with massive ipsilateral axillary lymph node invasion, without controlateral breast lesion or distant metastatic extent. Pathological examination of left mastectomy and axillary lymph node dissection showed a 40-mm (maximal diameter) invasive ductal carcinoma G3 of the left superior quadrants, with extensive peritumoral vascular invasion, retroareolar intraductal papilloma, and massive lymph node involvement (10 metastatic lymph nodes).

Teaching Points

The left axillary lymph node involvement is difficult to identify on MRI because of cardiac motion artefacts, but clearly visible on PET.

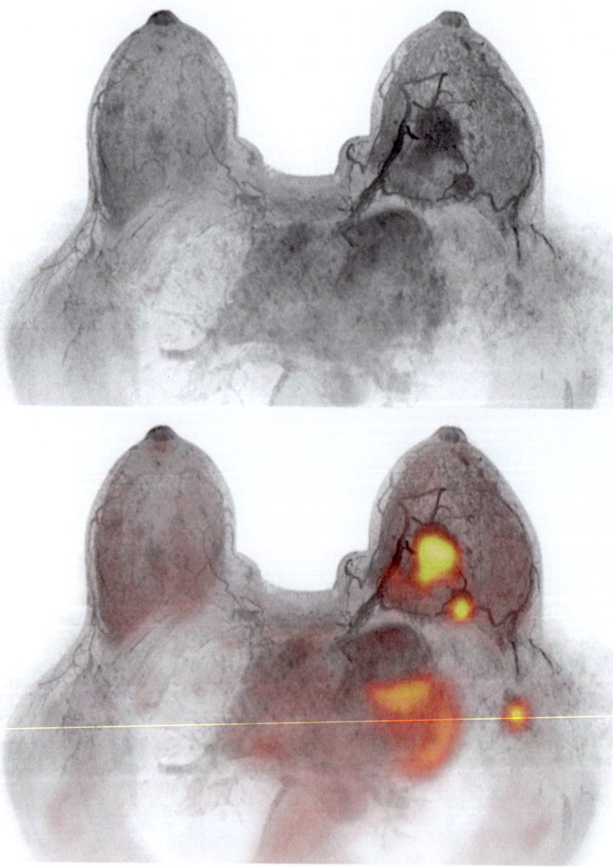

Fig. 6.11 Volume rendering of 3D arterial phase e-thrive MRI (*top*), fused with FDG-PET (*bottom*) showing multifocal tumor localization

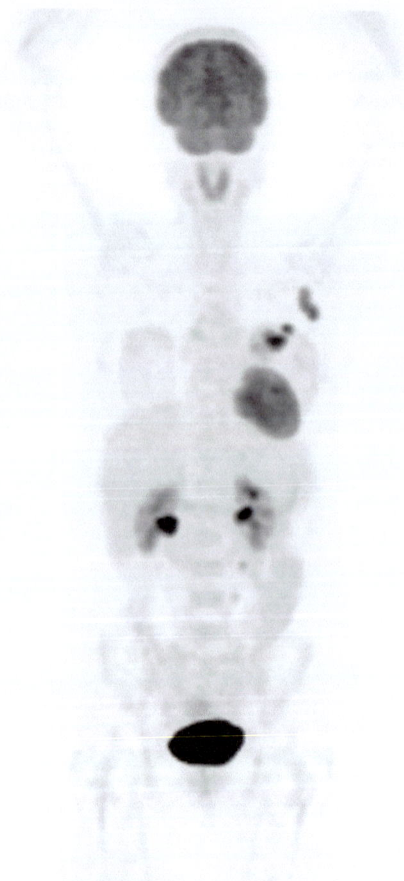

Fig. 6.12 Coronal view of the PET MIP acquired in prone position showing left breast tumor and axillary lymph node uptake of FDG

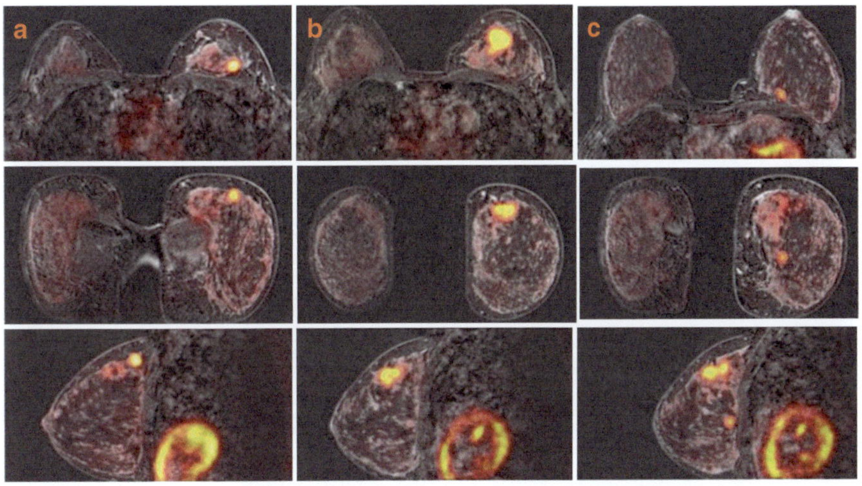

Fig. 6.13 (**a–c**) Three orthogonal planes of PET images fused with venous subtraction MRI sequence showing multiple primary lesions on three levels

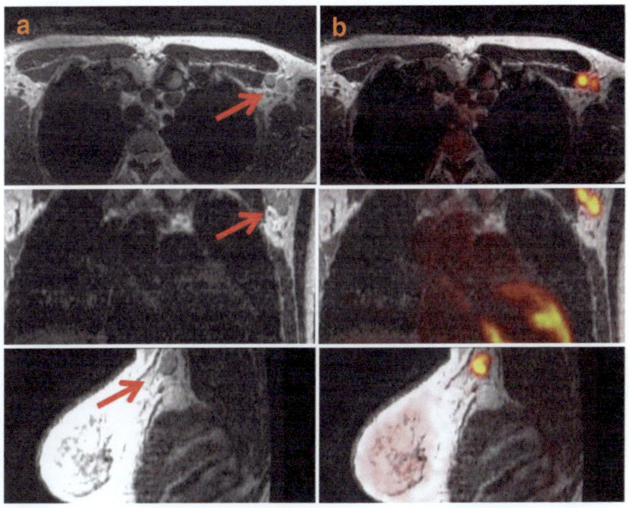

Fig. 6.14 Three orthogonal plane T2 TSE MRI sequences (**a**) and fused images with PET (**b**), showing positive axillary lymph nodes with tracer uptake (*arrow*)

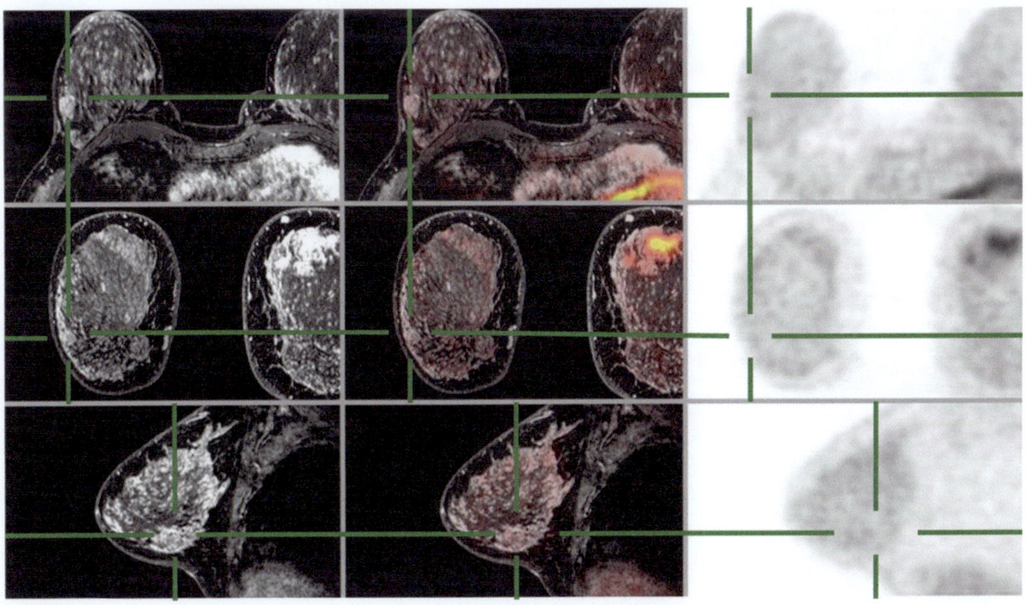

Fig. 6.15 Arterial phase of e-thrive MRI sequence showing a benign fibrocyst in the contralateral right breast with no significant FDG uptake

Bone Metastases of an IDC

Clinical History

Sixty-four-year-old patient with history of right breast invasive ductal carcinoma (IDC), diagnosed 10 years ago. Patient had bilateral mastectomy. Patient had whole body PET/MR for a suspicion of bone metastases.

Imaging Technique

Whole-body PET acquired 60 min after injection of 372 MBq of 18F-FDG, 62 kg/163 cm patient, with 4.8 mmol/L of fasting glycemia. Whole body atMR (T1 weighted), supine position.

T2 TSE axial, Total spine T1w and T2w TSE 3D e-thrive native, arterial and venous post-gadolinium, and breast PET in a SENSE breast-coil, prone position.

Findings

Whole body PET/MR showed several bone metastases including glenoid, sternum, pelvic bones and lumbar spine.

> **Teaching Points**
>
> Whole body PET helps confirming the presence of suspected bone metastases in different areas. Localized MRI can then be performed on suspicious areas.

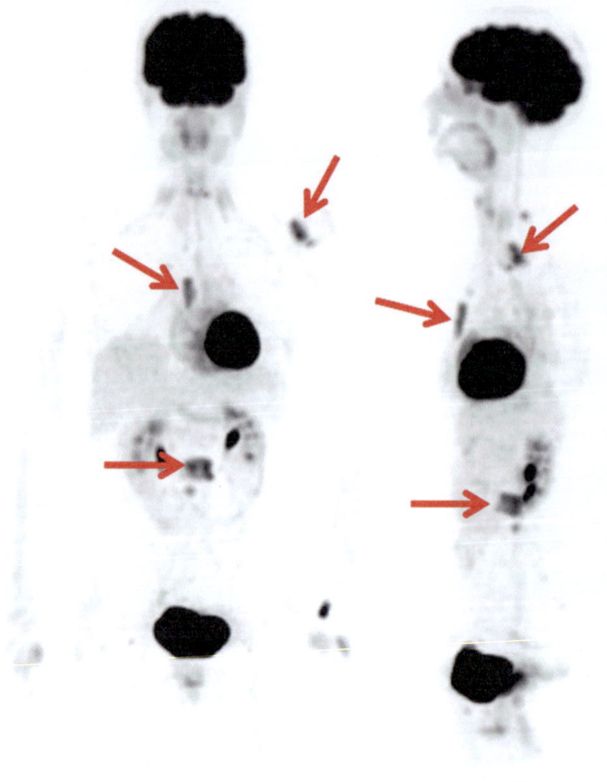

Fig. 6.16 Coronal and sagittal views of FDG-PET MIP, *arrows* showing the glenoid metastasis, sternal metastasis and lumbar vertebral metastasis

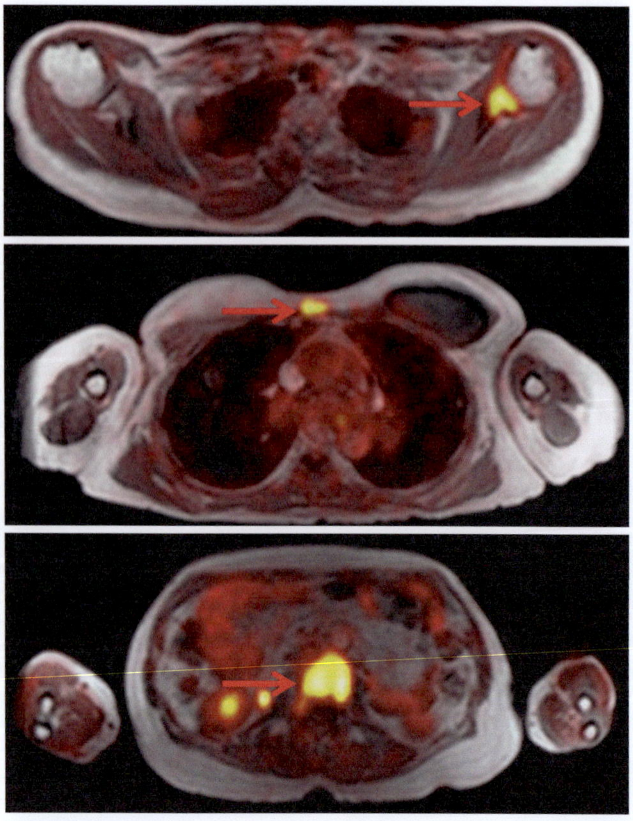

Fig. 6.17 Axial fused images of whole-body attenuation correction MRI and FDG-PET, showing the same lesions at the glenoid (*top arrow*), sternum (*middle arrow*) and L2 vertebra (*lower arrow*)

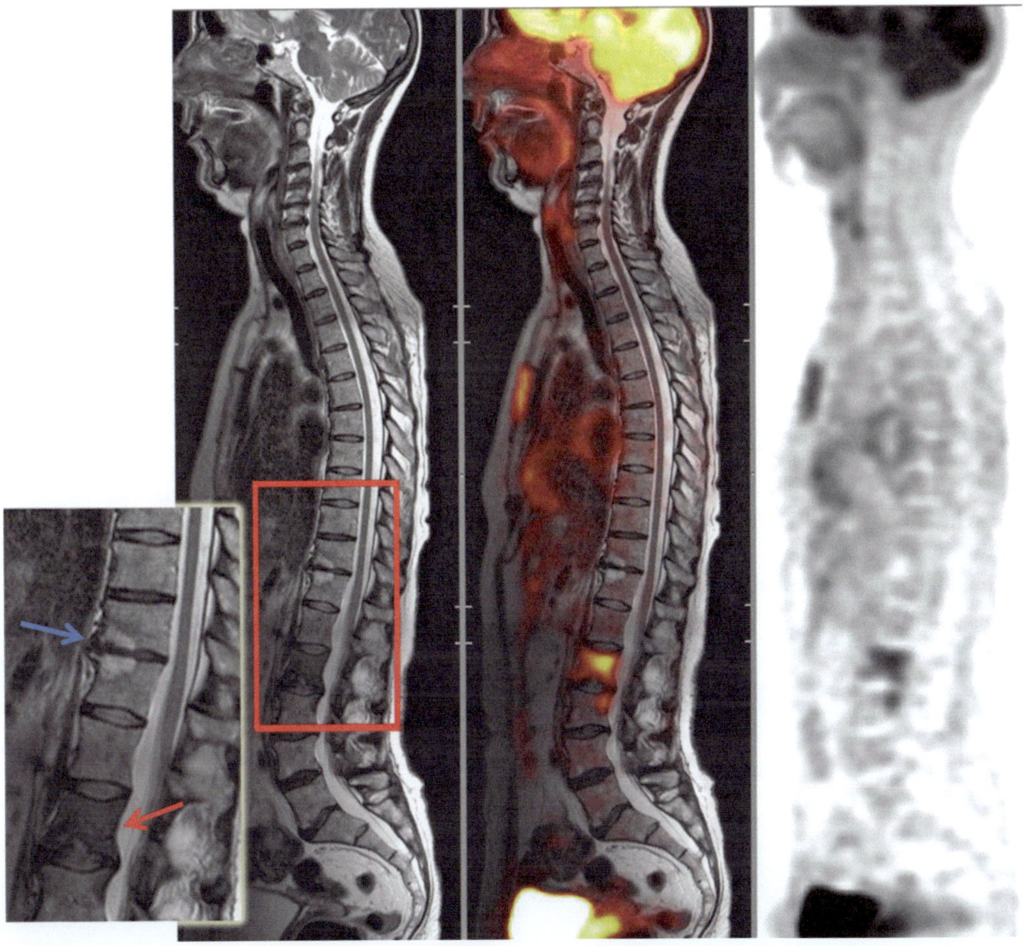

Fig. 6.18 T2W TSE MRI sequence showing vertebral metastases (*red arrow*). The *blue arrow* shows benign degenerative bone lesions with no significant FDG uptake on T11 and T12 vertebrae. The *red rectangle* shows the region that was enlarged in the inset image on the left

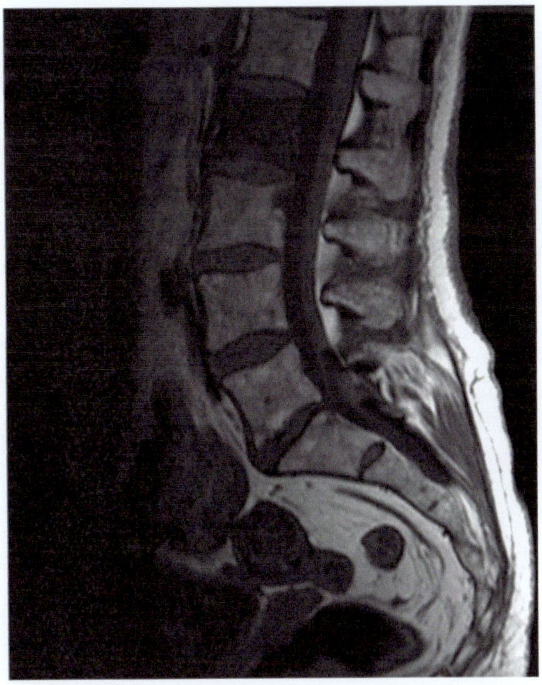

Fig. 6.19 T1W TSE sequence centered on the lower spine metastasis

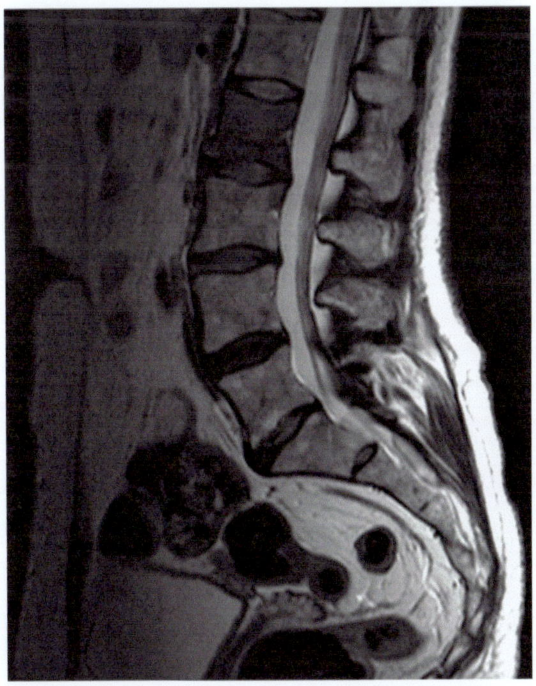

Fig. 6.20 T2W TSE MRI sequence centered on the lower spine metastasis

Metastatic Axillary Lymph Node

Clinical History

Forty-one-year-old patient with history of right skin-sparing mastectomy with advanced breast reconstruction surgery (DIEP) 7 years ago for ductal carcinoma in situ (DCIS). Invasive ductal carcinoma was found on core-needle biopsy (CNB) of a clinically suspicious right axillary lymph node.

Imaging Technique

Whole-body PET acquired 60 min after injection of 368 MBq of 18F-FDG, 64 kg/164 cm patient, with 5.1 mmol/L of fasting glycemia. Whole-body atMR (T1 weighted), supine position.

T2 TSE axial, 3D e-thrive native, arterial and venous post-gadolinium, and breast PET in a SENSE breast-coil, prone position.

Findings

No suspicious breast lesion was found on breast PET/MR. One suspicious right axillary lymph node on MRI and three suspicious lymph nodes on PET imaging were noted. Eight nodes among 17 were metastatic on subsequent pathological examination of right axillary node dissection. Three metastatic lymph nodes presented capsular disruption.

Teaching Points

Heterogeneous contrast-enhancement of non-tumoral left breast tissue was difficult to interpret on MRI alone, but PET showed no suspicious FDG uptake in that region excluding a tumor.

Right lymph node invasion was more clearly identified on PET compared to MRI.

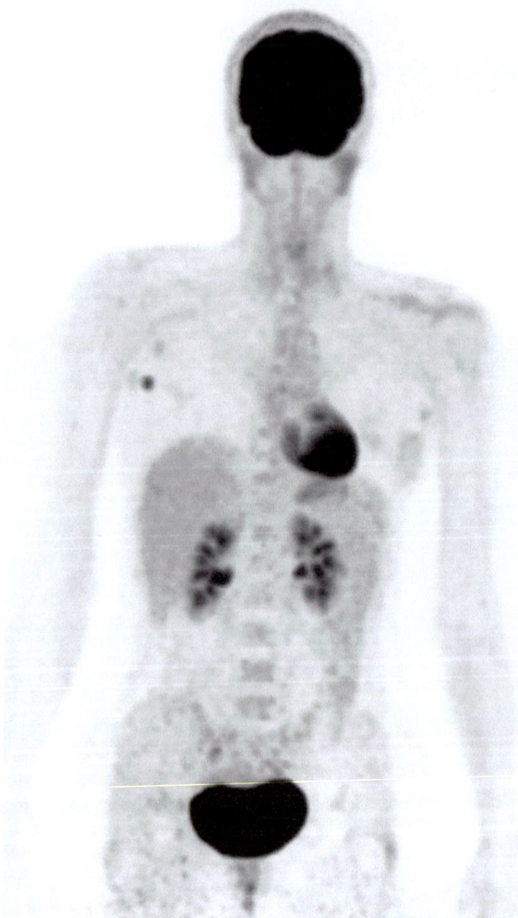

Fig. 6.21 Coronal whole body MIP of FDG PET study showing focal tracer uptake in the right axillary region

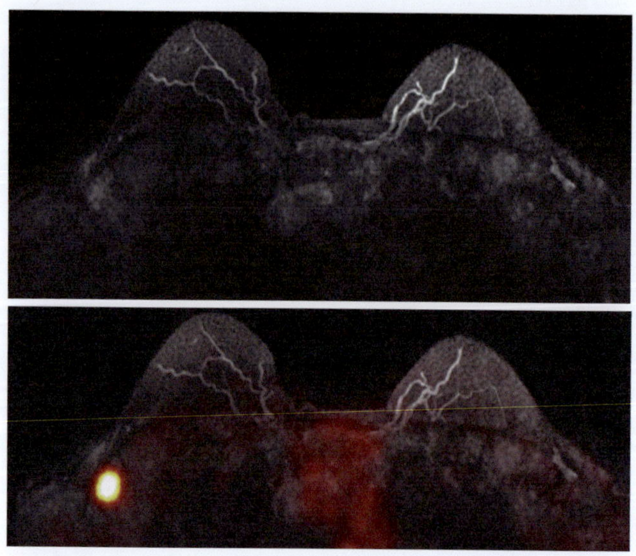

Fig. 6.22 Axial volume rendering of venous phase of MRI e-THRIVE sequence (*top*), fused with FDG-PET (*bottom*) showing absence of tracer uptake in the breast but focal uptake in the axillary region

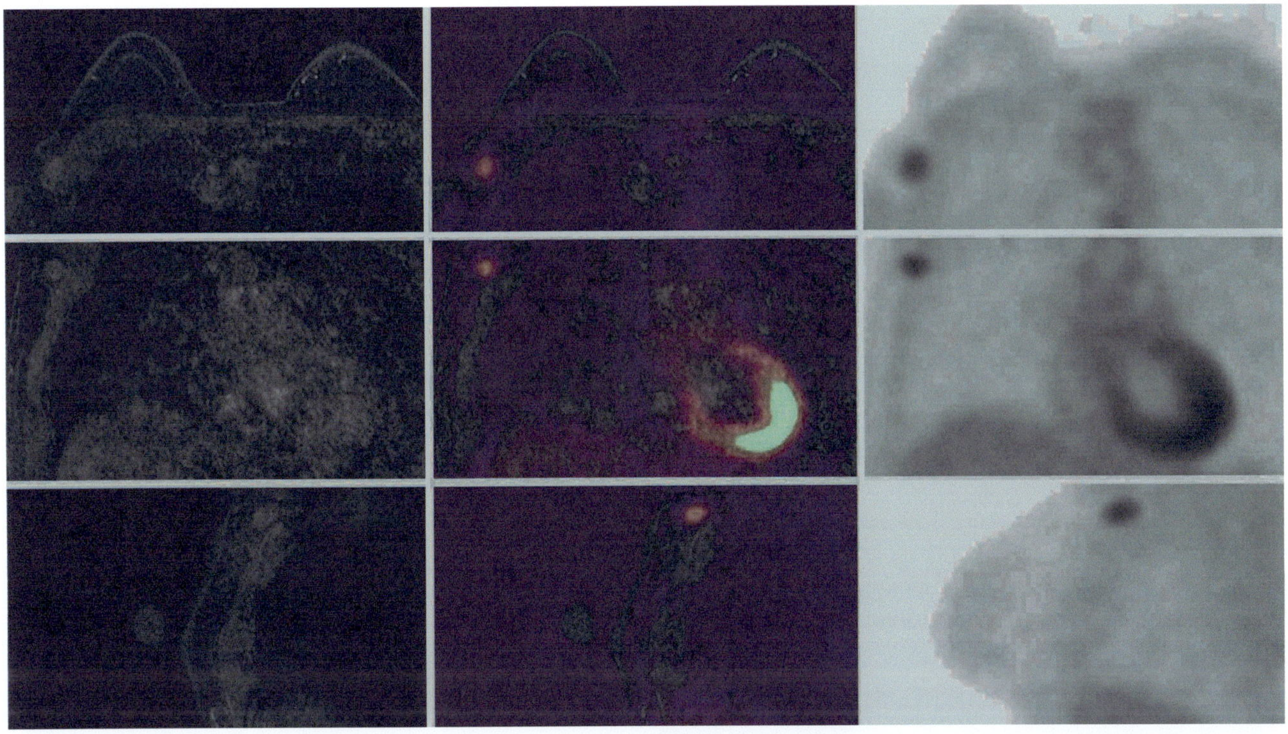

Fig. 6.23 Axial (*top*), coronal (*middle*) and sagittal (*bottom*) views of arterial phase e-THRIVE MRI sequence (*left*), fused with FDG-PET (*middle*), and FDG-PET alone (*right*), centered on the suspicious right axillary lymph node

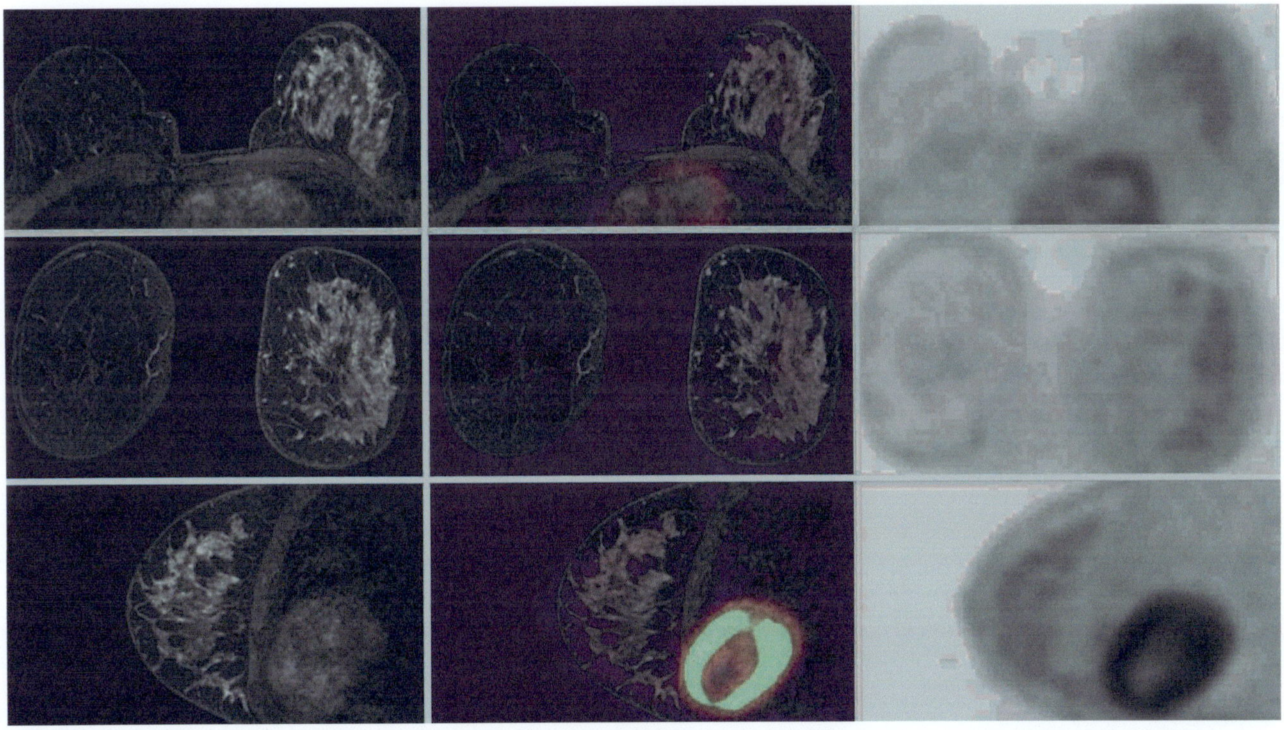

Fig. 6.24 Three orthogonal planes of T2 TSE MRI sequence (*left*) fused with FDG-PET (*middle*), and FDG-PET alone (*right*), showing no tracer uptake in the breasts, and dense left breast tissue compared to the right side, secondary to the DIEP performed 7 years earlier

Breast Implants

Clinical History

Forty-five-year-old patient with bilateral breast implants presenting with chronic inflammatory syndrome of unknown origin. Inflammatory or tumoral process was suspected.

Imaging Technique

Whole-body PET acquired 60 min after injection of 375 MBq of 18F-FDG, 58 kg/157 cm patient, with 6.5 mmol/L of fasting glycemia. Whole body atMR (T1 weighted), supine position.

T2 TSE axial, Silicone only T2w (achieved using STIR fat suppression and SPAIR water suppression) 3D e-thrive native, arterial and venous post-gadolinium, and breast PET in a SENSE breast-coil, prone position.

Findings

Breast PET/MR was interpreted as normal with no evidence of focal FDG uptake but with a small focal contrast enhancement on the right breast (see Fig. 6.27) corresponding to a benign lesion.

Teaching Points

MRI provides the high spatial and contrast resolution to assess breast implants. Small nodular contrast uptake at the retro-areolar glandular tissue is still difficult to interpret on MRI. The absence of metabolic activity in PET will help exclude the presence of a small malignant tumor.

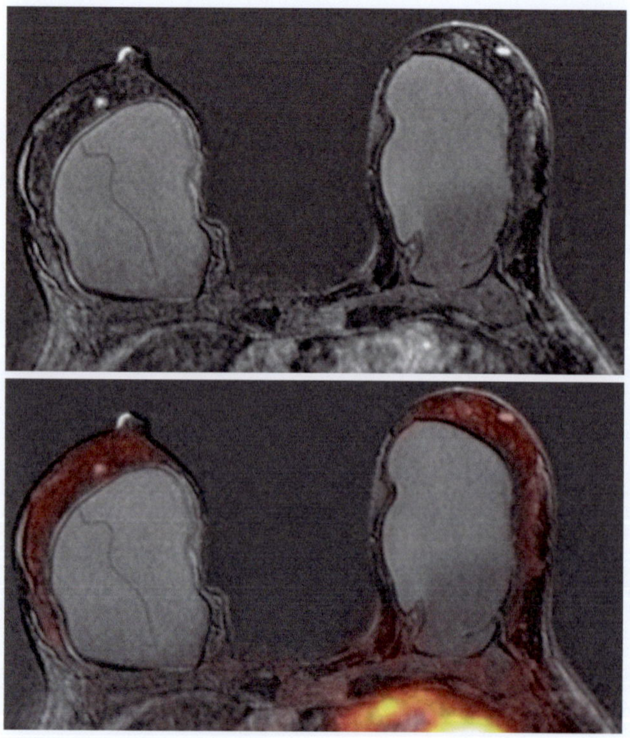

Fig. 6.25 Subtraction MRI sequence (*top*) fused with PET (*bottom*), showing neither suspicious uptake nor hypermetabolism

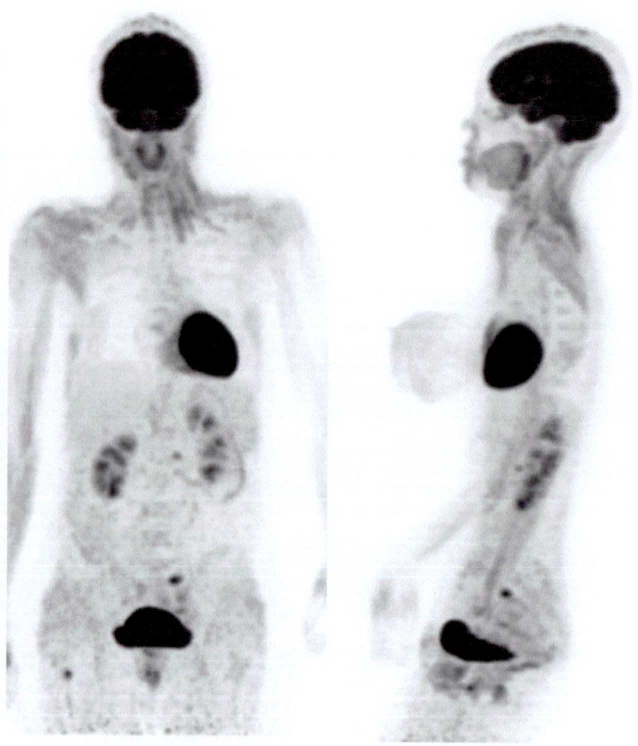

Fig. 6.26 Coronal and lateral views of the PET MIP

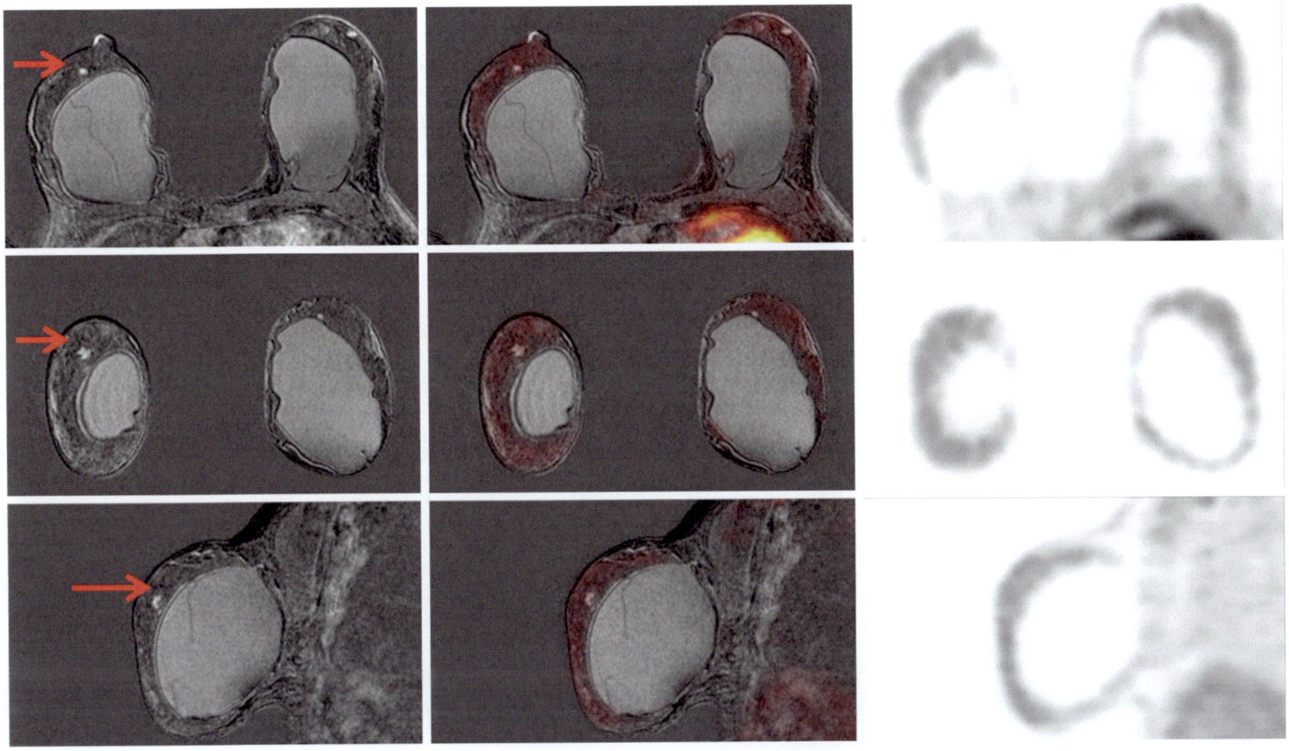

Fig. 6.27 Three orthogonal planes of subtraction e-thrive MRI sequence, fused with PET in the middle, and PET alone on the right showing small focal contrast enhancement on the right breast (*arrow*) with no significant metabolic tracer uptake

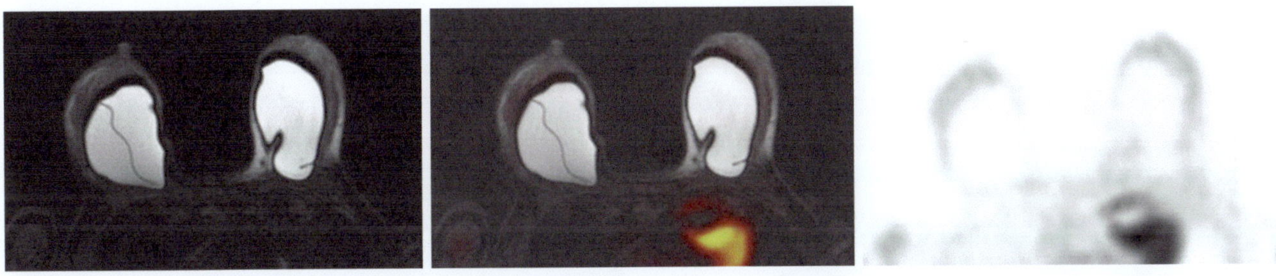

Fig. 6.28 Silicone only T2 weighted MRI sequence (*left*), fused with PET (*middle*), and PET alone (*right*)

Neuroendocrine Breast Tumor

Clinical History

18-F-DOPA PET for a 71-year-old patient with cT1 N0 neuroendocrine invasive carcinoma of the inferior outer quadrant of the left breast. Study requested for staging and evaluation of tumor extension.

Imaging Technique

Whole-body PET acquired 60 min after injection of 200 MBq of 18F-DOPA, 55 kg/158 cm patient. Whole body atMR (T1 weighted), supine position.

T2 TSE axial, 3D e-thrive native, arterial and venous post-gadolinium, and breast PET in a SENSE breast-coil, prone position.

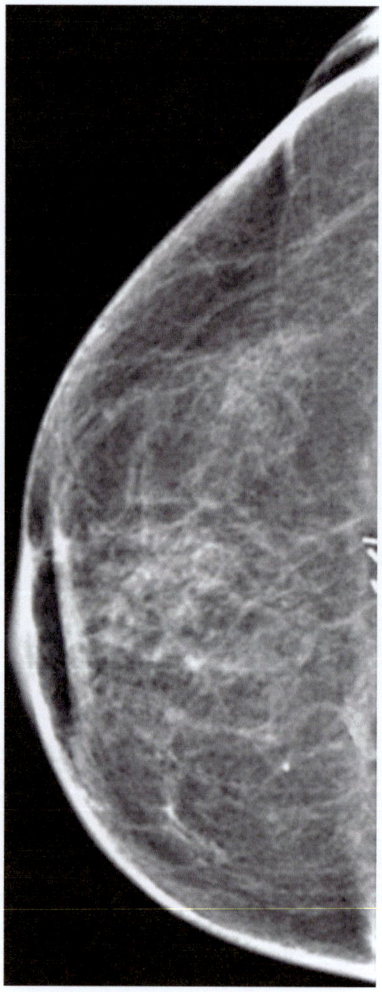

Fig. 6.29 Left mammography showing the left breast lesion

Findings

Breast PET/MR displayed a 25-mm single tumoral lesion of the left inferior outer quadrant. Subsequent pathological examination of lumpectomy showed a 30-mm diameter tumoral lesion. No metastasis was found on PET/CT and PET/MR. Sentinel lymph node biopsy was negative.

Teaching Points

This case demonstrates the effectiveness of 18F-DOPA in characterizing a rare breast tumoral lesion, with perfect correlation of PET and MRI findings in neuroendocrine tumor.

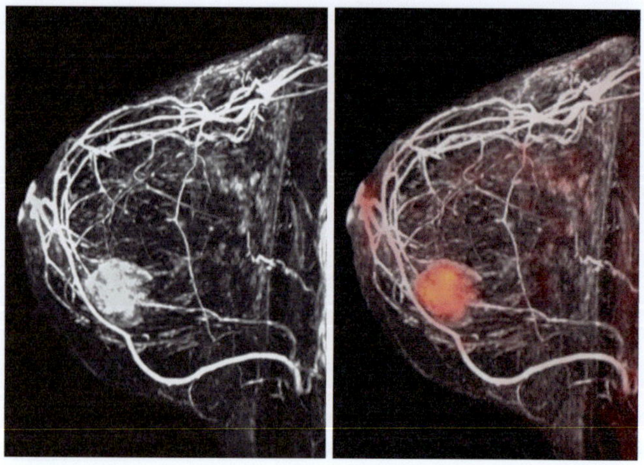

Fig. 6.30 Sagittal volume rendering of venous phase of e-thrive MRI sequence in 3D reconstruction showing the left breast lesion with 18-F DOPA uptake

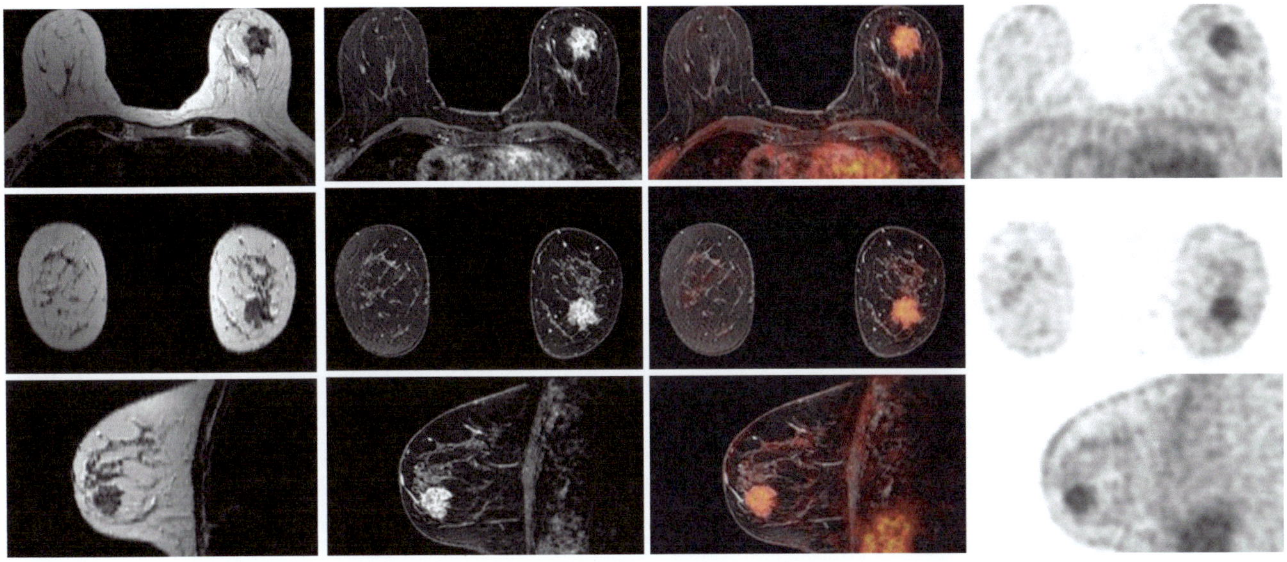

Fig. 6.31 Three orthogonal planes T2 TSE MRI (*far left*) and of venous phase of e-thrive MRI sequence after gadolinium injection (*left*), fused with PET (*middle*), and PET alone (*right*) showing gadolinium enhanced lesion with focal uptake of 18F-DOPA

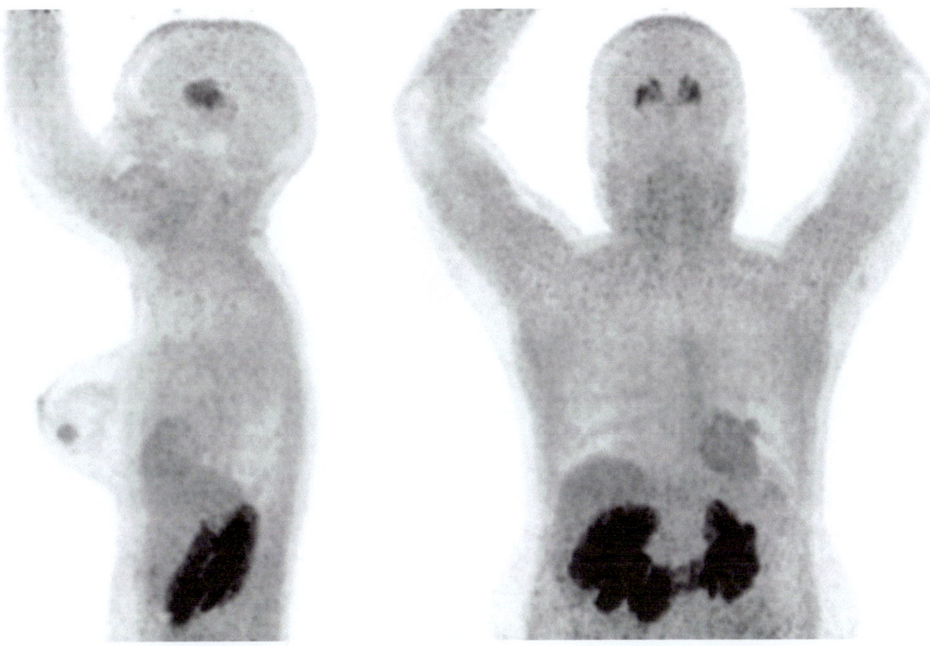

Fig. 6.32 Sagittal and coronal whole-body images of F18-DOPA study showing focal uptake of the left breast

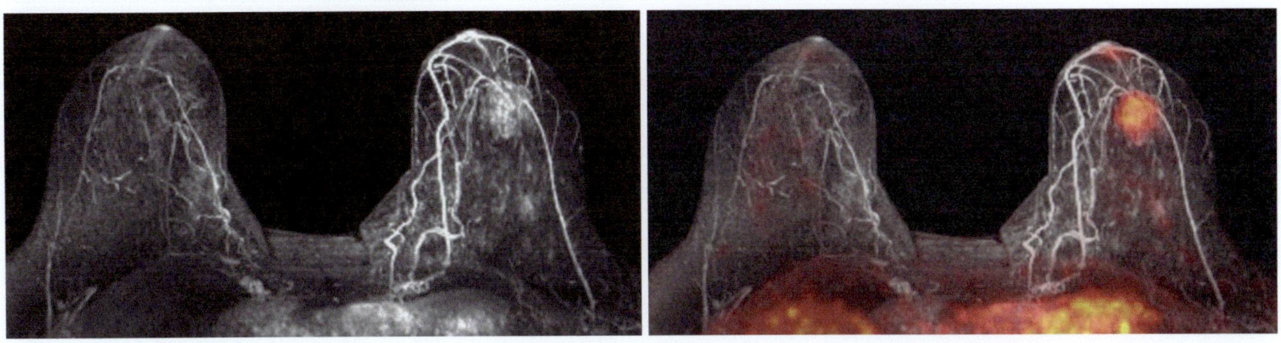

Fig. 6.33 Axial volume rendering of venous phase of e-thrive MRI sequence after gadolinium injection (*left*), and fused with 18F-DOPA PET (*right*) showing the location of left breast lesion

Multifocal IDC with Lymph Node Invasion

Clinical History

Forty-three-year-old patient with high grade (G3) cT2 N2 invasive ductal carcinoma (IDC) of the left breast. PET/MRI for staging disease was performed before neoadjuvant chemotherapy.

Imaging Technique

Whole-body PET acquired 60 min after injection of 375 MBq of 18F-FDG, 58 kg/157 cm patient, with 6.5 mmol/L of fasting glycemia. Whole body atMR (T1 weighted), supine position.

T2 TSE axial, 3D e-thrive native, arterial and venous post-gadolinium, and breast PET in a SENSE breast-coil, prone position.

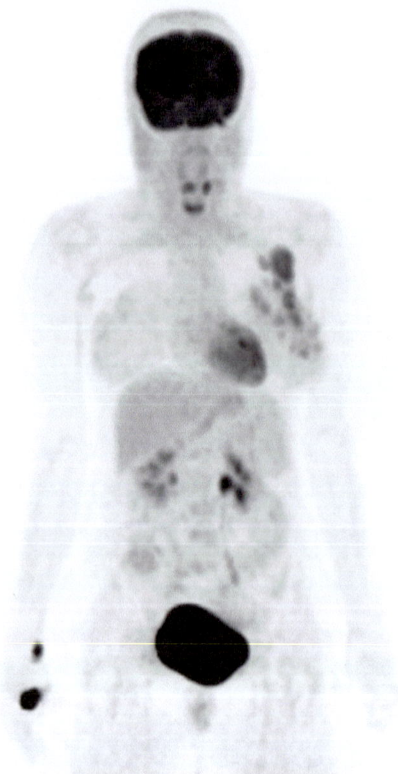

Fig. 6.34 MIP of the whole body PET, showing the left breast lesions with ipsilateral lymph node hypermetabolism

Findings

Whole body and breast PET/MR showed multifocal/multicentric hypermetabolic and enhanced tumoral extent of the left breast with massive ipsilateral axillar lymph node involvement, without controlateral breast lesion or distant metastasis.

Teaching Points

There is only very mild diffuse enhancement of the glandular tissue of the right breast. In the context of extensive tumor of the left breast, the absence of focal metabolic activity in the right breast PET makes the diagnosis of bilateral breast cancer very unlikely.

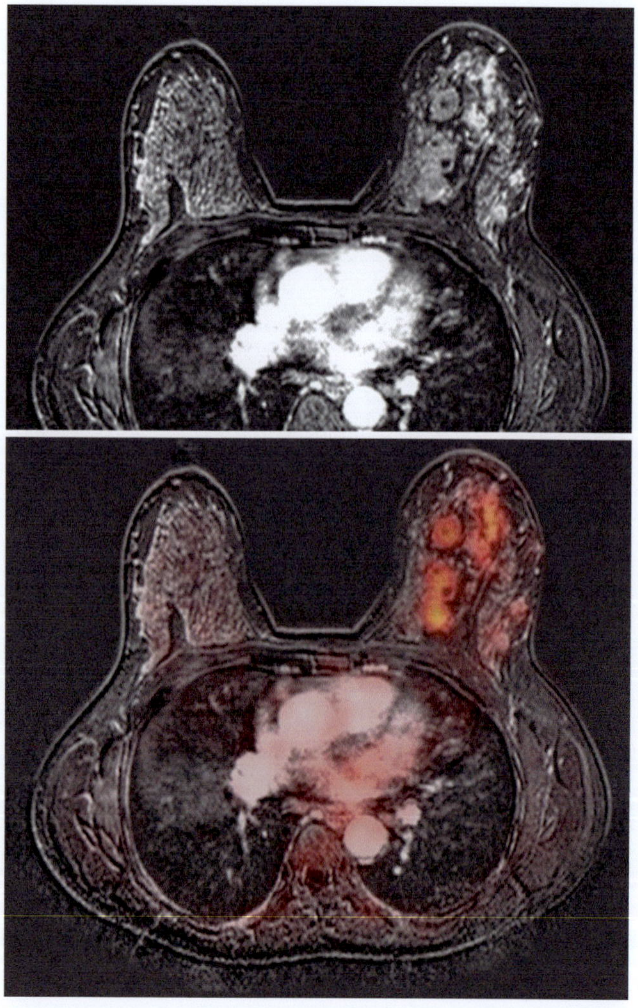

Fig. 6.35 E-thrive subtraction MRI sequence (*top*), fused with PET (*bottom*), both acquired in dedicated breast coil, showing the multifocal and multicentric left breast lesion, with important enhancement and hypermetabolism

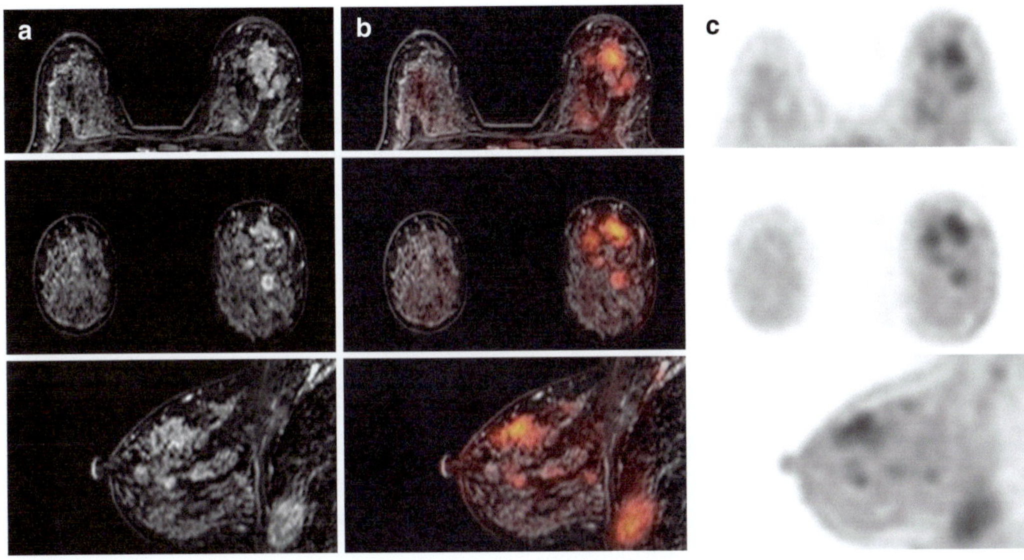

Fig. 6.36 *From left to right*, three orthogonal planes: (**a**) E-thrive subtraction MRI sequences, (**b**) fused PET/MRI, and (**c**) PET alone, acquired in the dedicated breast coil, showing the multifocal and multicentric left breast lesion, and axillary lymph node involvement

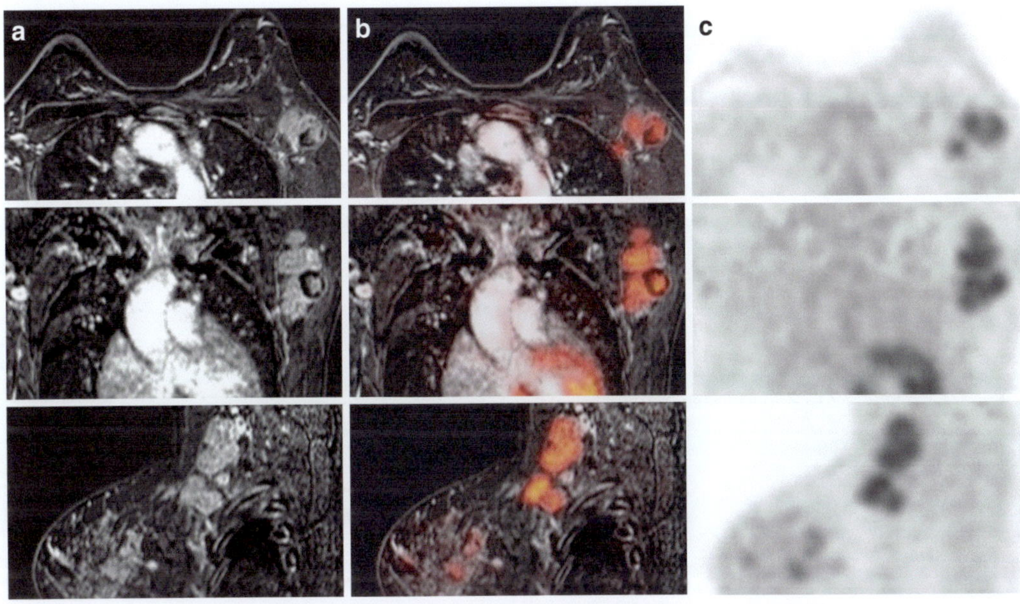

Fig. 6.37 E-thrive subtraction MRI sequence (**a**), fused PET/MRI (**b**), and PET alone (**c**), centered over the left axillar region showing the suspicious left axillar lymph nodes

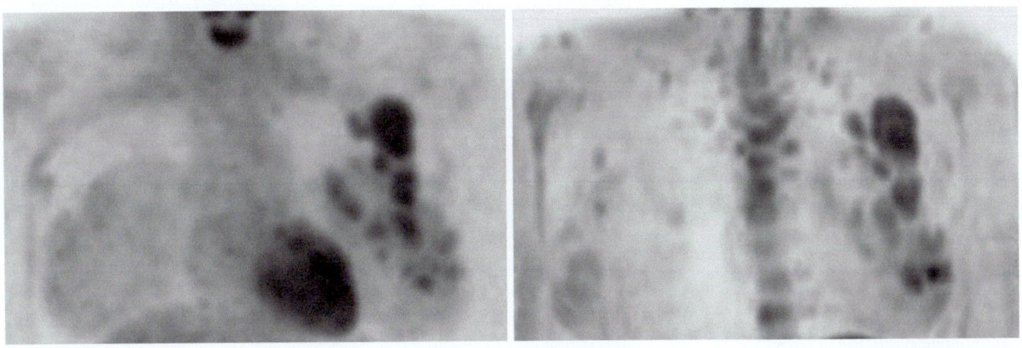

Fig. 6.38 Coronal views of the MIPS for PET on the *left*, vs Diffusion weighted (DWIBS) MRI sequence on the *right*, showing the multifocal tumor and suspicious axillary lymph nodes

Angiosarcoma of the Breast

Clinical History

Sixty-one-year-old patient with left breast carcinoma treated by lumpectomy and radiotherapy 10 years ago. Angiomatous lesions are noted on the skin at the junction of the inner quadrants of the left breast. Grade 2 angiosarcoma on CNB (core needle biopsy).

Imaging Technique

Whole-body PET acquired 60 min after injection of 375 MBq of 18F-FDG. Whole body atMR (T1 weighted), supine position.

3D e-thrive native, arterial and venous post-gadolinium, and breast PET in a SENSE breast-coil, prone position.

Findings

Breast MR showed suspected enhancement of the skin of the left inner inferior quadrant with 42-mm maximal diameter enhancement. PET images showed multifocal hypermetabolic lesions with the largest suspected lesion having a maximal diameter of 24 mm. Subsequent pathological examination of left mastectomy showed grade 2 angiosarcoma with 25 mm maximal size, dermal and hypodermal invasion.

Teaching Points

The area of contrast-enhancement on MRI is more extensive compared to the suspected lesion size. PET demonstrated more accurately the multifocal distribution and true tumor size. MRI could not separate the post radiation inflammatory component from undifferentiated tumor.

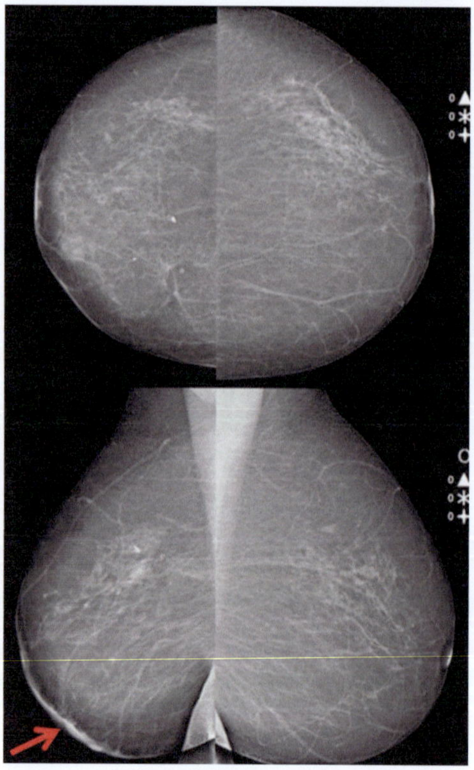

Fig. 6.39 Mammography of the right (*top*) and left (*bottom*) breast showing subcutaneous thickening at the location of the suspected lesion (*arrow*)

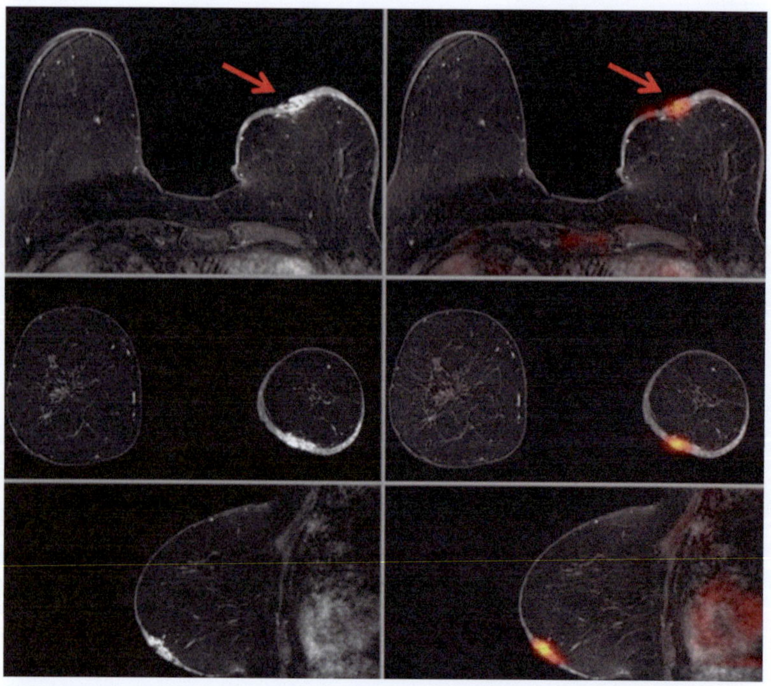

Fig. 6.40 Axial (*top*), coronal (*middle*) and sagittal (*bottom*) eThrive MRI images (*left*) fused with PET images (*right*) showing the multifocal distribution of the subcutaneous lesions (*arrows*)

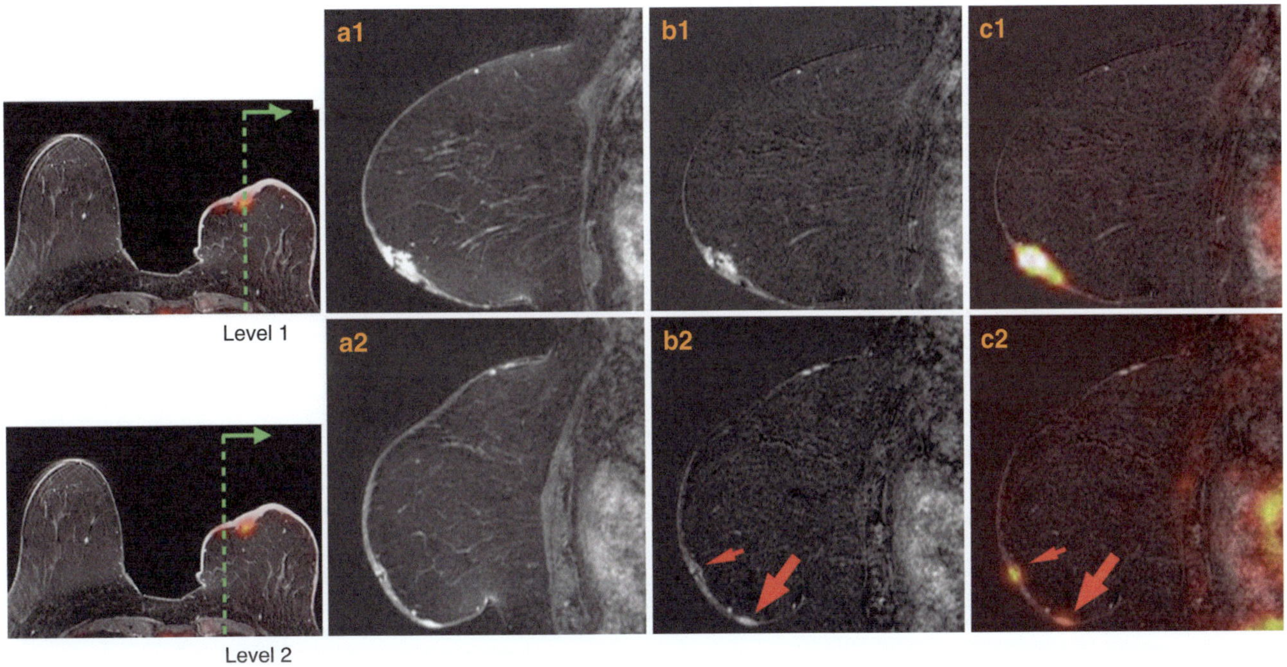

Fig. 6.41 Two levels of sagittal planes showing arterial (**a1**, **a2**), subtracted (**b1**, **b2**) and fused (**c1**, **c2**) images of the left breast showing the multifocal distribution of the lesions

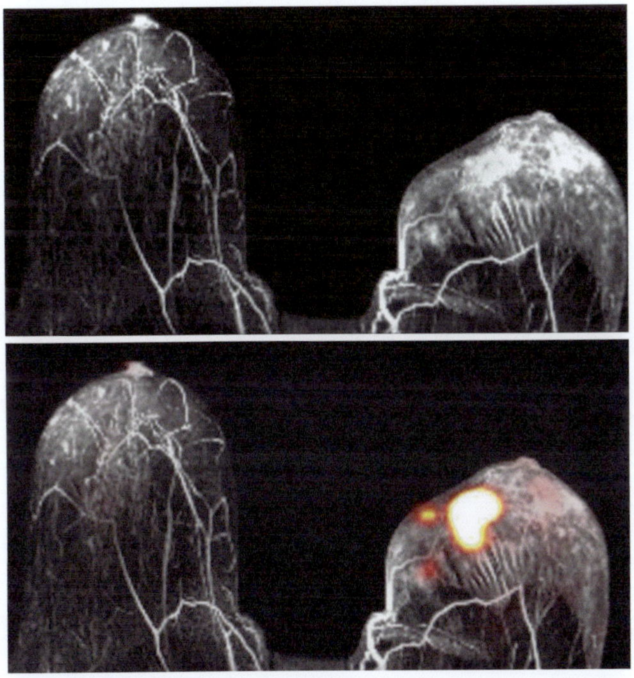

Fig. 6.42 Volume rendered images of contrast-enhanced MRI images (*top*) fused with PET images (*bottom*) of the left breast showing the multifocal distribution of the lesions

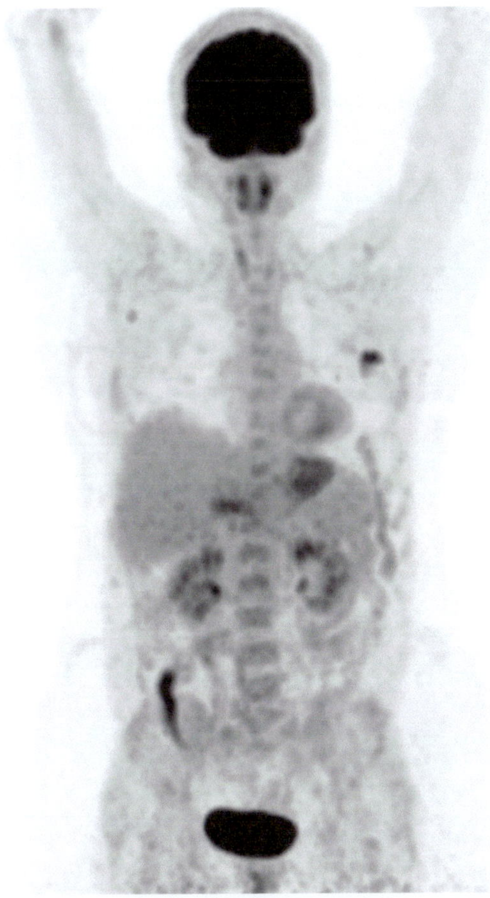

Fig. 6.43 Whole body MIP image of PET showing the left breast lesion but no other suspicious focal uptake of the tracer

Retroareolar ILC

Clinical History

Forty-five-year-old patient with retroareolar cT3 N1a invasive lobular carcinoma (ILC) grade 2 of the right breast. PET/MR was performed for staging.

Imaging Technique

Whole-body PET acquired 60 min after injection of 371 MBq of ^{18}F-FDG, 57 kg/157 cm patient, with 5 mmol/L of fasting glycemia. Whole body atMR (T1 weighted), supine position.

T2 TSE axial, 3D e-Thrive native, arterial and venous phase post-gadolinium, and breast PET in a SENSE breast-coil, prone position.

Findings

Breast PET/MR showed retroareolar, multicentric, 50 mm diameter tumor, with nipple invasion. Ipsilateral axillary lymphnode involvement was highly suspected on imaging. No contralateral breast lesion or distant metastatic extent was noted. Patient was treated by right mastectomy and axillary node dissection. On pathological examination, a 50-mm diameter invasive lobular carcinoma with dermal nipple showing the right breast retroareolar lesion with metastatic right axillary lymph nodes

> **Teaching Points**
>
> The glandular tissue of the right breast shows multinodular enhancement. In the context of contralateral tumor, the absence of high focal metabolic activity in PET in the left breast is an argument against the bilaterality of cancer. The hypermetabolism of right axillary lymph node was very suspicious, even though its diameter is <10 mm on MRI, which was found metastatic in pathological examination.

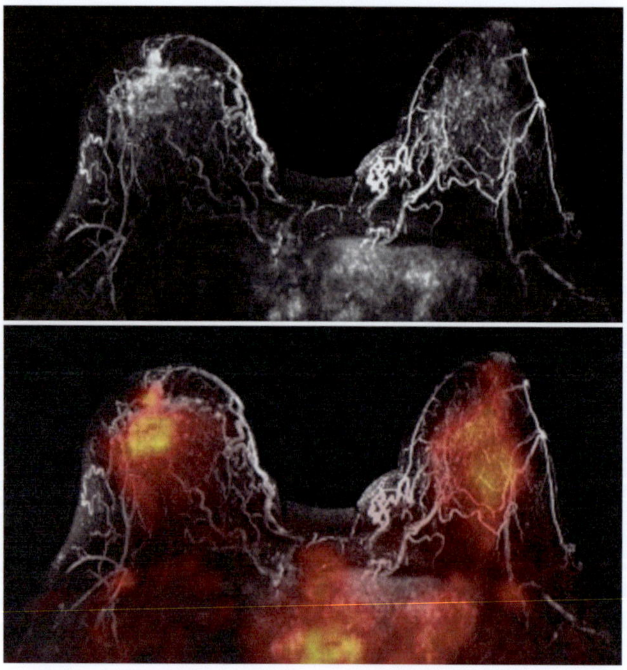

Fig. 6.44 3D reconstruction of arterial MRI e-Thrive sequence on the *top*, fused with FDG-PET at the *bottom*, showing the right breast retroareolar hypermetabolic lesion, with gadolinium uptake. This patient's breast tissues are dense, and therefore, there is a mild diffuse physiological FDG uptake in the opposite breast

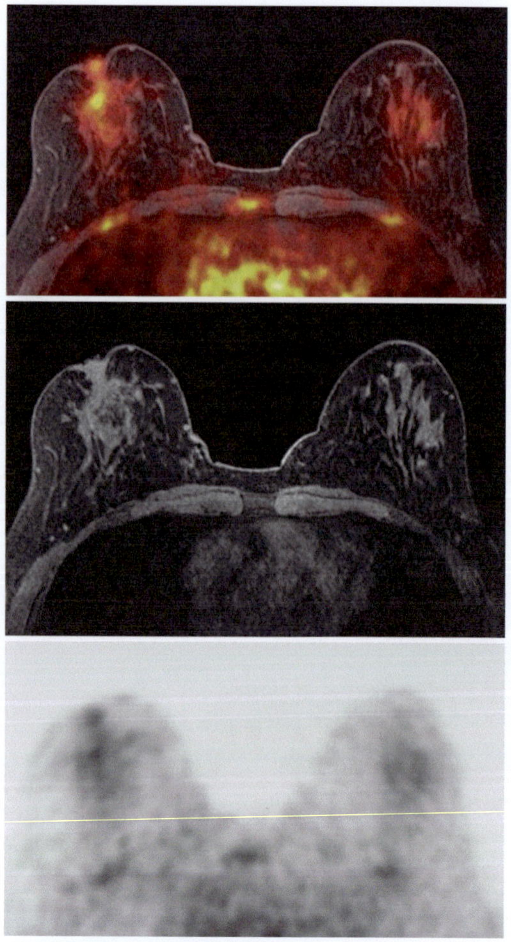

Fig. 6.45 *From the bottom to the top*, PET acquisition, native MRI e-Thrive sequence on the same level, and fusion of both modalities, showing the right breast lesion with nipple retraction

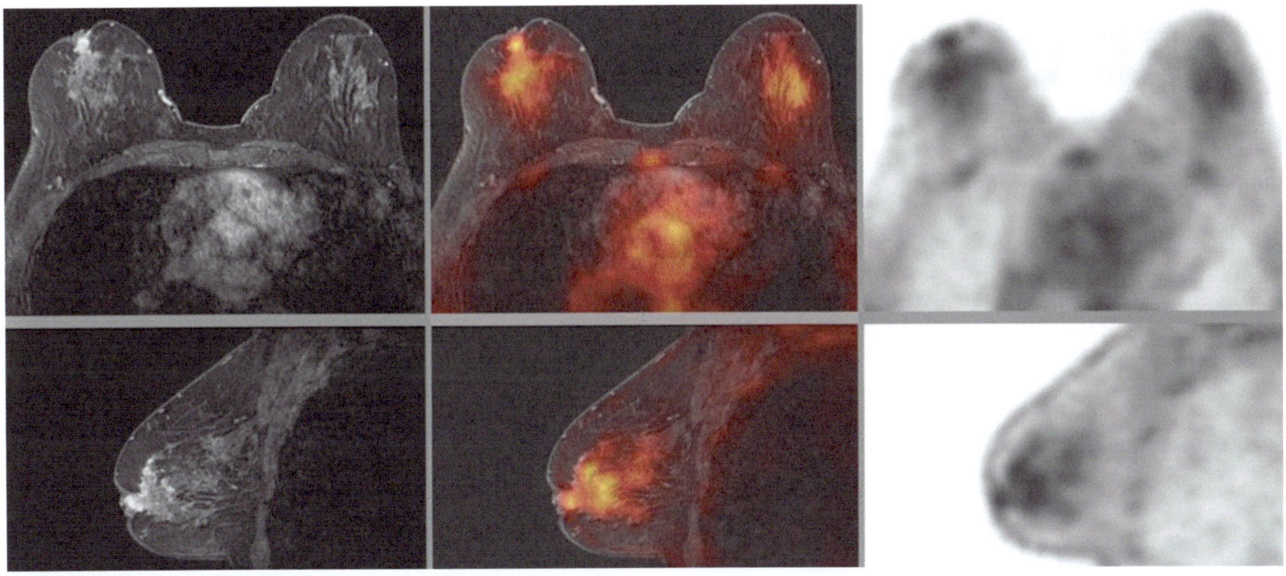

Fig. 6.46 Arterial MRI e-thrive sequence on the left, fused with the FDG-PET in axial (*top*) and sagittal (*bottom*) planes, showing the right breast retroareolar lesion

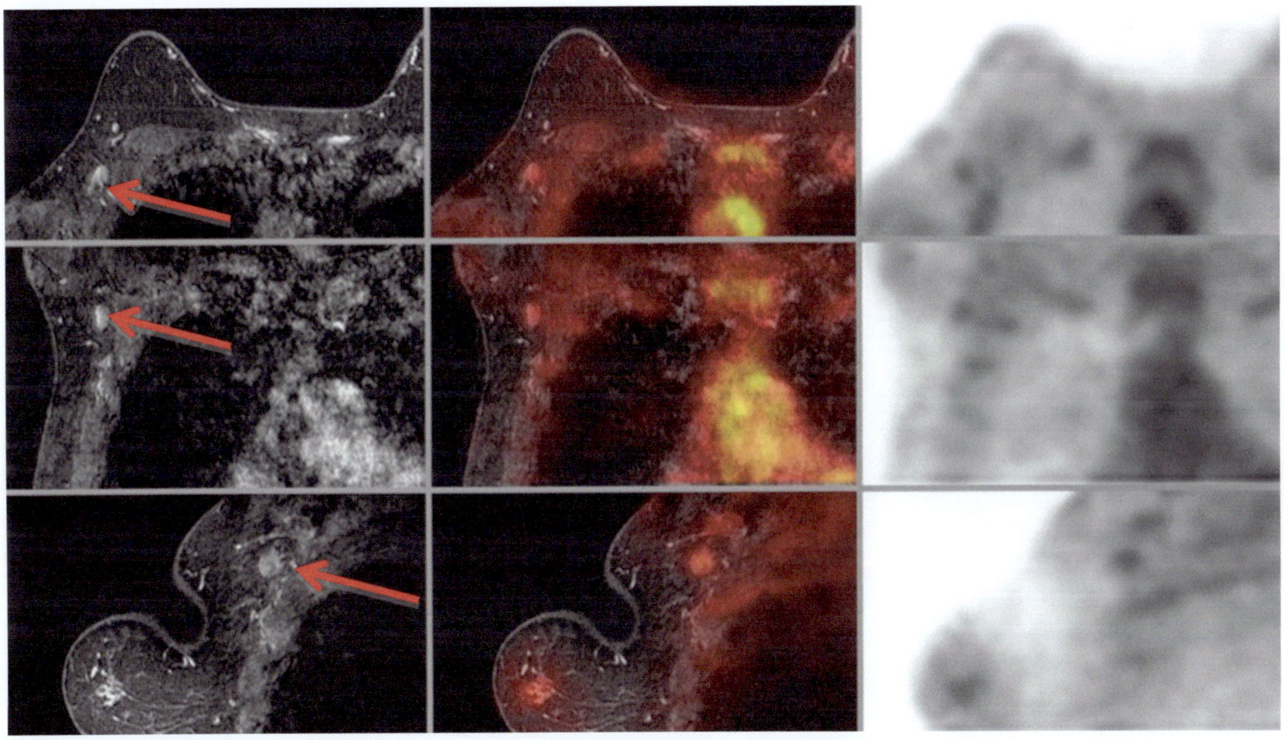

Fig. 6.47 Arterial phase e-thrive MRI sequence, fused with FDG-PET images in axial (*top*) coronal (*middle*) and sagittal (*bottom*) planes, showing one of the suspicious right axillary lymph nodes with mild to moderate PET uptake

Breast Cancer in Patient with Tuberculosis Clinical History

Sixty-six-year-old patient presenting with breast cancer. A conventional mammography performed at an outside institution showed the primary lesion in the left breast.

Imaging Technique

PET/MR images acquired 76 min after iv injection of 294 MBq F-18 FLT (fluorothymidine), 65 kg. 1 bed × 10 min together with axial T1 TSE, axial DWI, axial DCE (KWIC), ax T1 TSE+Gd, axial T1 VIBE+Gs

PET/CT images acquired 101 min after iv injection of 371 MBq F-18 FDG (fluoroglucose), 65 kg. 8 beds × 3 min with intravenous contrast

Findings

FLT-PET/MR and FDG-PET/CT for primary staging show a lesion in the left breast with high tracer uptake. In addition especially CT demonstrates multiple intrapulmonary lesions with positive uptake in the FLT and FDG-dataset. Due to previously known tuberculosis, the morphological appearance and the increased metabolism in PET the clinical suspicion was reactivated tubercular infiltration. The following biopsy confirmed reactivated tuberculosis.

Teaching Points

PET/MR imaging is suitable for whole body staging investigations. In this case both examinations (FDG-PET/CT and FLT-PET/MR) showed a good correlation between morphology and tracer uptake in the breast. However the FDG-PET/CT leads to a better morphological discrimination of the pulmonary lesions demonstrating the superiority of CT over MR for pulmonary pathologies.

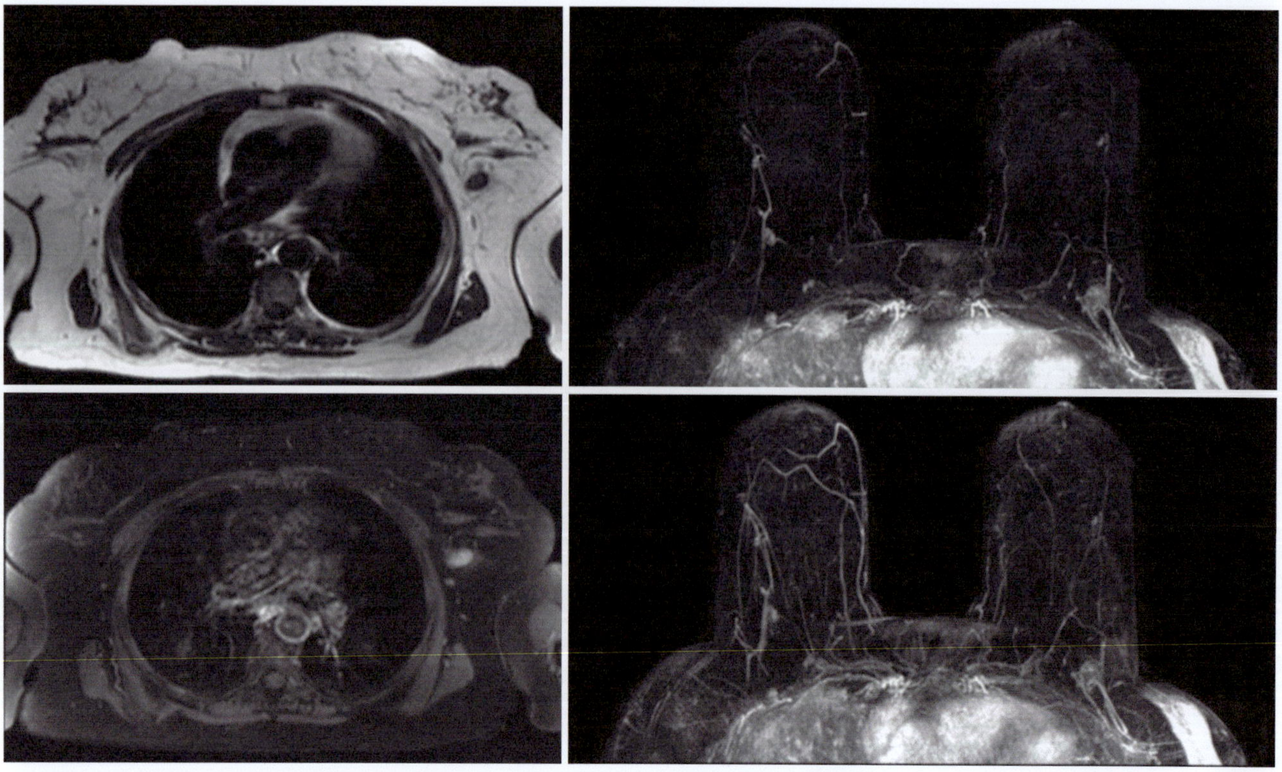

Fig. 6.48 *Left side*: Native T1w TSE demonstrates a nodular lesion in the left outer quadrant with intense enhancement in the T1w fs images. In addition several faint enhancing pulmonary lesions were found but difficult to discriminate on MR. *Right side*: Axial MIP projections nicely outline the whole breasts and demonstrate early as well as late contrast enhancement of the lesion

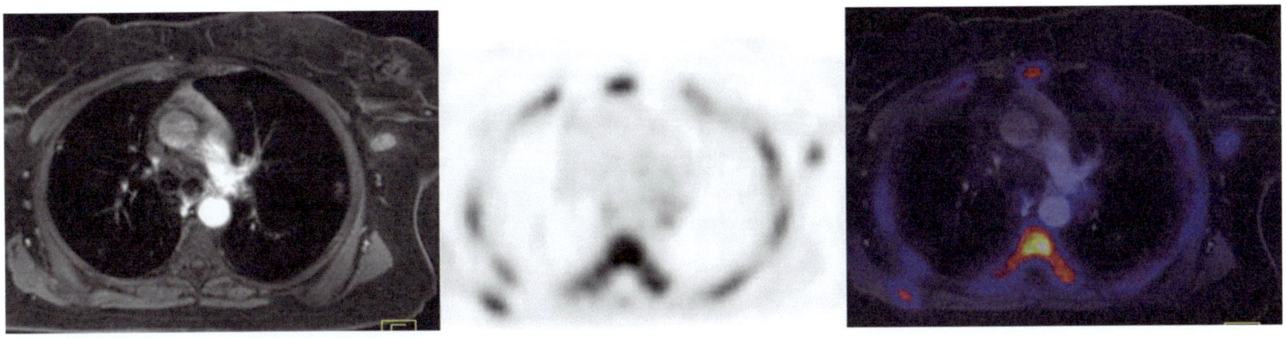

Fig. 6.49 *Left*: Contrast enhanced GRE fs-sequence in the arterial phase shows a hypervascularized lesion in the left outer quadrant; *middle*: moderate focal FLT-uptake is found in the corresponding area; *right*: fused PET/MR-image demonstrates a good co-registration between both datasets

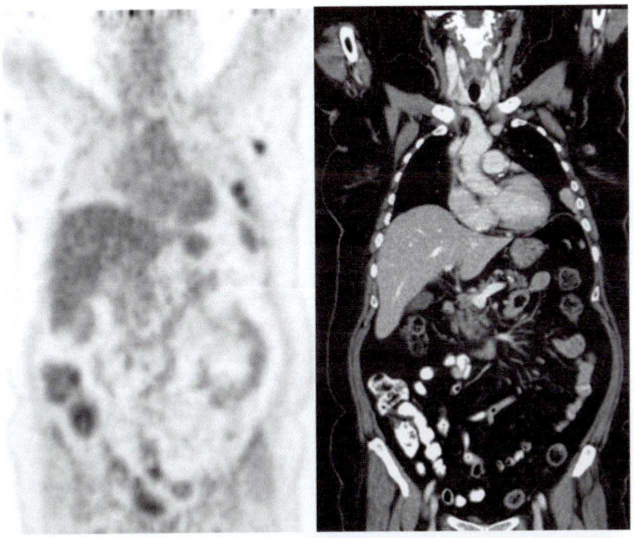

Fig. 6.50 FDG-PET and morphological contrast enhanced CT correlation shows the primary tumor of the left breast and in addition multiple pulmonary lesions, the biggest in the area of the basal left lung

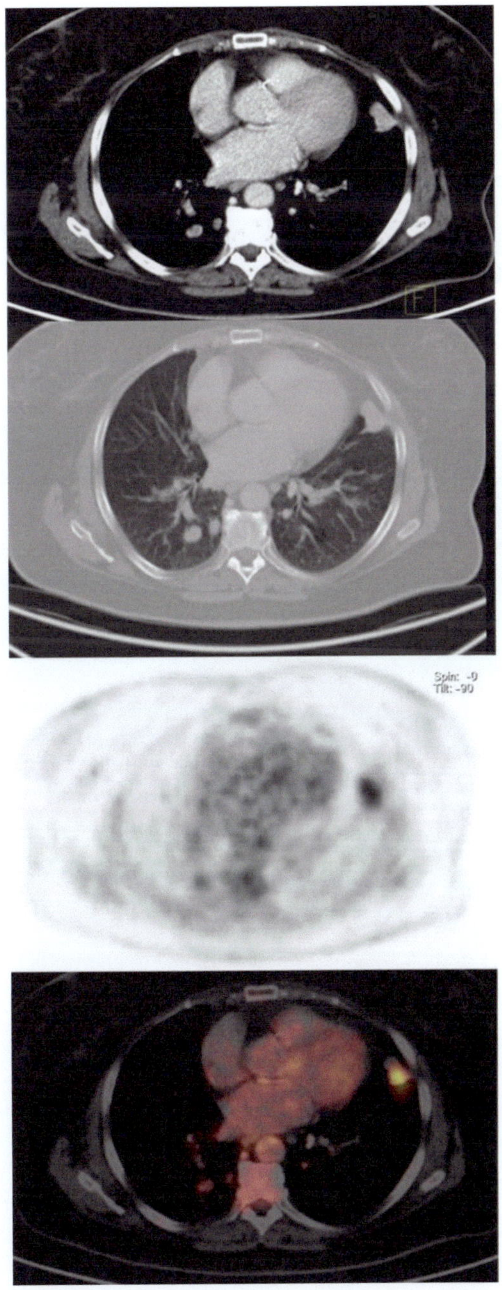

Fig. 6.51 *From top to bottom*: CT soft-tissue windows, CT lung window, axial PET, axial fused image: Clear anatomical outline of the pulmonary lesion is given by the CT dataset. The lesions show moderate focal uptake in FDG-PET indicating an active inflammatory process in known tuberculosis. However lung metastases could not be excluded in a patient with breast cancer

Triple-Negative Breast Cancer

Clinical History

Sixty-nine-year-old patient presenting with triple negative Breast Cancer on the right side. PET/MR indication: staging before neoadjuvant chemotherapy and early response imaging after first chemotherapy cycle.

Imaging Technique

First examination: Whole body PET/MR images acquired 79 min after iv injection of 316 MBq F-18 FLT (fluorothymidine), 72 kg.

Early response 2 weeks after the first cycle of chemotherapy: Whole body PET/MR images acquired 67 min after iv injection of 271 MBq F-18 FLT (fluorothymidine), 70 kg.

In both examinations 1 bed × 10 min together with axial T2 Haste fs, axial Vibe fs + Gd dynamic.

Findings

The staging examination shows high uptake of FLT in PET in the lower inner quadrant of the right breast. The MR images shows a pathological contrast enhancement of this lesion with a central radiopaque marker. Furthermore, a very low tracer uptake showed in projection on an enlarged lymph node in the area of the right internal mammary artery.

Early response imaging 2 weeks after first cycle of chemotherapy demonstrates a reduction of size in MRI and a significant decrease of tracer uptake of the primary lesion.

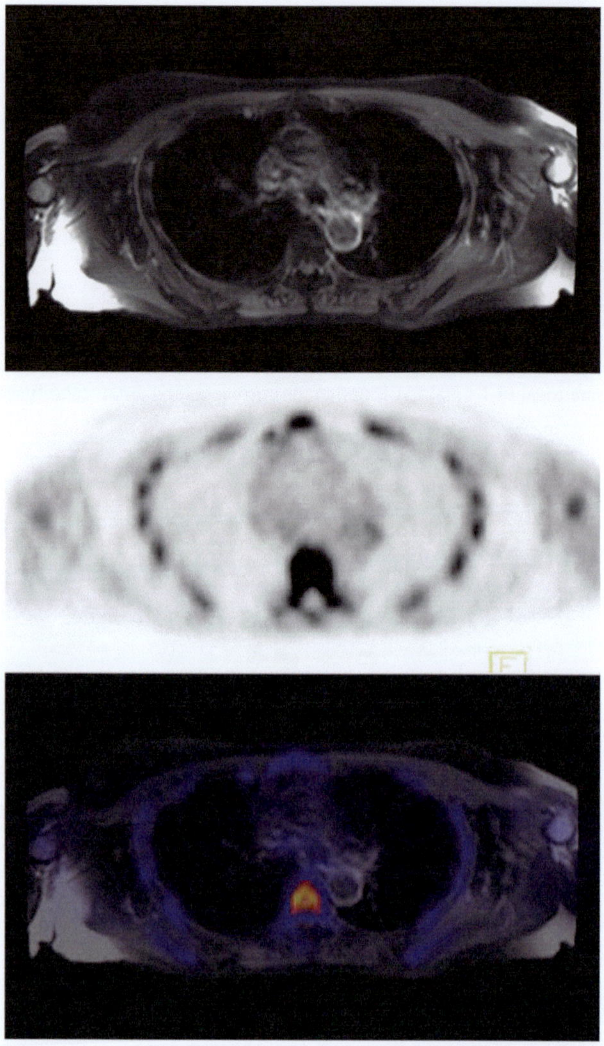

Fig. 6.52 Low FLT uptake of a lymph node in the area of the internal mammary artery to the right. The MR imaging (T1w fs + Gd) shows an enlarged lymph node with pathological contrast enhancement

Teaching Points

The combination of PET and MR imaging can lead to a more accurate discrimination of malignant lesions and their proliferation or metabolic activity. In this case, additional FLT-PET information shows a significant reduce of proliferation after one cycle of chemotherapy in correlation to the decrease in size in MRI in the sense of a good response to chemotherapy.

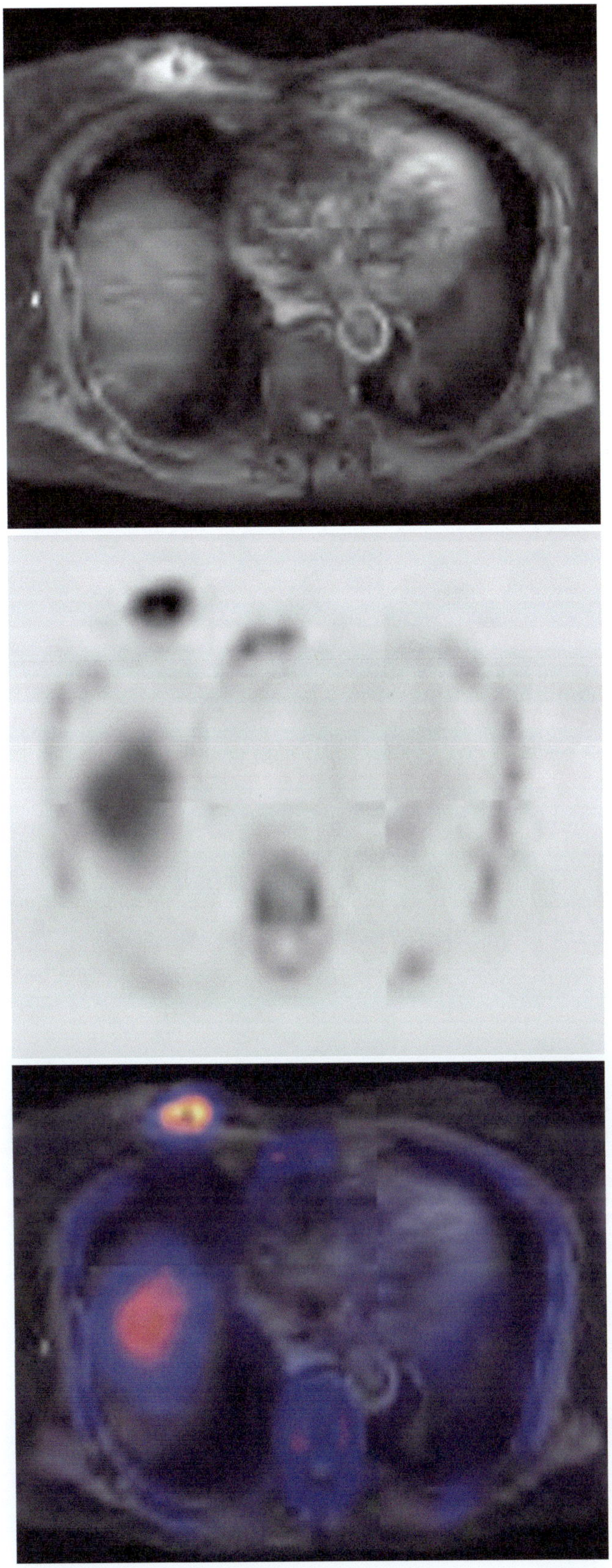

Fig. 6.53 Axial views. *From top to bottom*: MRI (ax T1w fs+Gd); FLT-PET Scan; PET/MR Fusion showing the staging images with a perfect co-registration of the lesion in the right breast before chemotherapy

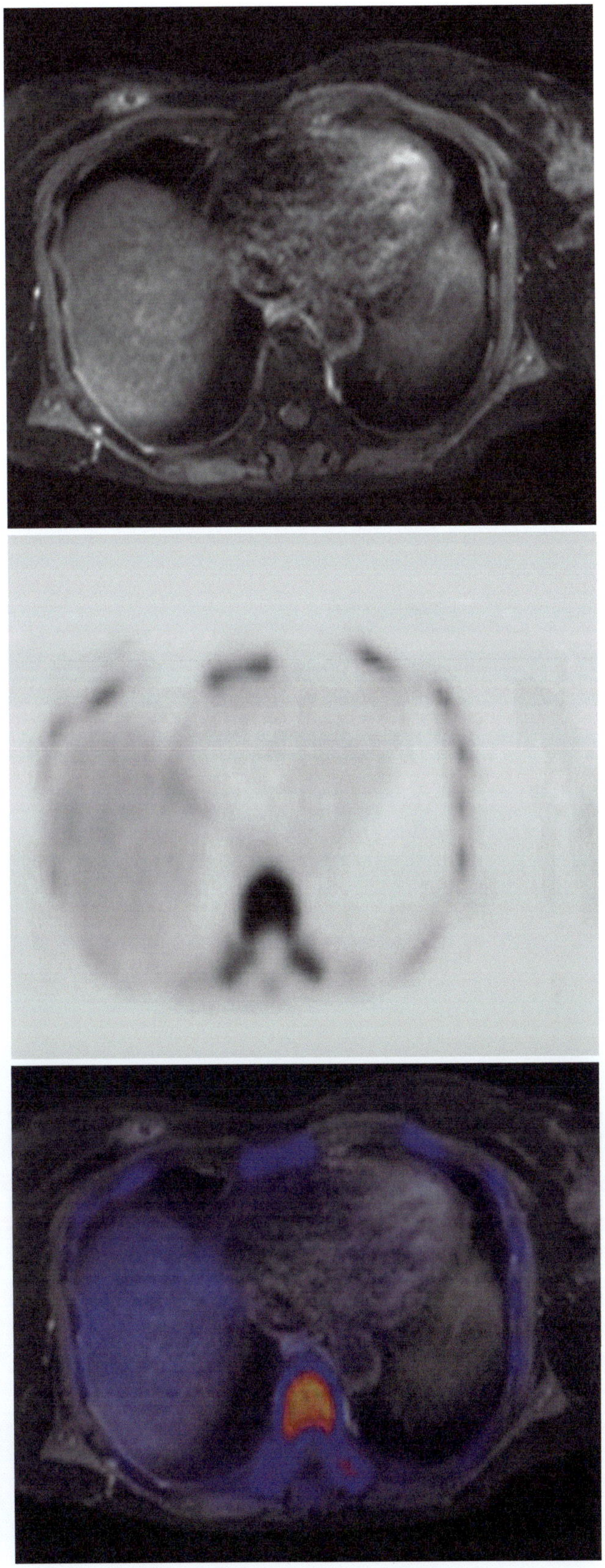

Fig. 6.54 Same sets of axial views acquired after chemotherapy shows no more or even a very low FLT uptake and a decrease of size 2 weeks after first cycle of chemotherapy

References

1. Kuhl C (2007) The current status of breast MR imaging. Part I. Choice of technique, image interpretation, diagnostic accuracy, and transfer to clinical practice. Radiology 244(2):356–378
2. Kuhl CK (2007) Current status of breast MR imaging. Part 2. Clinical applications. Radiology 244(3):672–91
3. Biglia N et al (2011) Role of MRI (magnetic resonance imaging) versus conventional imaging for breast cancer presurgical staging in young women or with dense breast. Eur J Surg Oncol 37(3): 199–204
4. Moy L et al (2010) Role of fusion of prone FDG-PET and magnetic resonance imaging of the breasts in the evaluation of breast cancer. Breast J 16(4):369–376
5. Koolen BB et al (2012) 18F-FDG PET/CT as a staging procedure in primary stage II and III breast cancer: comparison with conventional imaging techniques. Breast Cancer Res Treat 131(1):117–126
6. Alberini JL et al (2009) 18F-fluorodeoxyglucose positron emission tomography/computed tomography (FDG-PET/CT) imaging in the staging and prognosis of inflammatory breast cancer. Cancer 115(21):5038–5047
7. Carkaci S et al (2009) Retrospective study of 18F-FDG PET/CT in the diagnosis of inflammatory breast cancer: preliminary data. J Nucl Med 50(2):231–238
8. Pennant M et al (2010) A systematic review of positron emission tomography (PET) and positron emission tomography/computed tomography (PET/CT) for the diagnosis of breast cancer recurrence. Health Technol Assess 14(50):1–103
9. Ueda S et al (2011) Early metabolic response to neoadjuvant letrozole, measured by FDG PET/CT, is correlated with a decrease in the Ki67 labeling index in patients with hormone receptor-positive primary breast cancer: a pilot study. Breast Cancer 18(4): 299–308
10. Duch J et al (2012) PET/CT with [18F] fluorodeoxyglucose in the assessment of metabolic response to neoadjuvant chemotherapy in locally advanced breast cancer. Q J Nucl Med Mol Imaging 56(3):291–298
11. Duch J et al (2009) 18F-FDG PET/CT for early prediction of response to neoadjuvant chemotherapy in breast cancer. Eur J Nucl Med Mol Imaging 36(10):1551–1557
12. Vargas MI et al (2013) Approaches for the optimization of MR protocols in clinical hybrid PET/MRI studies. MAGMA 26(1):57–69

Gynecological Cancers

7

C. Tabouret-Viaud, A. Baskin, and P. Loubeyre

Contents

Gynecological Cancers

Cervical cancer is the second most common cancer in women worldwide. There are about 60,000 newly detected cases and 30,000 deaths each year in Europe.

18F-FDG-PET is already recommended to evaluate lymph node extension and was proven superior to MRI for detection of lombo-aortic lymph node extension, which is a major prognostic factor [1, 2]. Moreover, whole-body PET is able to detect distant metastases, and is recognized as having an interest in assessing treatment response 3 months after the completion of concurrent chemoradiation [3].

Given its excellent soft-tissue contrast, MRI plays an important role in the delineation of cervical lesions, and possible vaginal, parametrial, rectal or bladder invasion [4, 5]. Some MRI sequences such as dynamic contrast enhanced MRI can also provide additional information for the assessment of response to therapy [6].

Therefore, PET and MRI are complementary for cervical cancer local, loco-regional and distant staging and re-staging.

Thus, hybrid PET/MRI could be very useful for this indication, time-sparing for patients, and diminishing the total dose of radiation they receive in comparison with PET/CT.

C. Tabouret-Viaud (✉) • A. Baskin • P. Loubeyre
Department of Imaging, Division of Nuclear Medicine and Molecular Imaging, Geneva University Hospital, Rue Gabrielle Perret Gentil 4, 1211 Geneva 4, Switzerland
e-mail: claire.tabouretviaud@hcuge.ch

O. Ratib et al. (eds.), *Atlas of PET/MR Imaging in Oncology*,
DOI 10.1007/978-3-642-31292-2_7, © Springer-Verlag Berlin Heidelberg 2013

Squamous Cell Carcinoma of the Cervix

Clinical History

Fifty-one-year-old patient with FIGO IIIB squamous cell carcinoma of the cervix. Study requested for staging and evaluation of lymph-node extension for radiotherapy planning.

Imaging Technique

Whole-body PET acquired 60 min after injection of 369 MBq of ^{18}F-FDG, with 5.2 mmol/L of fasting glycemia. Whole body atMR (T1 weighted), supine position. TSE T2 weighted MRI sequences in sagittal, coronal and axial planes (TR: 3,400 ms; TE: 100 ms; NSA: 2; voxel: 0.7/0.7/3 mm), cardiac 32 CH coil. Supine position.

Findings

Forty-two-millimeter cervical lesion with serous invasion of the cervix, involvement of 2/3 of the vagina, and numerous retroperitoneal metastatic lymph nodes. This patient was not eligible for surgical treatment and underwent chemoradiotherapy.

Teaching Points

PET clearly demonstrates diffuse iliac and retroperitoneal lymph node invasion. In particular, para-aortic suprarenal lymph nodes are invaded, which is important information to know before determining the radiation field (usually, the radiation field does not extend above the renal veins in cervical cancer).

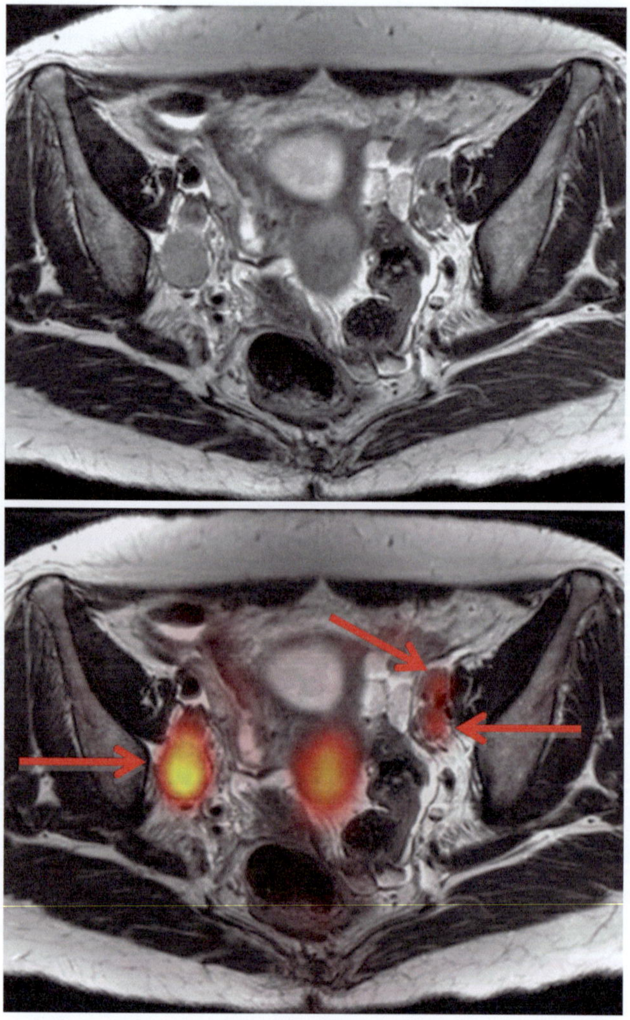

Fig. 7.1 T2 weighted TSE axial MRI sequence (*top*), fused with PET images (*bottom*), showing right and left metastatic iliac lymph nodes (*arrows*)

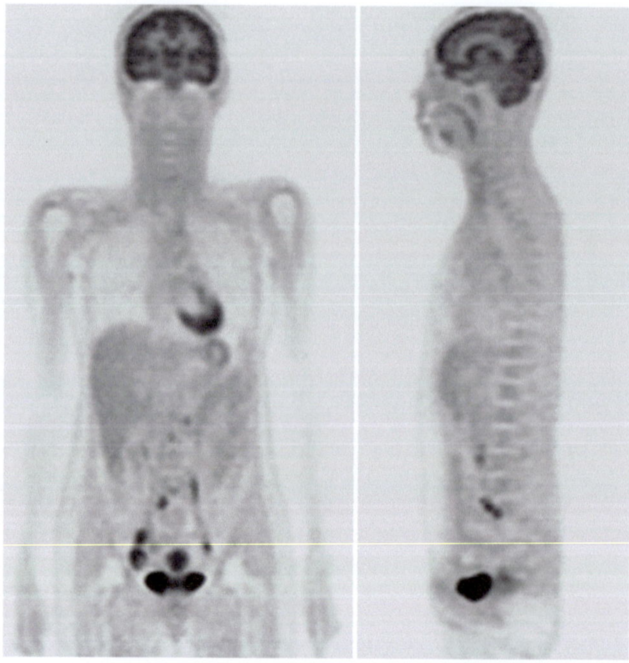

Fig. 7.2 Frontal and lateral views of the whole-body PET MIP, showing hypermetabolism of the cervical lesion and lymph nodes invasion

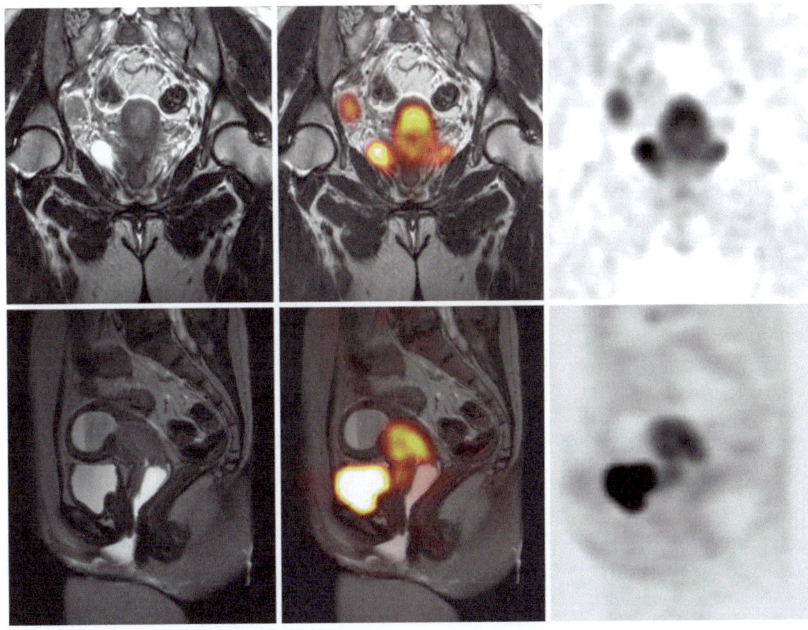

Fig. 7.3 Coronal and sagittal T2 weighted TSE MRI sequences (*left*), fused with PET (*middle*) and PET (*right*), showing the hypermetabolic cervical lesion with invasion of the 2/3 of the anterior and superior wall of the vagina, with liquid retention above the lesion, in the uterine cavity. Two hypermetabolic metastatic lymph nodes can also be seen on the coronal views

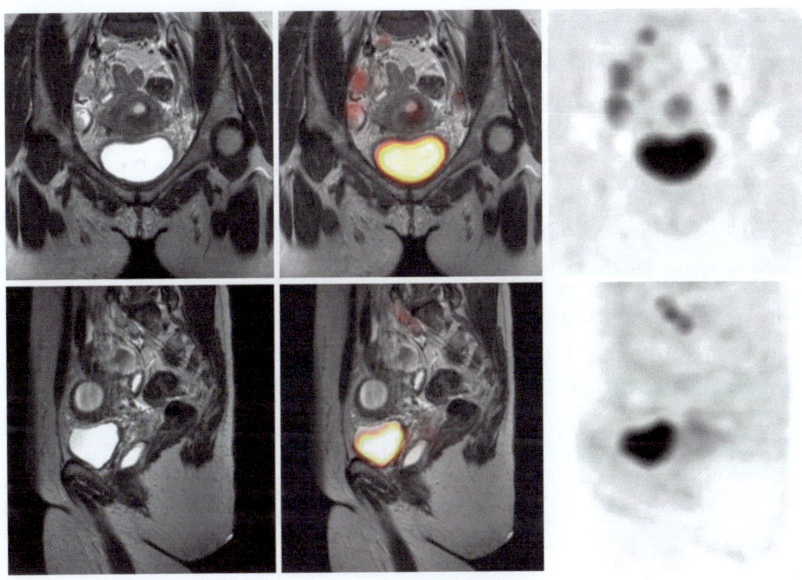

Fig. 7.4 Coronal and sagittal T2 weighted TSE MRI sequences on the *left*, fused with PET in the *middle* and PET alone on the *right*, showing hypermetabolic metastatic bilateral iliac lymph nodes

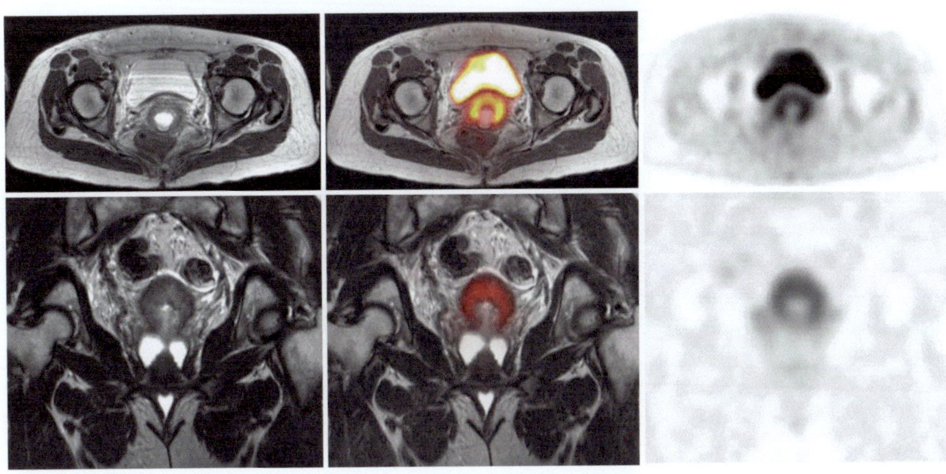

Fig. 7.5 Axial and coronal T2 weighted TSE MRI sequences on the *left*, fused with PET in the *middle* and PET alone on the *right*, showing the hypermetabolic cervical cancer

Cervical Cancer Post Surgery

Clinical History

Twenty-two-year-old patient with FIGO IIA1 squamous cell carcinoma of the cervix. Positive surgical margins on pathological examination of cervical conization. PET/MR was requested for staging prior to further therapeutic decision.

Imaging Technique

Whole-body PET acquired 60 min after injection of 374 MBq of ^{18}F-FDG, with 3.9 mmol/L of fasting glycemia. Whole body atMR (T1 weighted), supine position. TSE T2 weighted MRI sequences in sagittal, coronal and axial planes (TR: 3,400 ms; TE: 100 ms; NSA: 2; voxel: 0.7/0.7/3 mm), STIR and eThrive sequences Supine position.

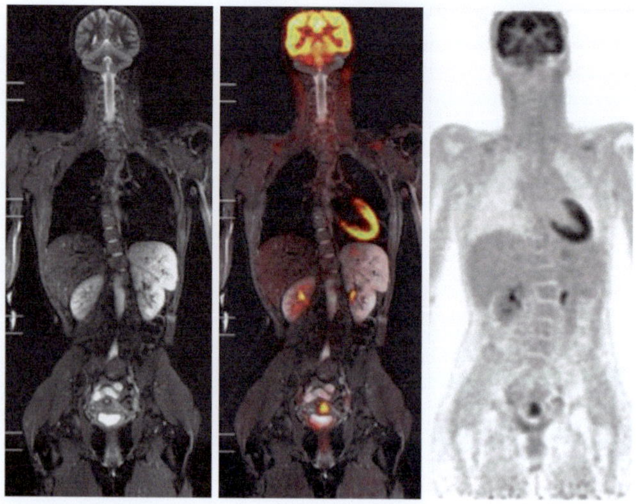

Fig. 7.6 Coronal whole-body STIR sequence on the *left*, fused with PET on the *middle*, and PET alone on the *right*, showing the hypermetabolic cervical cancer

Findings

Twenty-five-millimeter maximal diameter cervical tumoral process with left serous effraction and minor left parametrial invasion. Surgical treatment is contraindicated and the patient is proposed for chemo-radiotherapy.

> **Teaching Points**
>
> PET helps identify the extent of the disease. No retroperitoneal lymph node invasion was found on PET. Radiation fields were thus limited to pelvic lymph nodes.

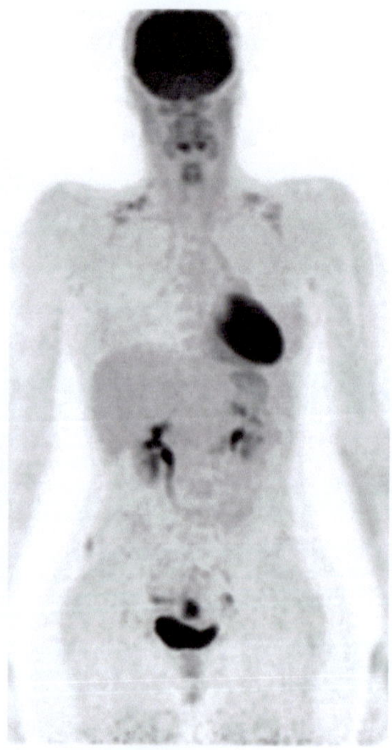

Fig. 7.7 Coronal MIP rendering of FDG-PET study, showing mild hypermetabolism in both supra-clavicular regions, due to physiological brown fat uptake in this young patient

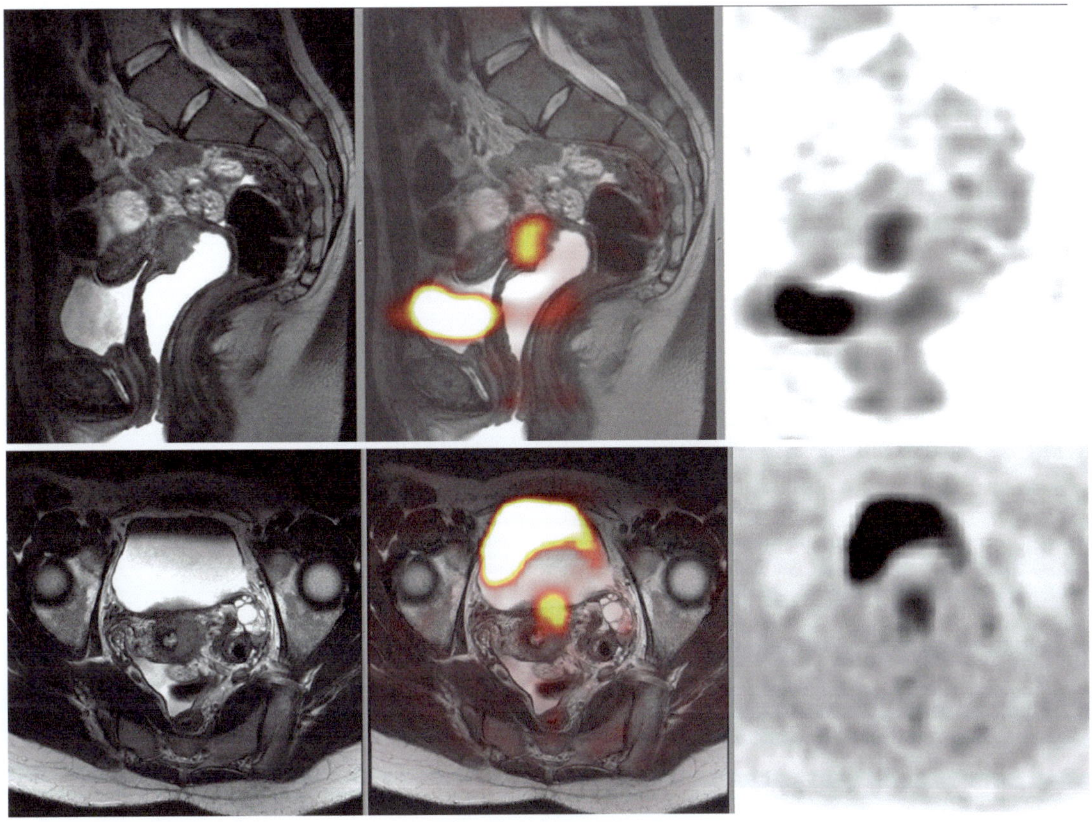

Fig. 7.8 T2 TSE sagittal and axial MRI sequences on the *left*, fused with PET on the *middle*, and PET alone on the *right*, showing the hypermetabolic cervical cancer. The contrast agent in the vagina helps to delineate the cervical lesion

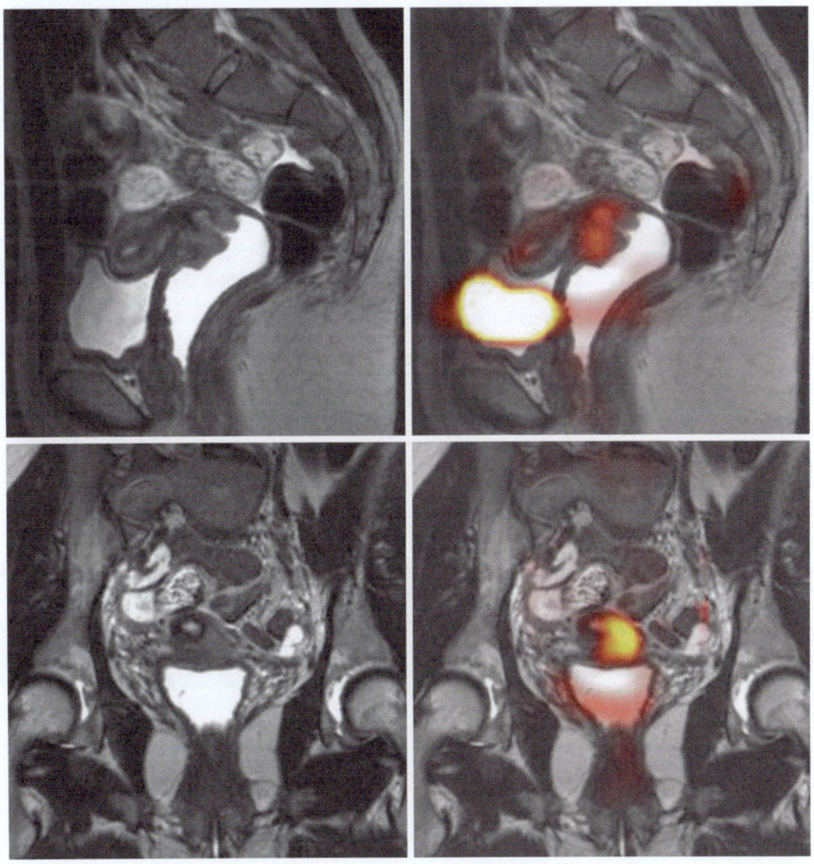

Fig. 7.9 T2 TSE sagittal and coronal MRI sequences on the *left*, fused with PET on the *right*, showing the topographic distribution of the hypermetabolic cervical cancer

Squamous Cell Cervical Carcinoma

Clinical History

Forty-two-year-old patient with FIGO IIB squamous cell carcinoma of the cervix. Study requested for staging prior to surgery.

Imaging Technique

Whole-body PET acquired 60 min after injection of 376 MBq of 18F-FDG, with 5.7 mmol/L of fasting glycemia. Whole body atMR (T1 weighted), supine position. TSE T2 weighted MRI sequences in sagittal, coronal and axial planes (TR: 3,400 ms; TE: 100 ms; NSA: 2; voxel: 0.7/0.7/3 mm), cardiac 32 CH coil. Supine position.

Findings

Sixty-two-millimeter cervical tumor with serous effraction and vaginal involvement on MRI. Bilateral iliac lymph node involvement found on PET/MR. This patient was subsequently scheduled for chemo-radiotherapy.

Teaching Points

The patient had clearly positive lymph nodes on PET/MR: this is a contraindication for surgery. Therefore, PET/MR helped to plan the treatment and the patient had chemo-radiotherapy.

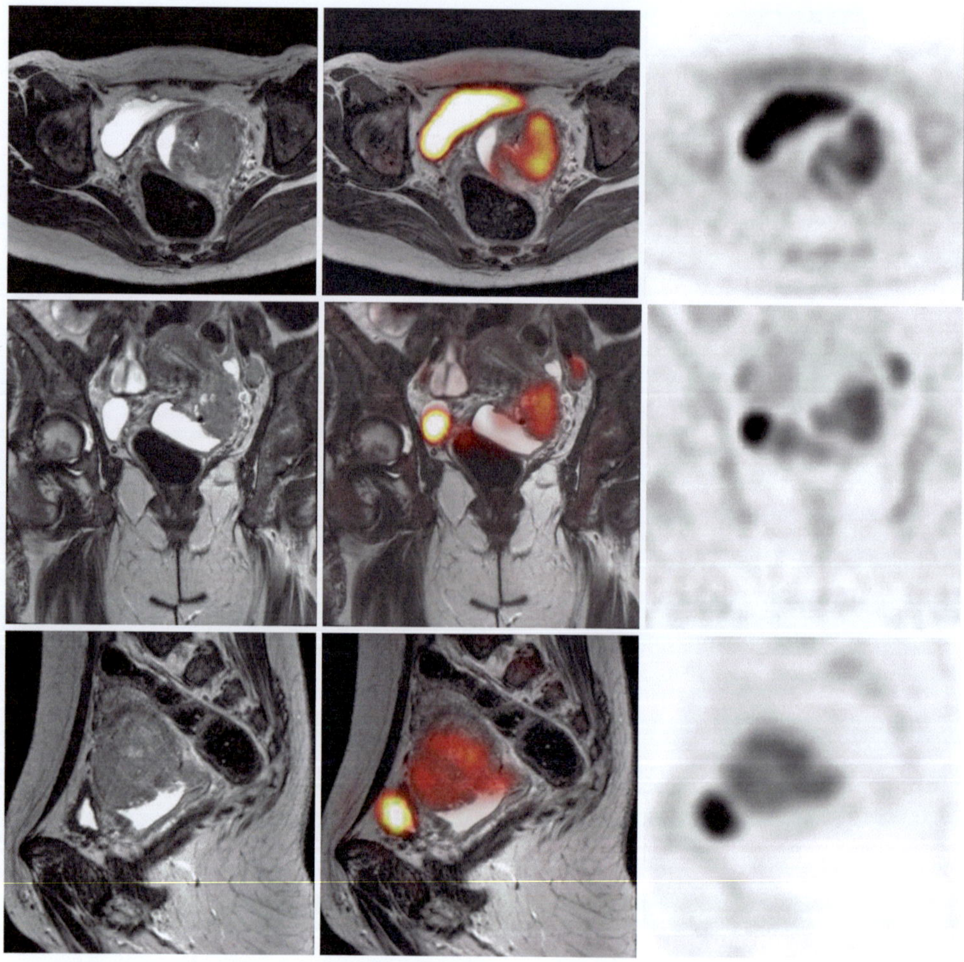

Fig. 7.10 T2 TSE axial, frontal and sagittal SENSE MRI sequences *from top to bottom on the left*, fused with PET on the *middle*, and PET alone on the *right*, showing the large hypermetabolic and heterogeneous cervical tumor

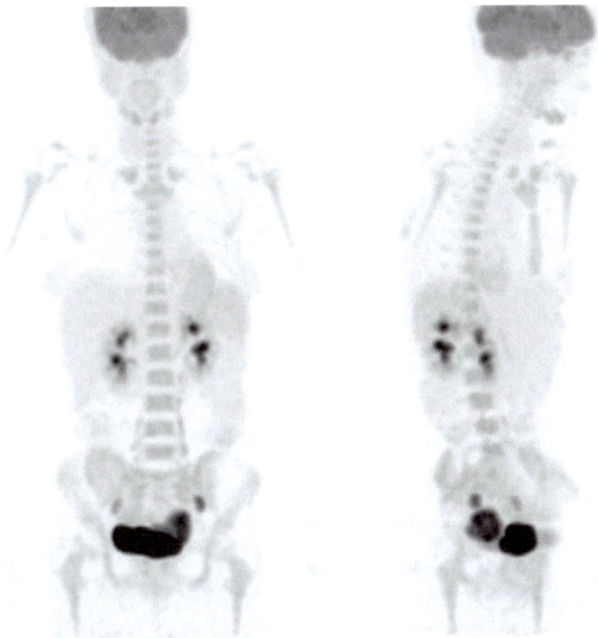

Fig. 7.11 Coronal and left postero-lateral views of the whole-body FDG-PET showing the large hypermetabolic cervical tumor, and bilateral iliac focal uptake in lymph nodes

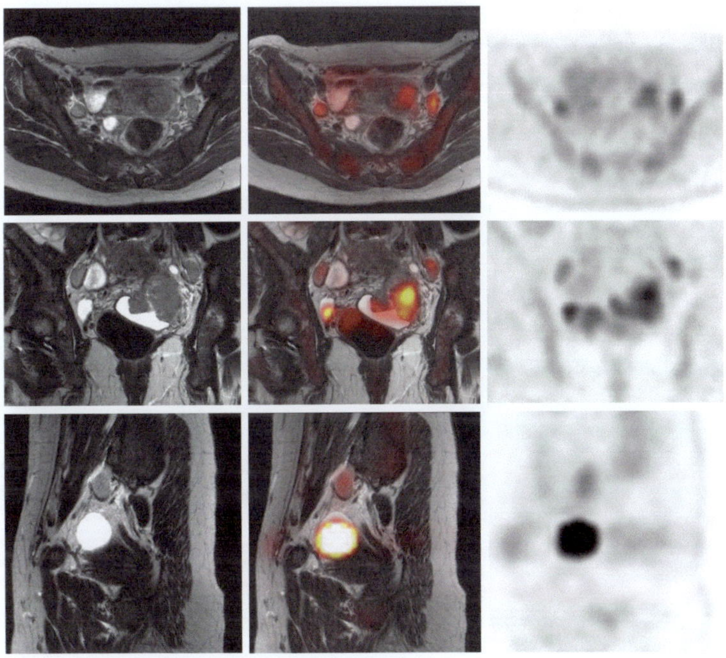

Fig. 7.12 T2 TSE axial (*top*), coronal (*middle*) and sagittal (*bottom*) MRI sequences on the *left*, fused with PET on the *middle*, and PET alone on the *right*, showing bilateral iliac lymph nodes with FDG uptake, therefore suspicious of metastatic dissemination

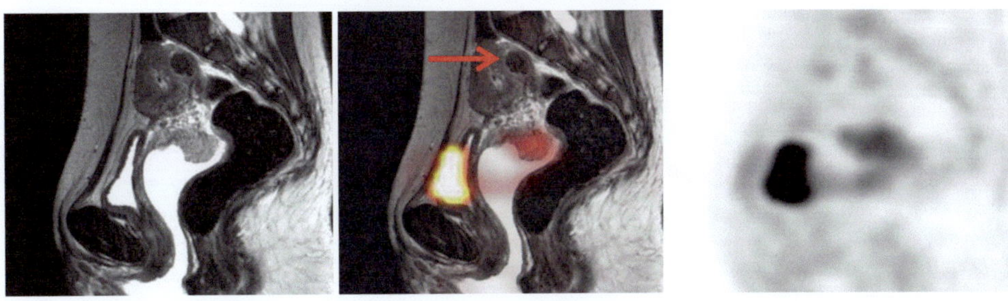

Fig. 7.13 T2 TSE sagittal SENSE MRI sequences on the *left*, fused with PET on the *middle*, and PET alone on the *right*, showing no significant FDG tracer uptake on this uterine lesion, in hyposignal T2, corresponding to a myoma (*arrow*)

References

1. Choi HJ et al (2006) Comparison of the accuracy of magnetic resonance imaging and positron emission tomography/computed tomography in the presurgical detection of lymph node metastases in patients with uterine cervical carcinoma: a prospective study. Cancer 106(4):914–922
2. Reinhardt MJ et al (2001) Metastatic lymph nodes in patients with cervical cancer: detection with MR imaging and FDG PET. Radiology 218(3):776–782
3. Schwarz JK et al (2009) The role of 18F-FDG PET in assessing therapy response in cancer of the cervix and ovaries. J Nucl Med 50(Suppl 1):64S–73S
4. Hricak H et al (2007) Early invasive cervical cancer: CT and MR imaging in preoperative evaluation - ACRIN/GOG comparative study of diagnostic performance and interobserver variability. Radiology 245(2):491–498
5. Sahdev A et al (2007) The performance of magnetic resonance imaging in early cervical carcinoma: a long-term experience. Int J Gynecol Cancer 17(3):629–636
6. Kinkel K et al (1997) Differentiation between recurrent tumor and benign conditions after treatment of gynecologic pelvic carcinoma: value of dynamic contrast-enhanced subtraction MR imaging. Radiology 204(1):55–63

Brain Tumors

8

V. Garibotto, A. Baskin, M. Essler, S. Foerster, A. Drzezga, S. Haller, L. Merlini, T. Pyka, M.-I. Vargas, and D. Weber

Contents

V. Garibotto(✉)
Division of Nuclear Medicine and Molecular Imaging, Department of Medical Imaging, Geneva University and Geneva University Hospitals, Geneva, Switzerland
e-mail: valentina.garibotto@hcuge.ch

A. Baskin
Department of Imaging, Division of Nuclear Medicine and Molecular Imaging, Geneva University Hospitals, Geneva, Switzerland

M. Essler • S. Foerster • T. Pyka
Department of Nuclear Medicine, Technische Universität München, Munich, Germany

A. Drzezga
Department of Nuclear Medicine, University Hospital of Cologne, Cologne, Germany

S. Haller • M.-I. Vargas
Division of Neuroradiology, Department of Medical Imaging, Geneva University and Geneva University Hospitals, Geneva, Switzerland

L. Merlini
Division of Pediatric Radiology, Department of Medical Imaging, Geneva University and Geneva University Hospitals, Geneva, Switzerland

D. Weber
Division of Radiation Oncology, Department of Medical Imaging, Geneva University and Geneva University Hospitals, Geneva, Switzerland

Brain Tumors

Because of its high soft-tissue contrast, MRI is the method of choice for the assessment of brain tumors. Conventional MRI sequences provide excellent visualization of the lesions, but still have limitations for the accurate definition of lesion boundaries and for differentiating some treatment related changes and tumor recurrence. MRI techniques such as diffusion-weighted imaging, perfusion-weighted imaging and MR spectroscopy have the potential to provide powerful additional information.

PET, on the other hand, targets specific biochemical and metabolic processes. In particular, PET with specific amino acid tracers, such as 18F-Fluoroethyl-L-thyrosine (18F-FET) is an established diagnostic tool in the clinical management and treatment planning of cerebral gliomas. This technique can be used to guide biopsy in heterogeneous tumors, to determine tumor extent and differentiate it from the edema typically surrounding a mass lesion, and it may also guide treatment planning, specifically radiation therapy. Furthermore, PET imaging might contribute to the differentiation of post-therapeutic alterations and tumor recurrence.

Thus, hybrid PET/MRI might represent the modality of choice to investigate, in a single imaging session, tracer uptake and perfusion metabolic changes shown by MRI in the neoplastic tissue. The current research with this new hybrid modality will allow testing the added value of the combination of PET and MRI parameters for the characterization of tumor tissue and the differentiation between tumor tissue and therapy-induced changes in the brain. In particular, we expect a diagnostic gain in clinically challenging areas such as the early assessment of response to anti-angiogenic therapies and the differential diagnosis of tumor recurrence and radiation necrosis.

O. Ratib et al. (eds.), *Atlas of PET/MR Imaging in Oncology*,
DOI 10.1007/978-3-642-31292-2_8, © Springer-Verlag Berlin Heidelberg 2013

Oligodendroglioma

Clinical History

Thirty-four-year-old F with oligodendroglioma (WHO grade II) of the right temporal pole, surgically removed 8 years earlier, with newly appeared Gd-enhanced lesions on the last MR scan. PET/MR indication: restaging before chemotherapy.

Imaging Technique

Brain PET images acquired 30–50 min after iv injection 213 MBq 18F-Fluoroethyltyrosine (FET), head MRI (T2 turbo spin echo, fluid attenuated inversion recovery, arterial spin labeling, conventional perfusion, diffusion tensor imaging T1W 3D with Gadolinium administration; SENSE Head-8 coil).

Findings

Brain PET shows an intense radiotracer uptake extending from the surgical resection cavity to the ipsilateral frontal and temporal lobe and thalamus.

The 18F-FET distribution shows clearly the neoplastic lesion: in this case, the area of significant uptake is larger than the focal lesions showing significant contrast enhancement.

Teaching Points

The combination of 18F-FET PET and MR images in one acquisition allows identifying tumor recurrence and the extent of the metabolically active tumor components.

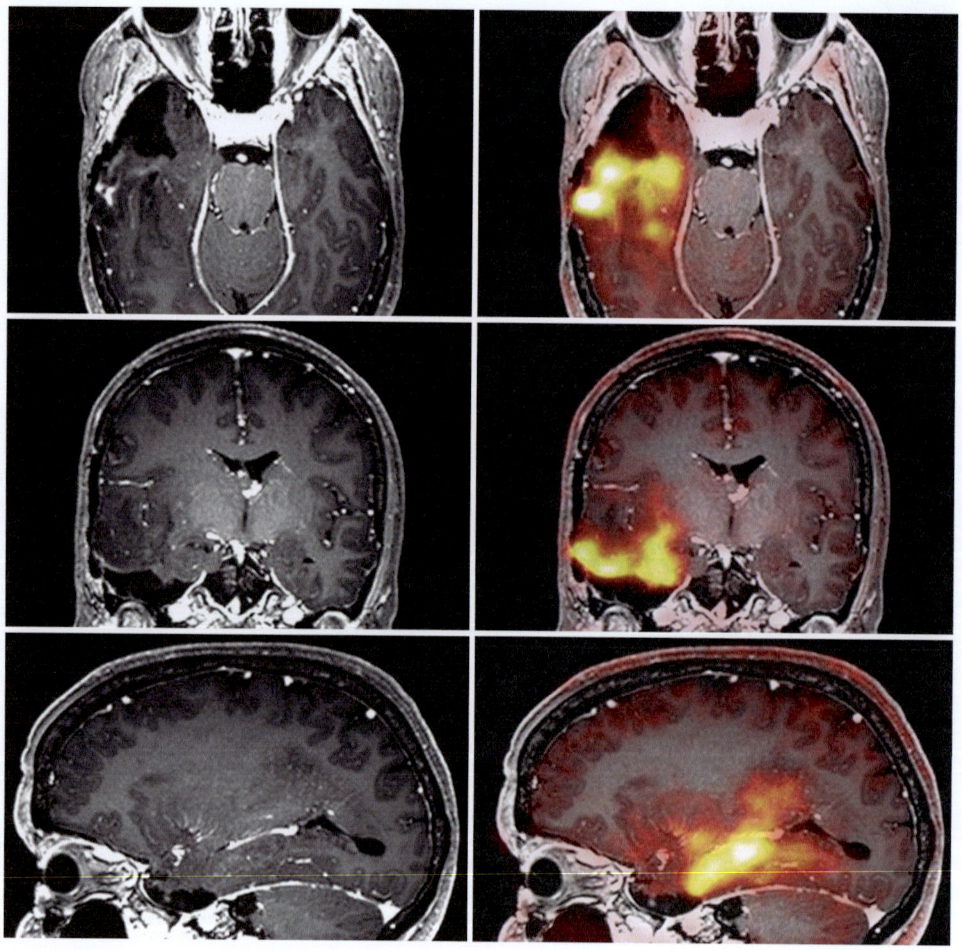

Fig. 8.1 Fused 18F-FET (*on the right*) and T1w Gd images (*on the left*) showing the surgical sequelae and tumor infiltration in the temporal pole, associated with a significant tracer uptake

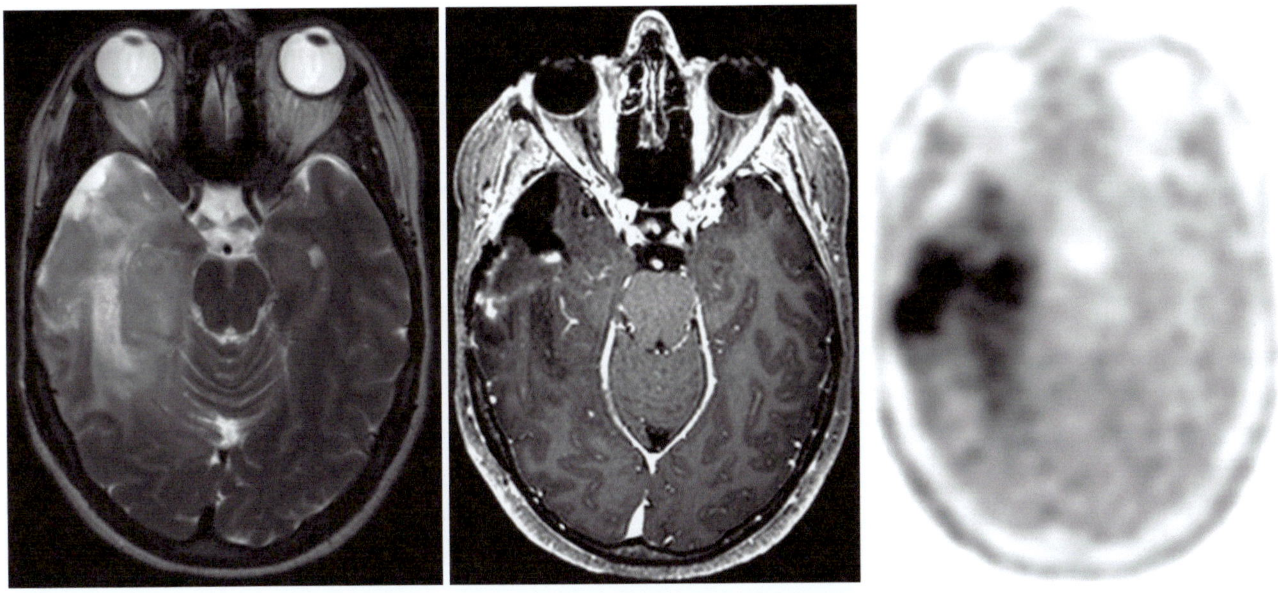

Fig. 8.2 T2 images (*left*), T1 3D images after Gd administration (*middle*), and 18F-FET images (*right*). The three modalities allow visualizing different components of the tumoral lesion

Fig. 8.3 Fusion image 18F-FET and T1Gd MR

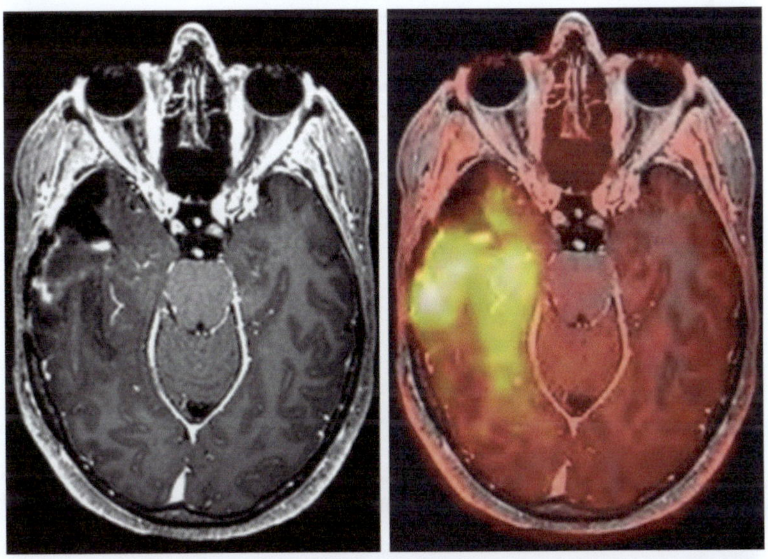

Fig. 8.4 Fusion images 18F-FET and FLAIR MR, showing concordant pathological findings of the thalamus, internal capsule and temporal lobe

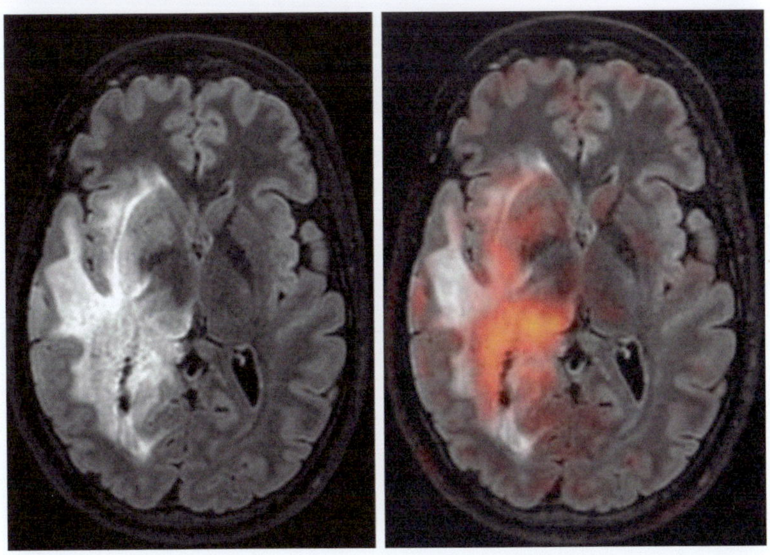

Glioblastoma: Staging

Clinical History

Fifty-three-year-old M with newly diagnosed brain mass, presumably a glioblastoma.

PET/MR indication: staging and biopsy planning.

Imaging Technique

Brain PET images acquired 30–50 min after iv injection 213 MBq 18F-Fluoroethyltyrosine (FET), head MRI (T2W turbo spin echo, fluid attenuated inversion recovery, arterial spin labeling, conventional perfusion, diffusion tensor imaging T1W 3D with Gadolinium administration; SENSE Head-8 coil).

Findings

Brain PET/MR shows a mass centered on the corpus callosum with involvement of both frontal lobes, a "butterfly glioma". The biopsy was done at level of contrast enhancement and focal tracer uptake. The biopsy of this area showed a glioblastoma (WHO grade IV).

Teaching Points

PET/MR allows identifying MR lesions with a high metabolic activity and significant enhancement, helping selecting the best target for biopsy.

In addition PET/MR allows acquiring parameters which are relevant for patient staging and surgery planning, such as fiber involvement by diffusion tensor imaging.

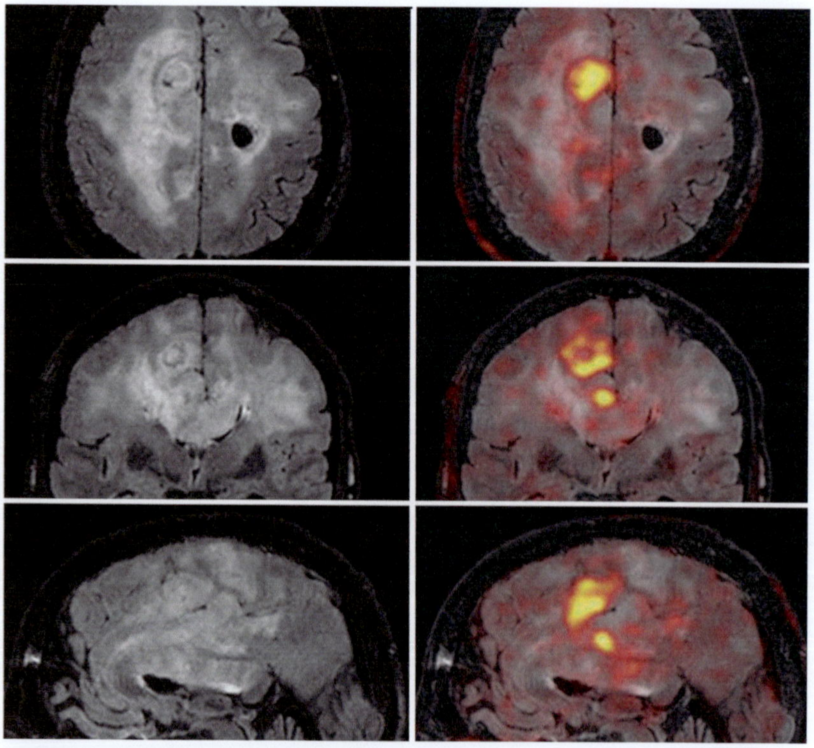

Fig. 8.5 Fused 18F-FET and FLAIR images showing two uptake foci of the right frontal lobe and corpus callosum in axial (*top*), coronal (*middle*) and sagittal (*bottom*) planes

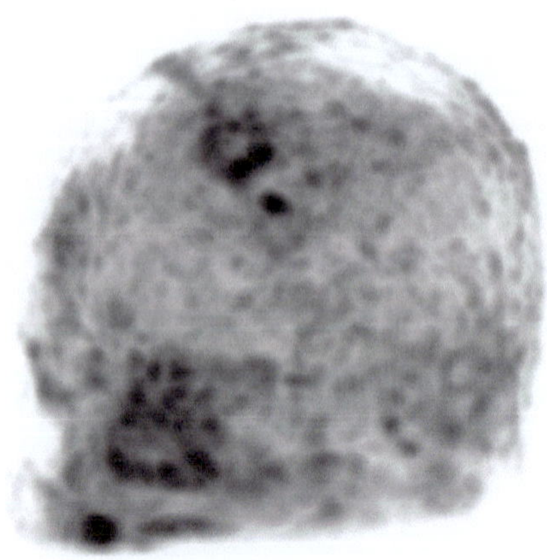

Fig. 8.6 MIP image showing two significant foci of 18F-FET uptake

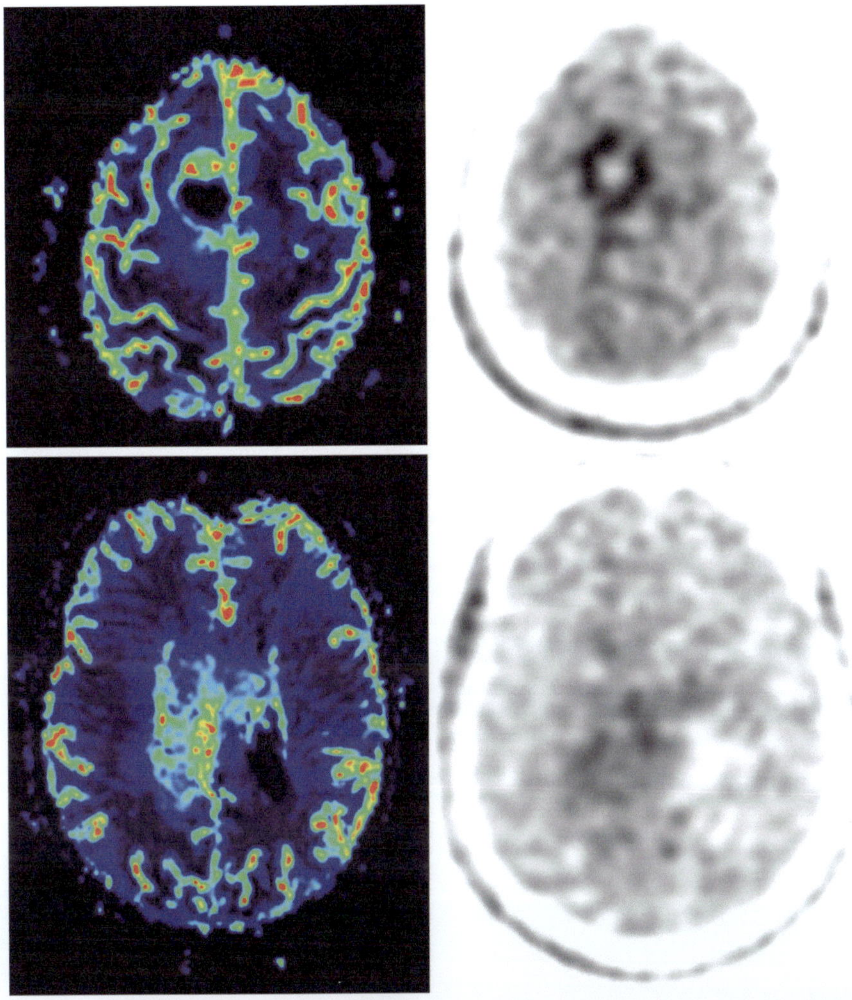

Fig. 8.7 Perfusion images and 18F-FET images showing concordant hyperperfusion (*left*) and tracer uptake (*right*)

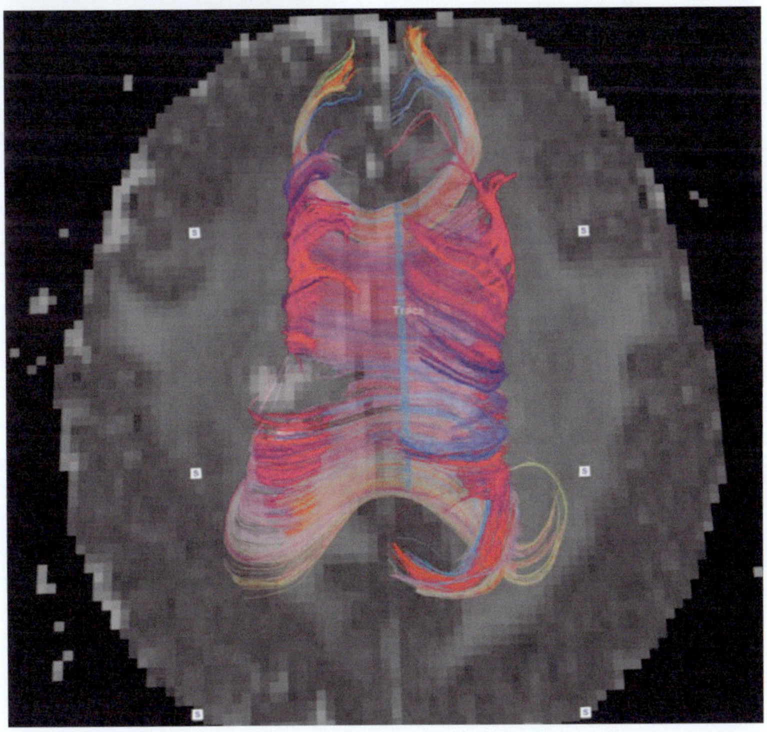

Fig. 8.8 Diffusion tensor imaging shows that corpus callosum fibers are globally preserved, except for the area corresponding to the focal contrast uptake

Brain Tumors – Glioblastoma

Clinical History

Sixty-eight-year-old M with newly diagnosed glioblastoma (WHO grade IV). PET/MR indication: staging and radiation therapy planning.

Imaging Technique

Brain PET images acquired 30–50 min after iv injection 213 MBq 18F-Fluoroethyltyrosine (FET), head MRI (T2 turbo spin echo, fluid attenuated inversion recovery, arterial spin labeling, conventional perfusion, diffusion tensor imaging T1W 3D with Gadolinium administration; SENSE Head-8 coil).

Findings

Brain PET shows a focal lesion of the right thalamus with central hypoactivity, corresponding to a ring-enhancing lesion on MR, extending to the internal capsule and to the ipsilateral temporoparietal white matter. The images were fused with the CT images used for radiation therapy planning in order to realize intensity-modulated radiation therapy.

Teaching Points

Brain PET/MR allows better definition of MR contrast enhancement and tumor FET uptake in a single imaging session, identifying the most active lesion components and allowing accurate radiation therapy planning.

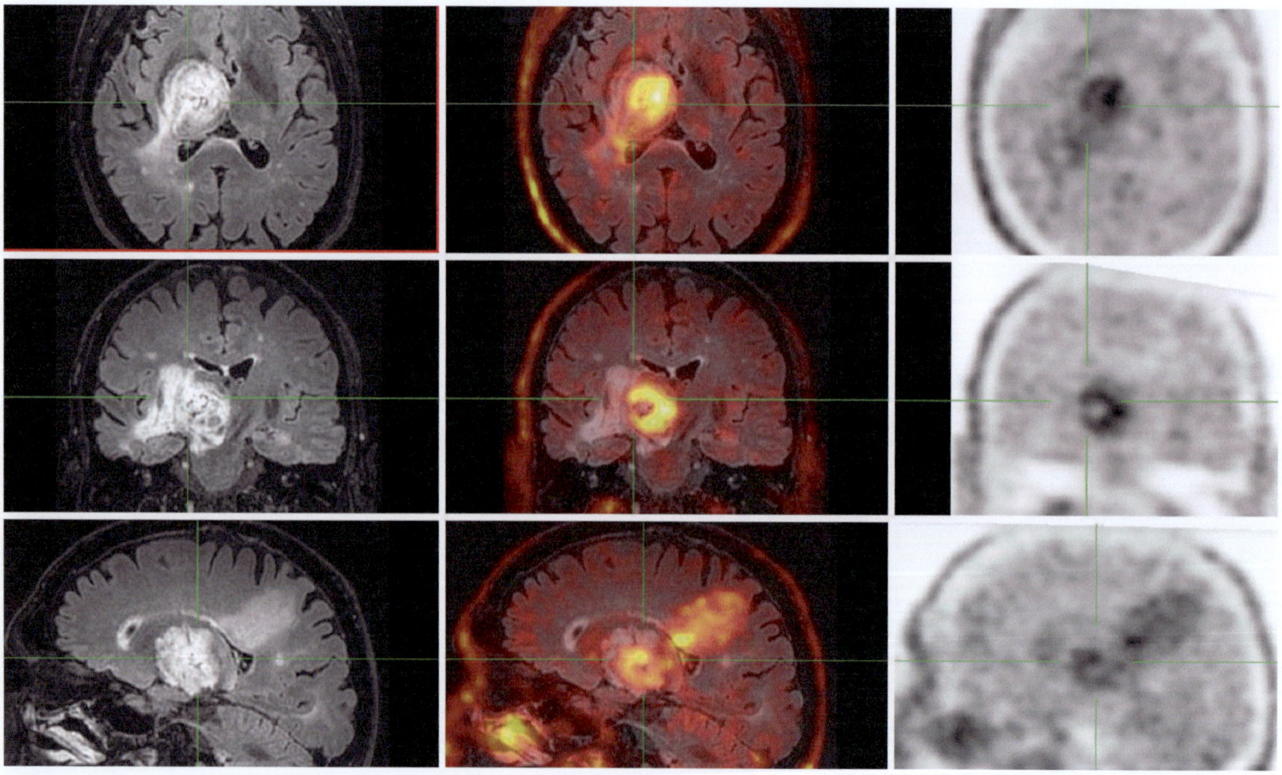

Fig. 8.9 Fused 18F-FET and FLAIR images showing the thalamic mass, with a hypometabolic centre and a temporo-parietal ipsilateral extension

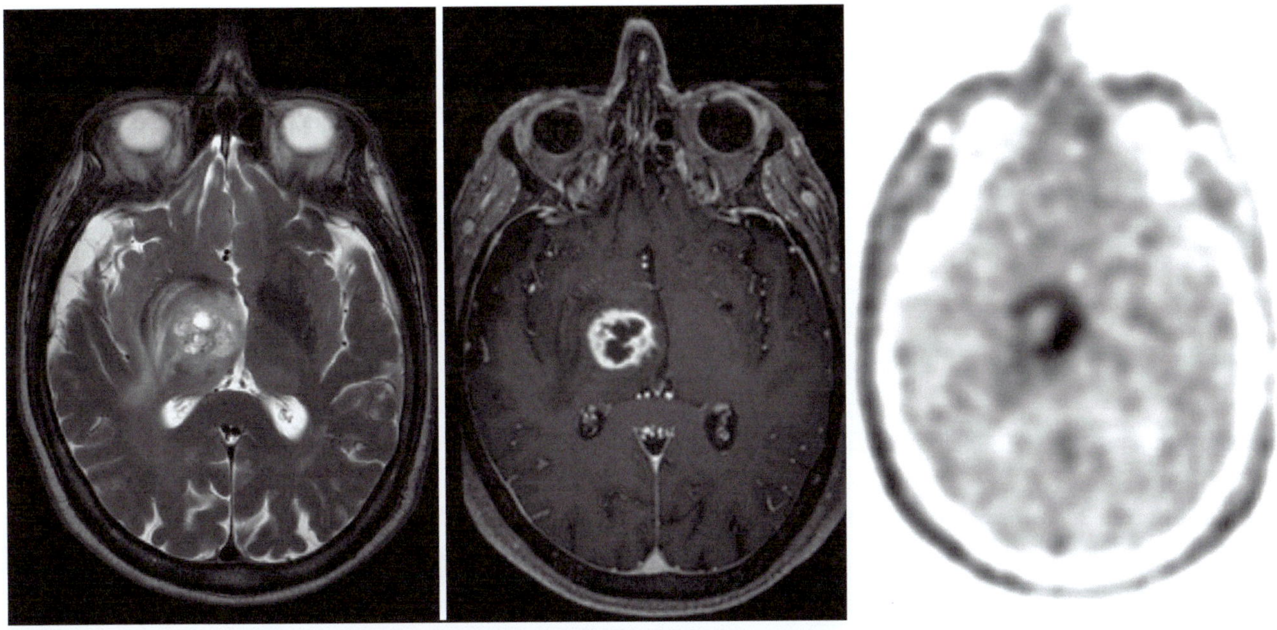

Fig. 8.10 From *left* to *right*: T2w, T1Gd and 18F-FET PET images of the thalamic lesion, showing the concordance between the gadolinium ring enhancement and the tracer uptake

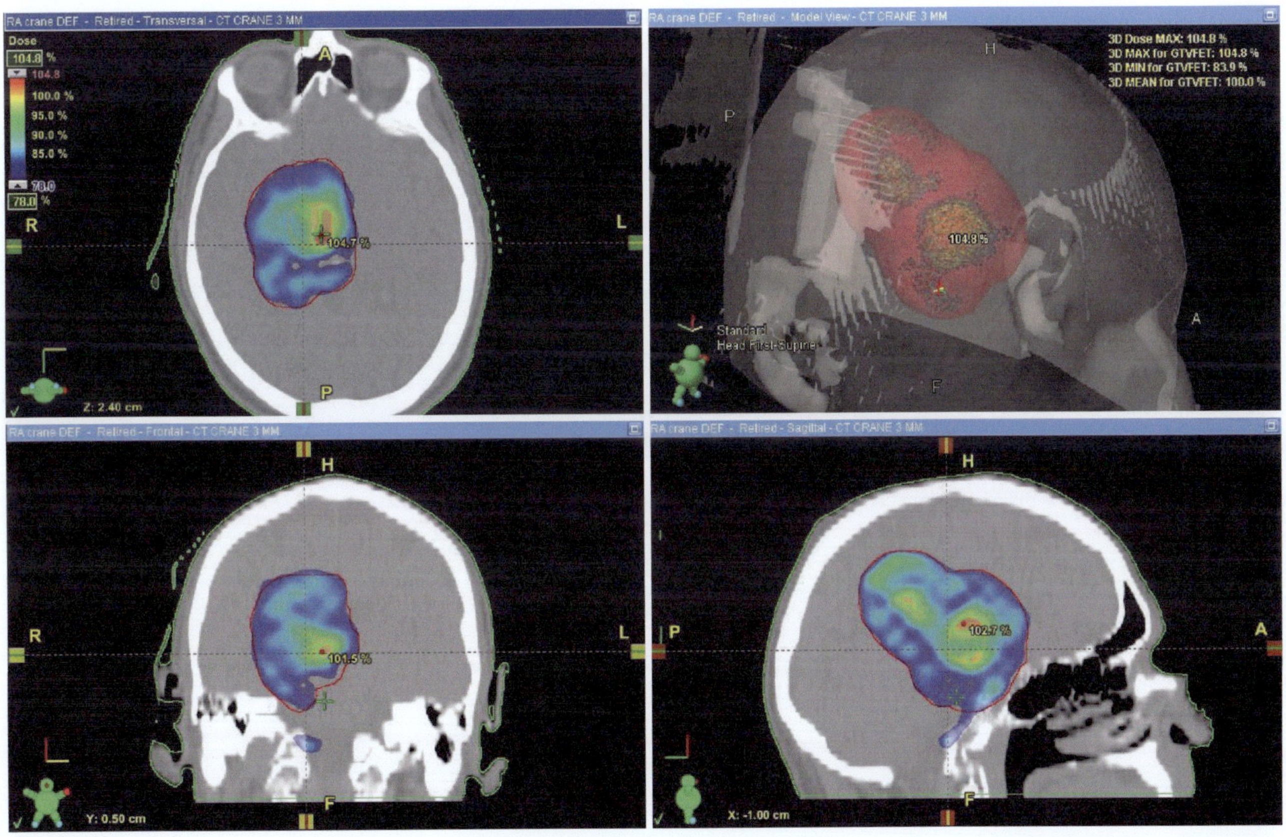

Fig. 8.11 Radiation therapy volume definition, identifying gross tumor volume and the most active tumor components to be treated with a simultaneous integrated boost

Brain Tumors – Follow Up

Clinical History

Ten-year-old F followed up for medulloblastoma treated by surgery and chemo-radiotherapy. PET/MR indication: restaging.

Imaging Technique

Brain PET images acquired 30–50 min after iv injection 213 MBq 18F-Fluoroethyltyrosine (FET), head MRI (T1W 3D with Gadolinium administration, T2W turbo spin echo, fluid attenuated inversion recovery, arterial spin labeling, diffusion tensor imaging; SENSE Head-8 coil).

Findings

Brain PET/MR shows surgical sequelae, and no focal MR alteration or focal 18F-FET uptake.

Teaching Points

Brain PET/MR can be realized as a one-stop diagnostic procedure for the follow-up of brain tumors, providing an accurate evaluation of various morphological and metabolic parameters and avoiding the radiation dose CT-related of the PET/CT.

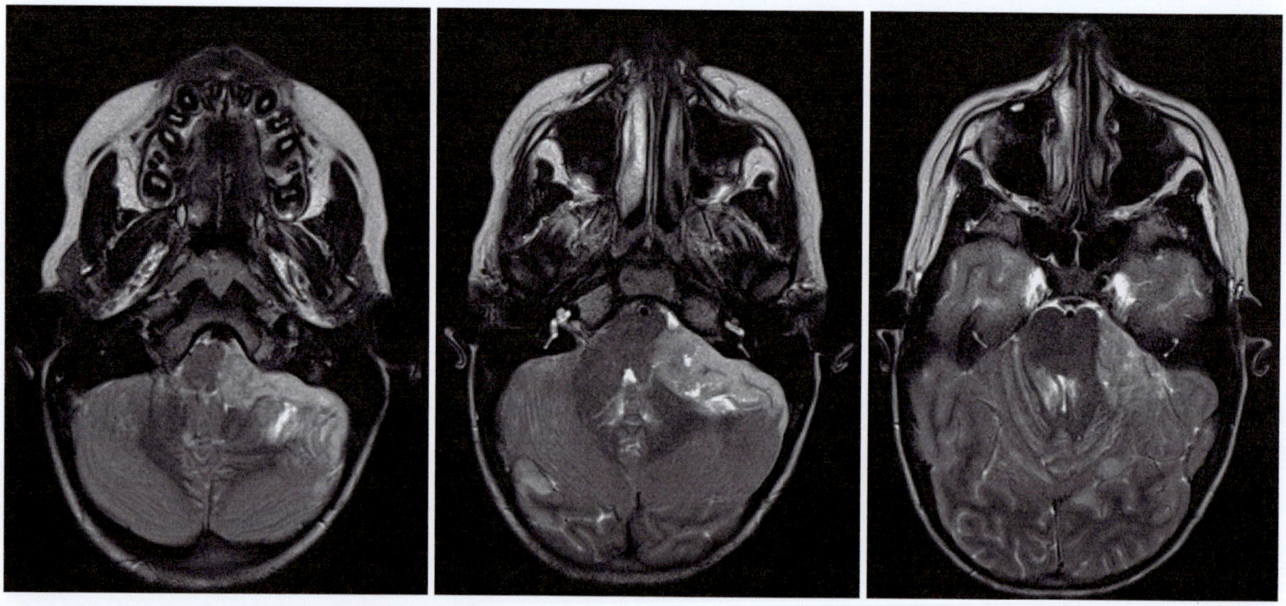

Fig. 8.12 MRI realized at diagnosis, showing a large mass centered on the left ponto-cerebellar cistern

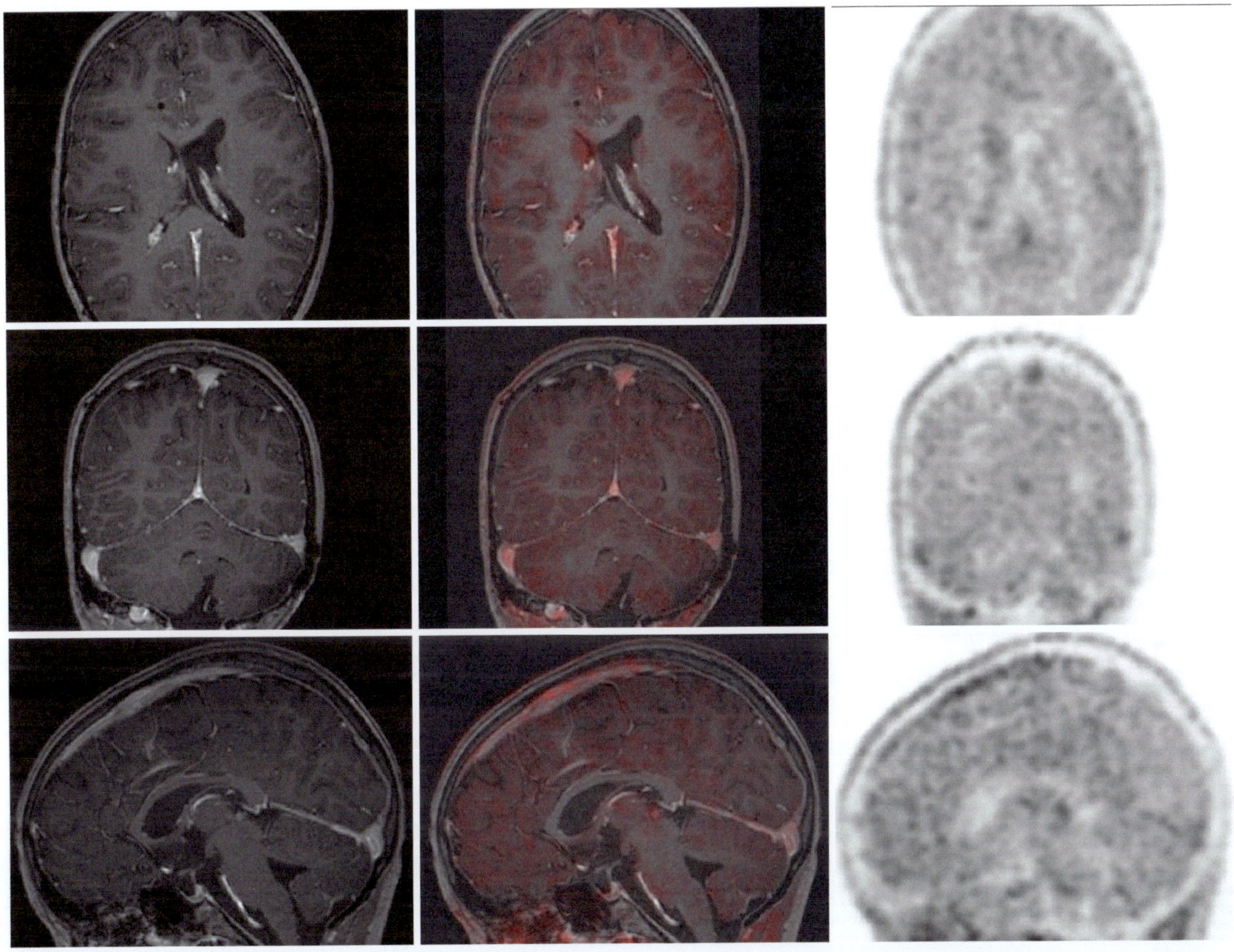

Fig. 8.13 Fused 18F-FET and T1w Gd enhanced images showing the surgical sequelae in the left posterior fossa and the ventriculo peritoneal drain, but no findings indicating tumor recurrence

Brain Lesions – Radiation Necrosis

Clinical History

Thirty-four-year-old M with treated 2 years earlier by surgery and proton-therapy for a chordoma of the clivus. MR follow-up shows the appearance of an intra-axial left mesiotemporal lesion. PET/MR indication: differentiation between radiation necrosis and tumor recurrence.

Imaging Technique

Brain PET images acquired 30–50 min after iv injection 213 MBq 18F-Fluoroethyltyrosine (FET), head MRI (T1W 3D with Gadolinium administration, T2W turbo spin echo, fluid attenuated inversion recovery, diffusion weighted imaging, spectroscopy; SENSE Head-8 coil).

Findings

Brain PET shows a significant uptake in the MR-enhancing intraaxial left mesiotemporal lesion. The uptake is moderate to high and does not allow differentiating radiation necrosis from tumor extension. The lesion has a significant contrast enhancement. The radiological follow-up showed lesion regression in the absence of any treatment supporting the benign origin of these findings.

Teaching Points

Brain PET/MR might show significant enhancement and 18F-FET uptake for an active radiation necrosis lesion: this finding highlights the importance of interpreting with caution these imaging findings after radiation therapy. A follow-up examination might be required in the case of positive findings.

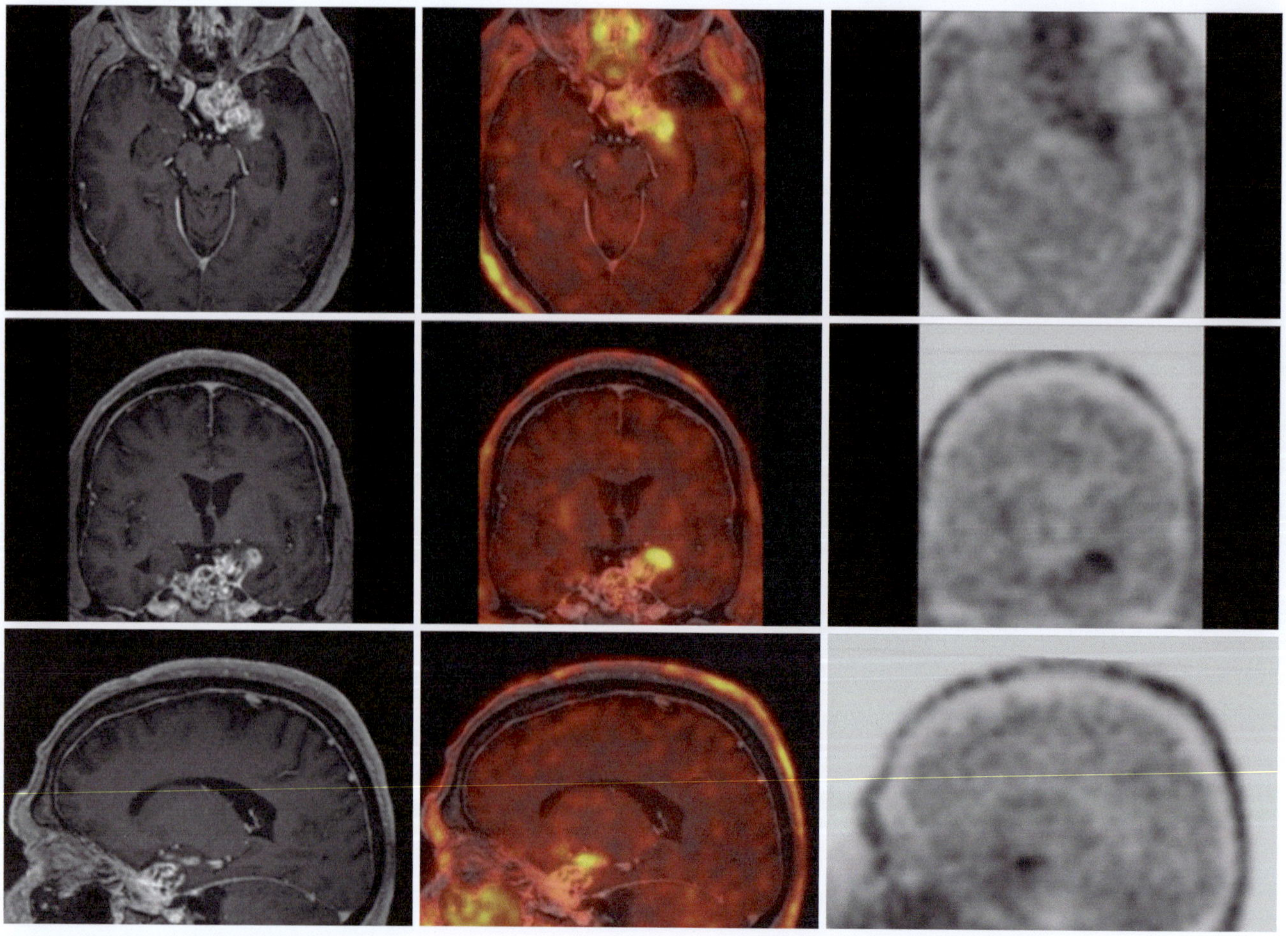

Fig. 8.14 Fused 18F-FET and T1w Gd images showing the clivus mass, the mesiotemporal left lesion and a millimetric contrast enhancement on the right mesiotemporal cortex

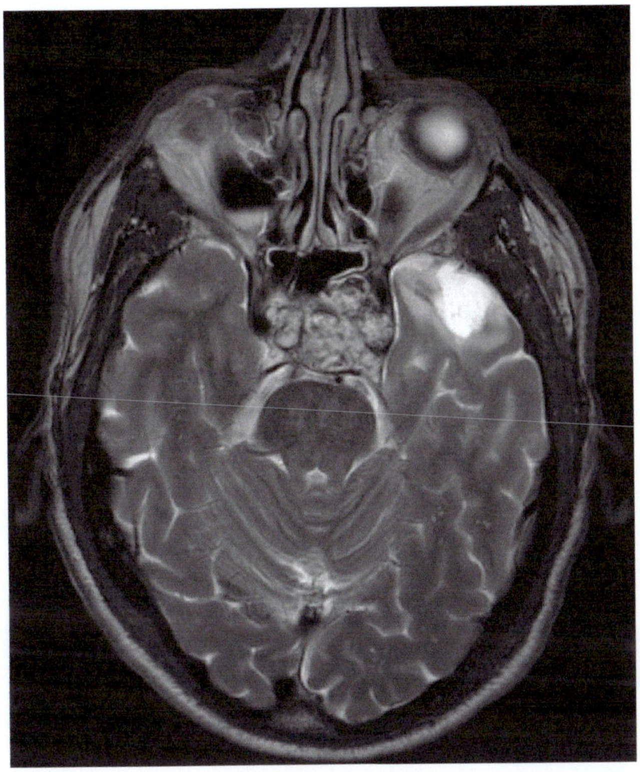

Fig. 8.15 T2w image showing the chordoma of the clivus and a temporo-polar surgical sequela

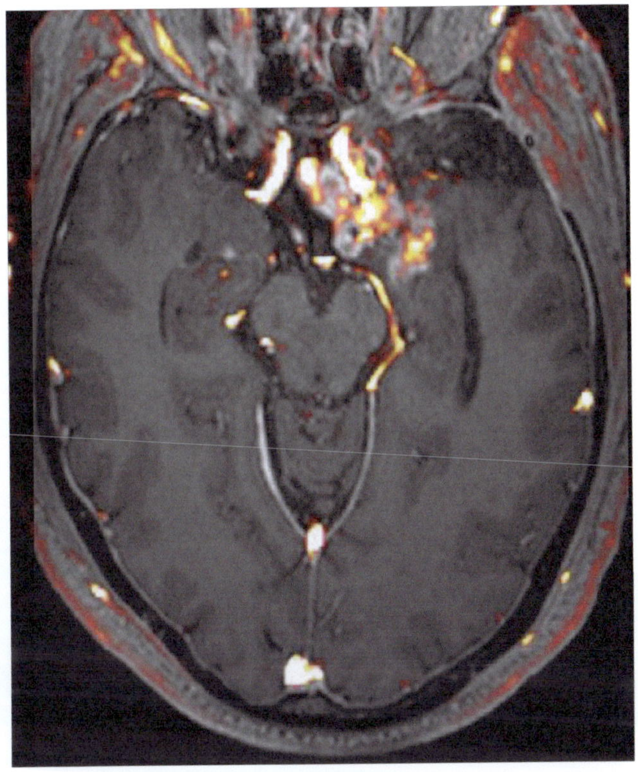

Fig. 8.16 Fused T1w and ASL images showing perfusion of the chordoma of the clivus and of the temporomesial lesion

Fig. 8.17 MR spectroscopy of the left mesiotemporal lesion

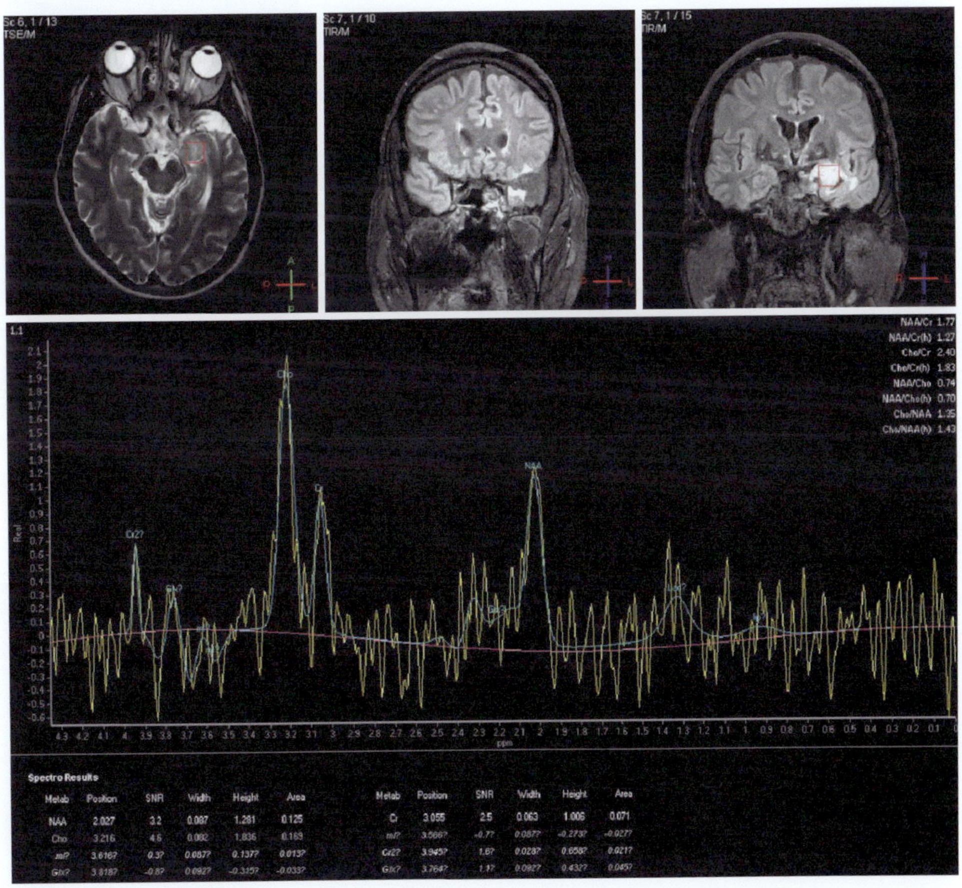

Skull Base Meningioma

Clinical History

Fifty-six year old patient scheduled for stereotactic radiation therapy presenting with meningioma of the right sphenoid bone adjacent to the carotid artery.

Imaging Technique

PET/MR images of the head were acquired 18 min after iv injection 67 MBq 68Ga-DOTANOC.

T1 VIBE Dixon for attenuation correction. Axial T1 MPRAGE+CM, axial FLAIR, axial T2 dark-fluid.

Findings

T1w MRI shows a highly enhancing formation in the region of the right cavernous sinus which correlates with a focal DOTANOC accumulation in PET. The findings are consistent with a skull base meningioma. T2 dark-fluid MRI shows encasement of the artery by the tumor but no indirect signs of obstruction.

Teaching Points

68Ga-DOTANOC detects meningiomas with high sensitivity and excellent tumor to background ration. MRI provides information about adjacent critical structures as required for radiation therapy planning.

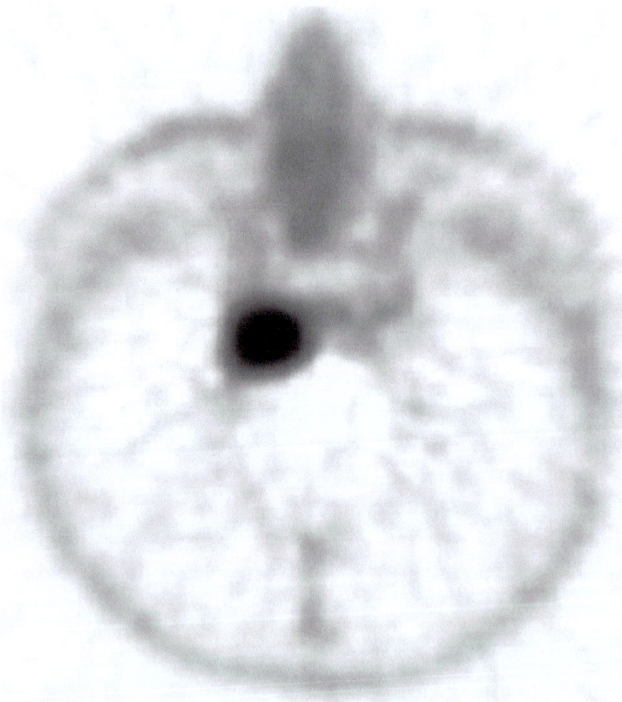

Fig. 8.18 Axial Ga68-DOTANOC PET image shows high intensity focal uptake in the region of the right cavernous sinus

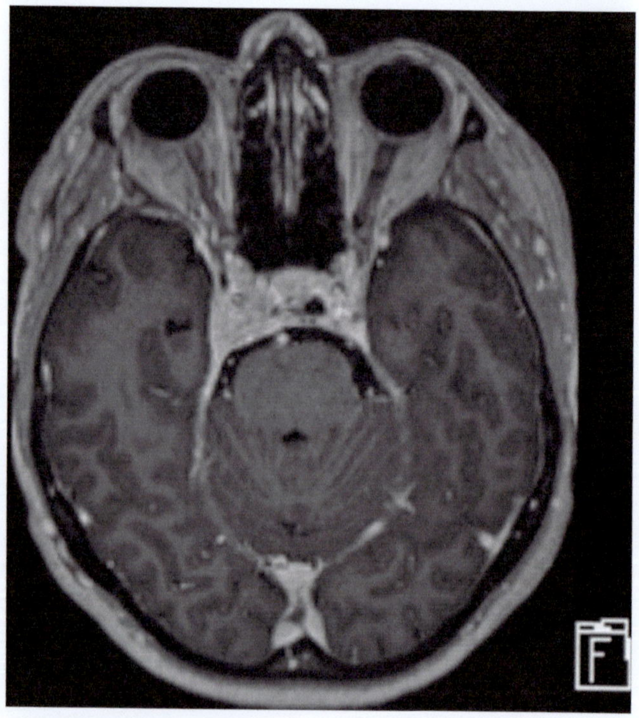

Fig. 8.19 Axial T1w MRI after Gadolinium injection anatomically outlines of the meningioma in the sphenoid bone

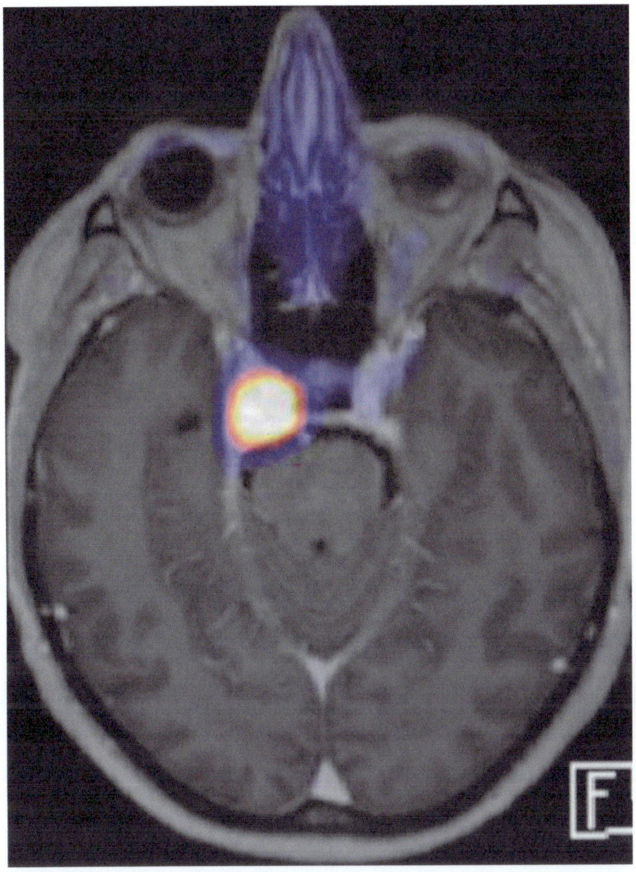

Fig. 8.20 Fusion of PET and T1w MRI demonstrates perfect coregistration of DOTANOC-uptake and MRI

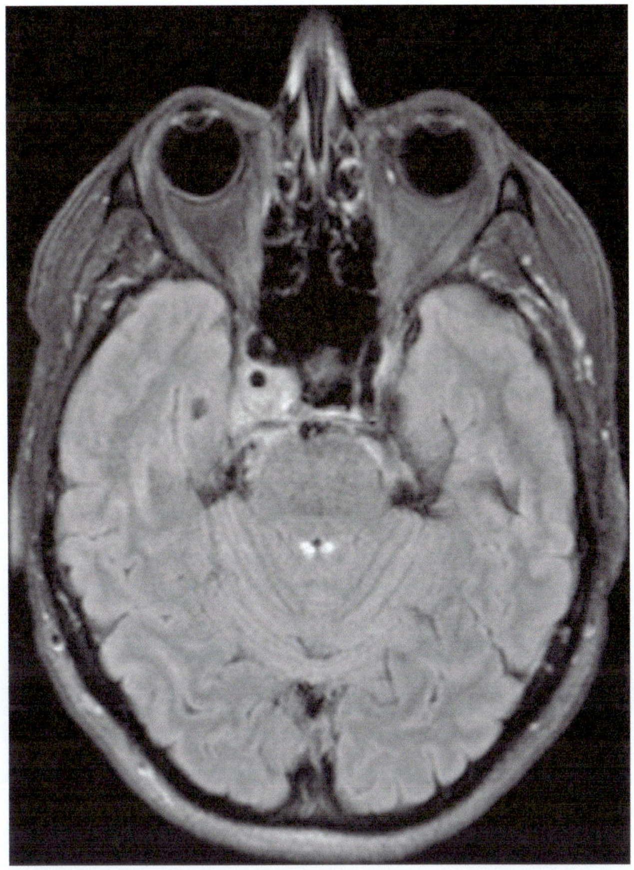

Fig. 8.21 Axial T2 dark-fluid MRI shows encasement of the carotid artery by the meningioma. Note that the flow-void of the vessel lumen is preserved

Convexity Meningioma

Clinical History

Seventy-nine year old female patient scheduled for stereotactic radiation therapy of a recurrent convexity meningioma.

Imaging Technique

Injection of 95 MBq 68Ga-DOTANOC. Start of acquisition after 25 min, 1 bed position. T1 VIBE Dixon for attenuation correction. 3D-MPRAGE + Gd.

Findings

Intense DOTANOC-uptake corresponding to a moderately enhancing structure seen in MRI consistent with a convexity meningioma. Physiologic DOTATOC-uptake is seen in the pituitary gland.

Teaching Points

Coregistration of DOTATOC-PET and MRI allows differentiation of scar tissue from somatostatin-receptor expressing tumor tissue in recurrent meningioma as required for radiation therapy planning.

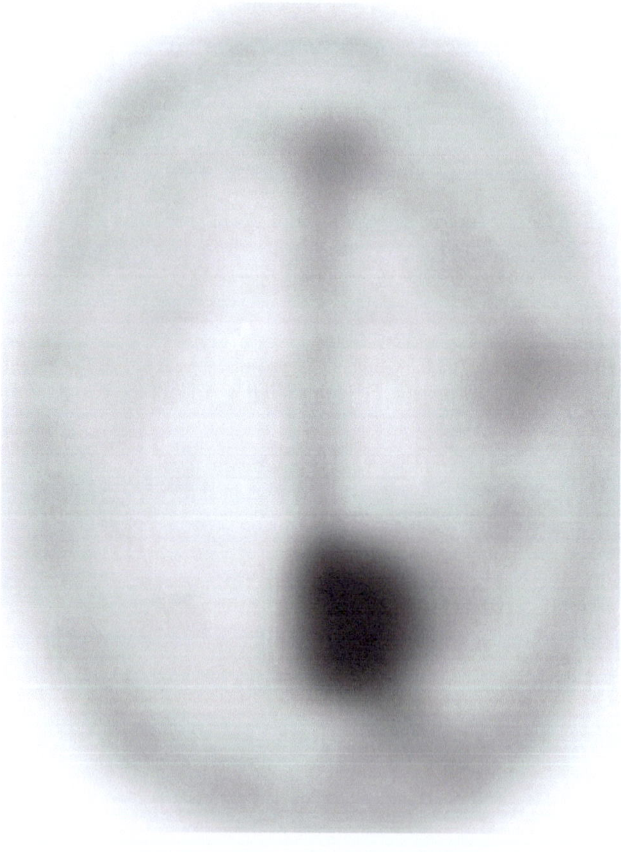

Fig. 8.22 Axial PET image shows intense DOTATOC accumulation indicating somatostatin-receptor expression

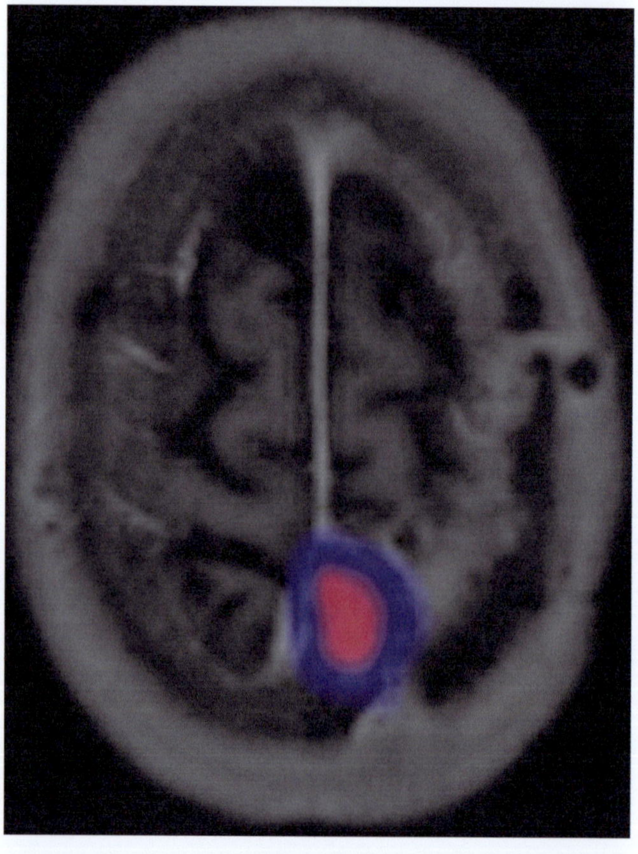

Fig. 8.23 Fusion of axial MPRAGE after contrast media from MRI and PET. The trepanation defect due to a recent operation can be seen in MRI

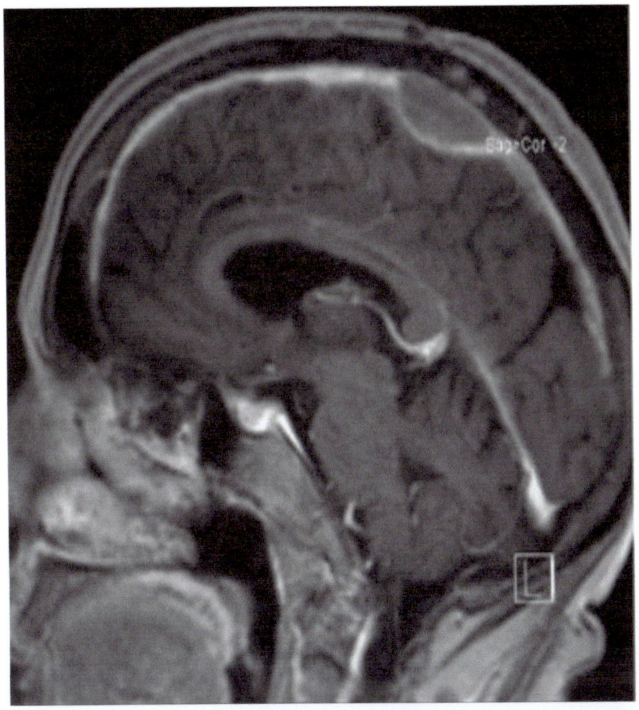

Fig. 8.24 Sagittal fusion of MPRAGE after contrast media from MRI and PET. The trepanation defect due to a recent operation can be seen. Physiologic tracer accumulation in the pituitary gland

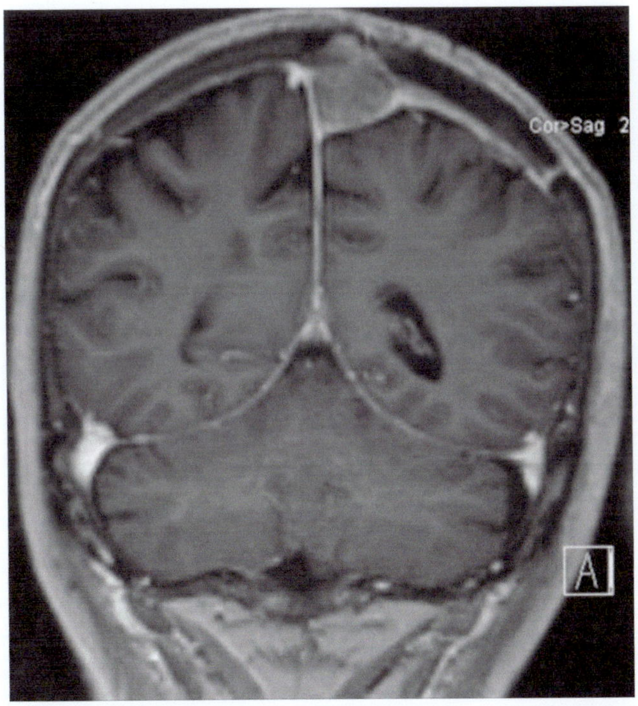

Fig. 8.25 Coronal MPRAGE after contrast media

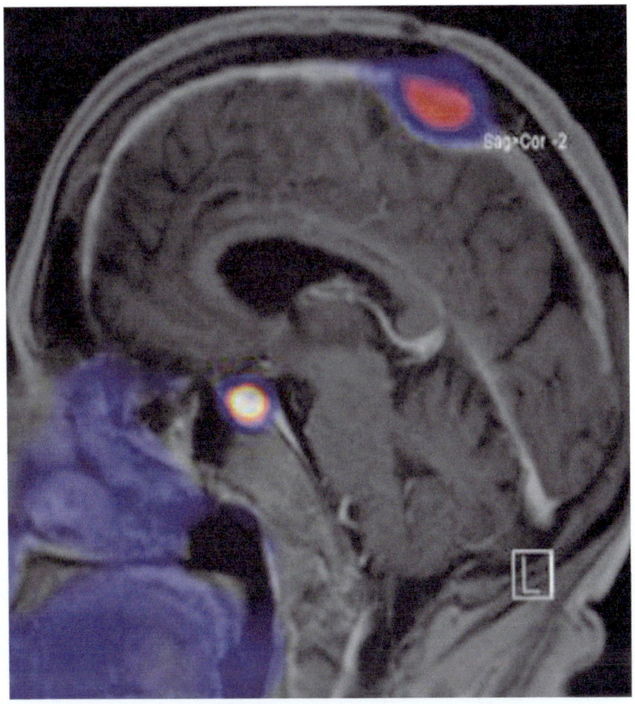

Fig. 8.26 Sagittal MPRAGE MRI. The trepanation defect due to a recent operation can be seen

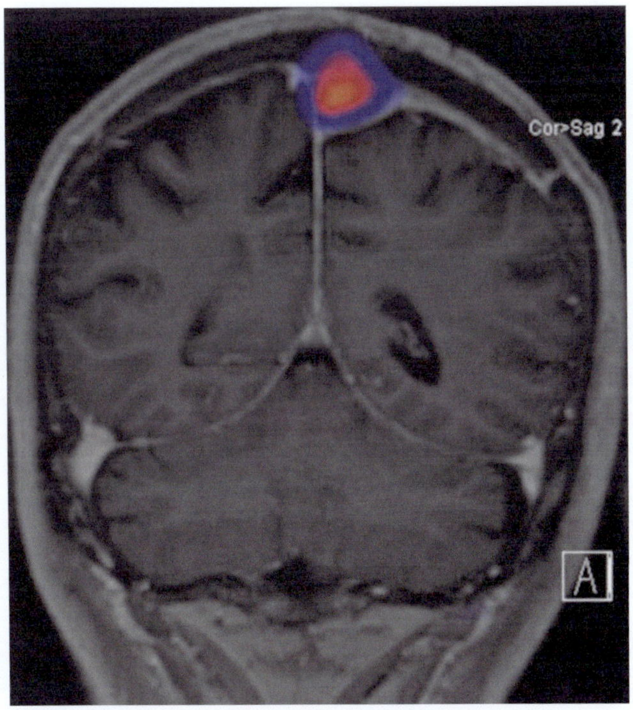

Fig. 8.27 Fusion of PET with coronal MPRAGE after contrast media

Recurrent Glioblastoma

Clinical History

Forty-nine-year-old patient with glioblastoma resection in right parietal lobe 2 years ago and adjuvant radio-chemotherapy. Tumor recurrence or posttherapeutic changes?

Imaging Technique

PET measurement started 42 min after injection of 128 MBq [18F]FET. Simultaneous acquisistion of MRI sequences (Dixon, T1, T2, CE T1 and T2 FLAIR).

Findings

Two foci of increased amino acid uptake, in the right parietal lobe adjacent to the resection cavity and in the right anterior cingulate gyrus, suggest viable tumor recurrence. Only the large parietal lesion shows contrast enhancement in T1w MRI as well as clear T2 FLAIR hyperintensity.

Teaching Points

Compared to conventional MRI alone, FET-PET may increase diagnostic specificity in the detection of recurrent glioma.

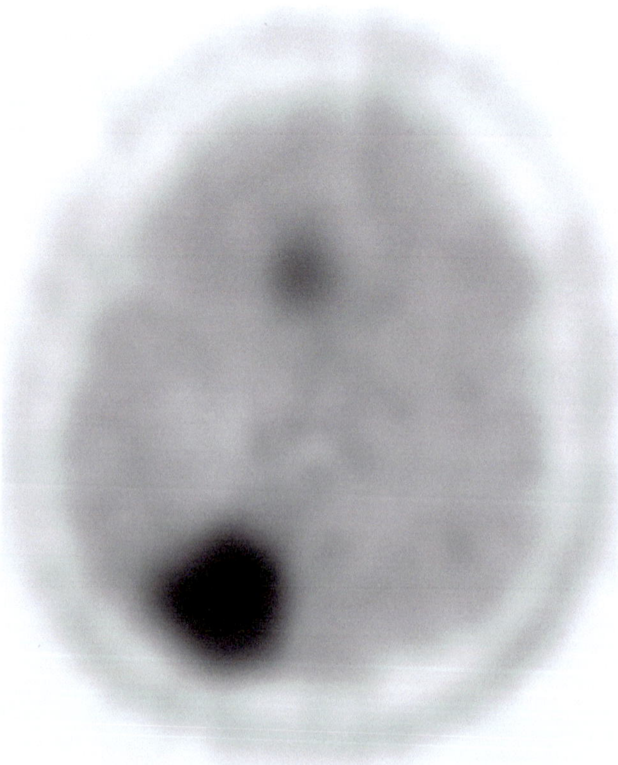

Fig. 8.28 [18F]FET PET study showing Two foci of increased amino acid uptake, suggesting viable tumor recurrence

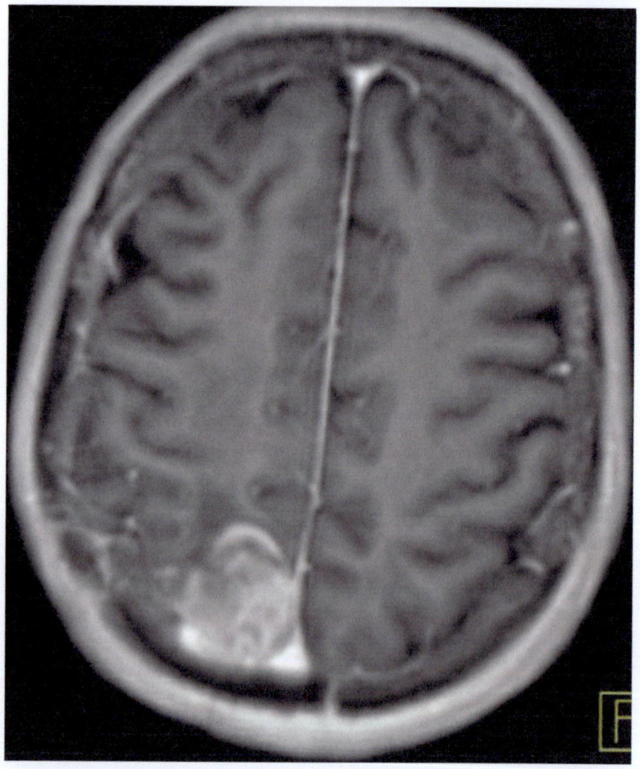

Fig. 8.29 T1 (CE) MRI sequence showing the localization of the posterior lesion in the right parietal lobe adjacent to the resection cavity

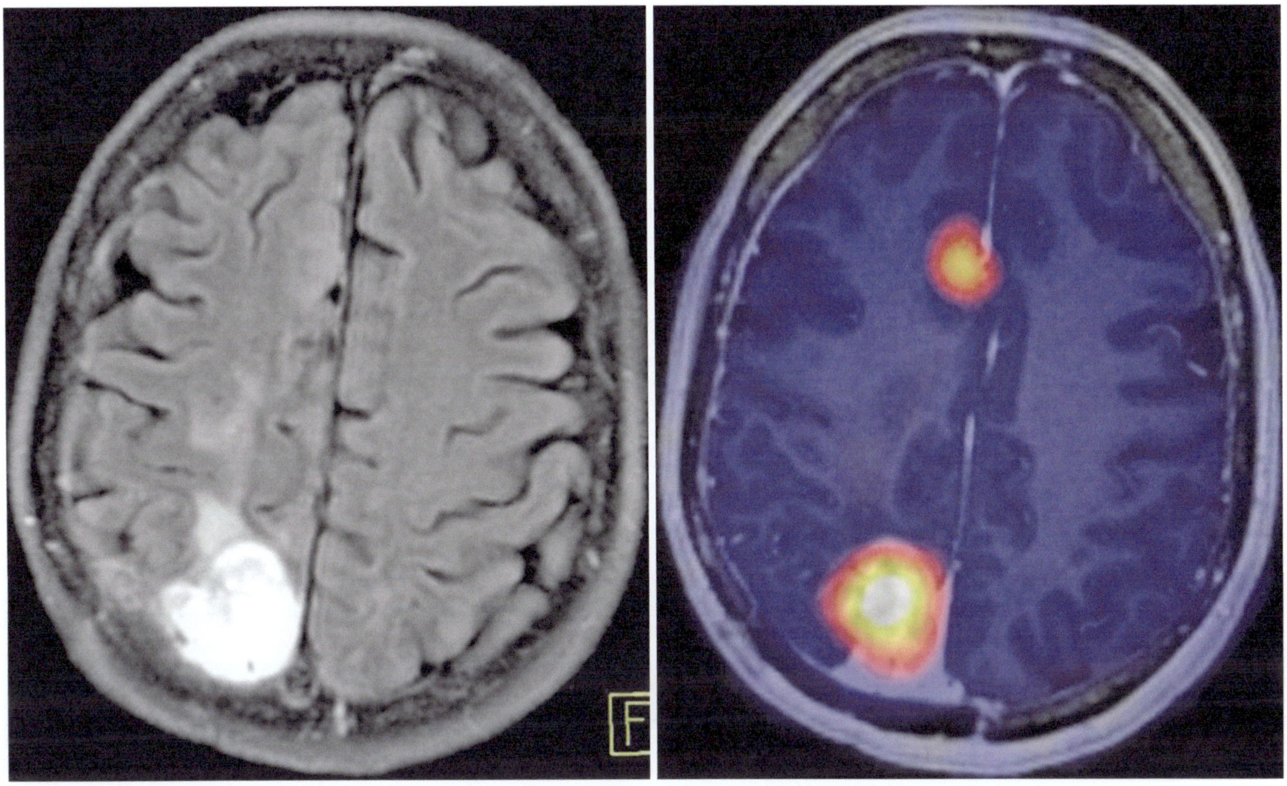

Fig. 8.30 T2-FLAIR MRI (*left*) and fused PET MR image (*right*) allowing a better localization of the recurrent tumor lesions

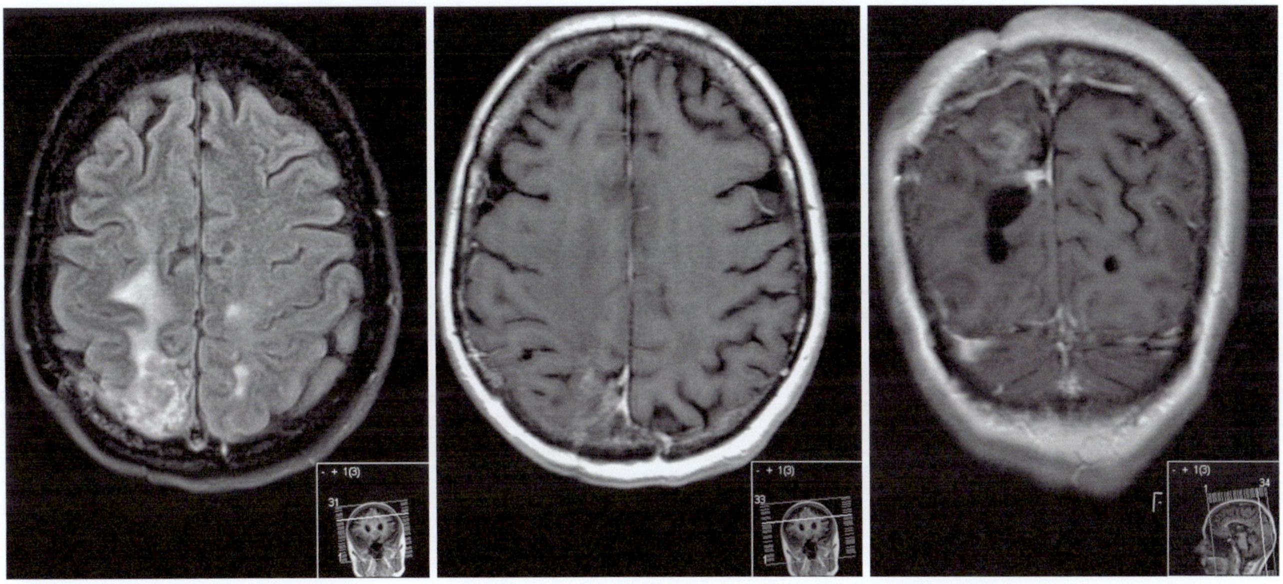

Fig. 8.31 MR follow-up after 3 months Avastine treatment showing decreased contrast enhancement of the parietal lesion in T1w image axial (*middle*) and coronal image (*right*) and decreasing size of the lesion in Flair image (*left*) confirming the response to therapy

Meningioma

Clinical History

Seventy-three-year-old patient with newly diagnosed meningioma.

Imaging Technique

PET measurement started 47 min after injection of 95 MBq [68Ga]-DOTANOC. Simultaneous acquisistion of MRI sequences (Dixon, T1, T2, CE T1 and T2 FLAIR).

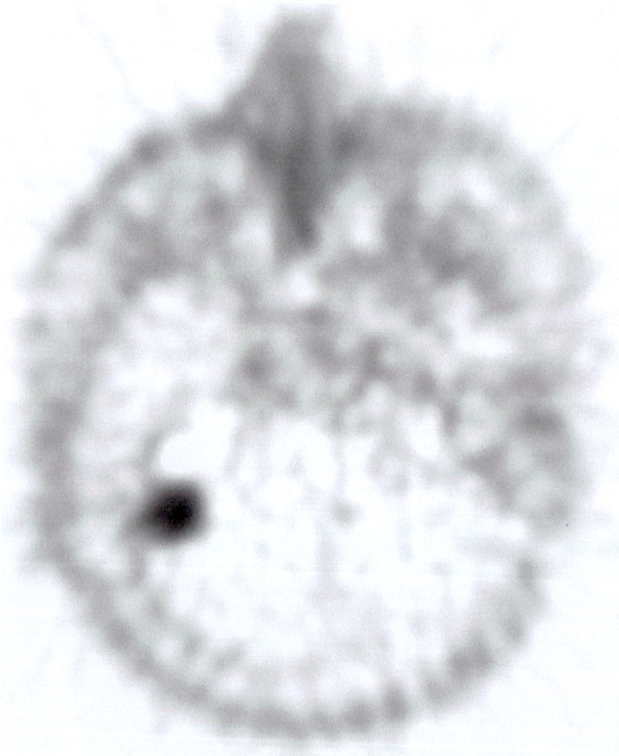

Fig. 8.32 [68Ga]-DOTANOC PET image shows a posterior focal tracer uptake identifying tumor with somatostatin receptor expression

Findings

Intense somatostatin receptor expression in the FLAIR hyperintense lesion adjacent to ventrolateral right cerebellar hemisphere, transverse/sigmoid sinus and petrous bone. The lesion shows typical strong contrast enhancement in the T1w image.

> **Teaching Points**
>
> DOTANOC PET/MR may be useful for accurate tumor delineation in the therapy planning of meningioma.

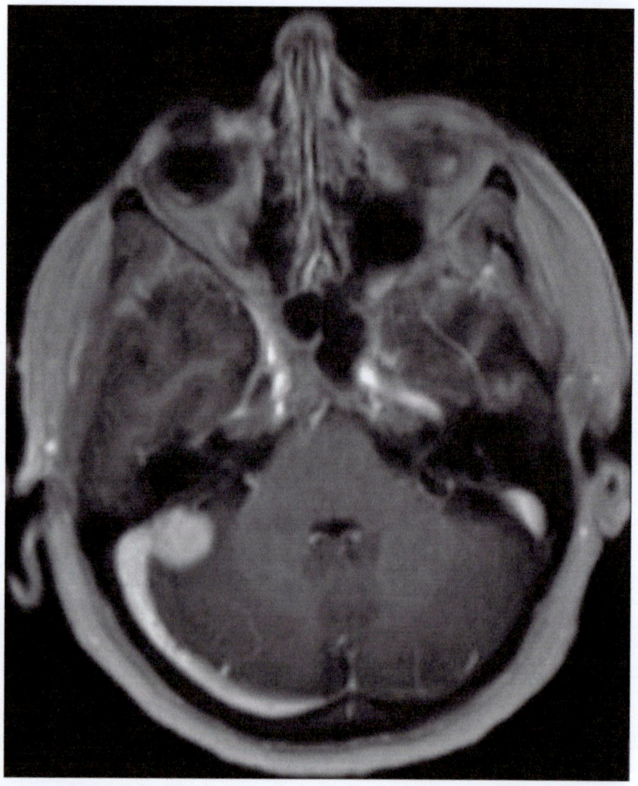

Fig. 8.33 T1 weighted (CE) MR image showing typical strong contrast enhancement in the tumoral lesion

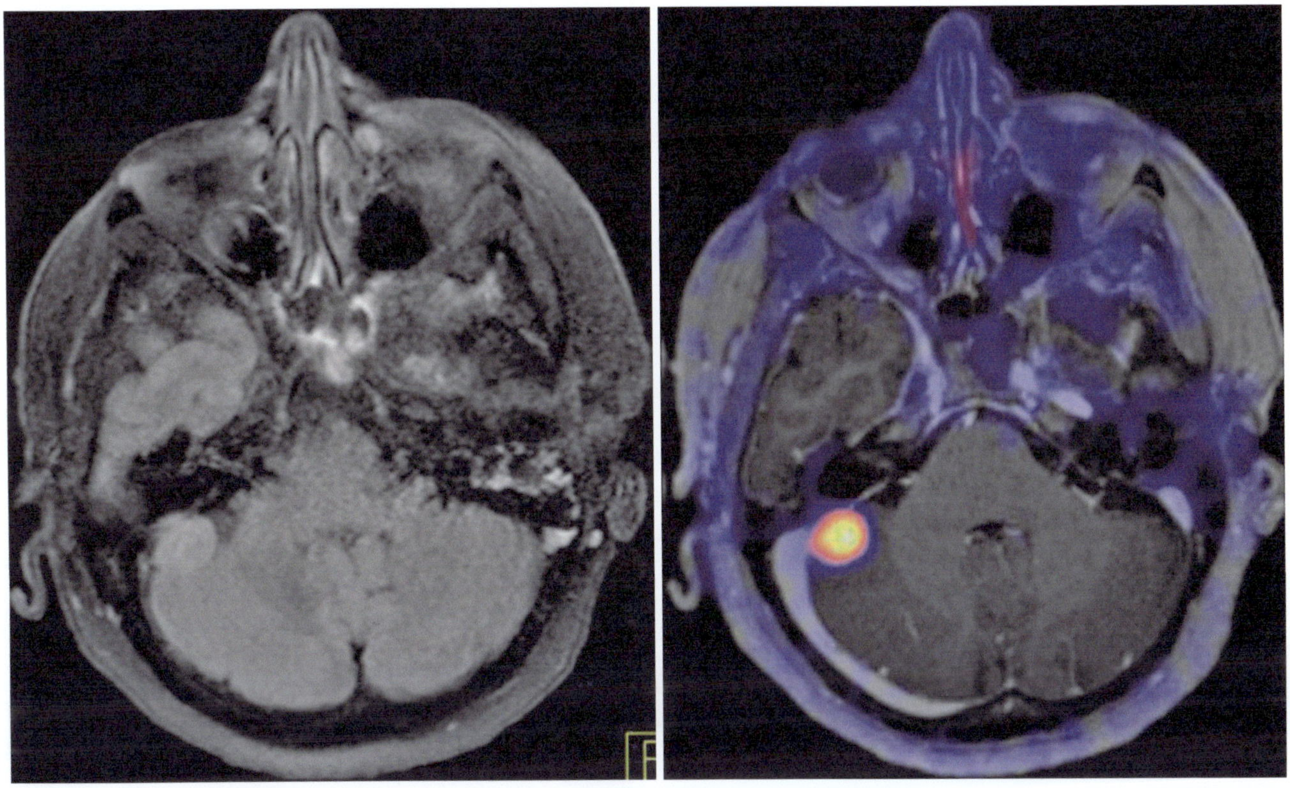

Fig. 8.34 T2 weighted (FLAIR) MR image and PET/MR fusion image for more accurate localization of tumor tissue

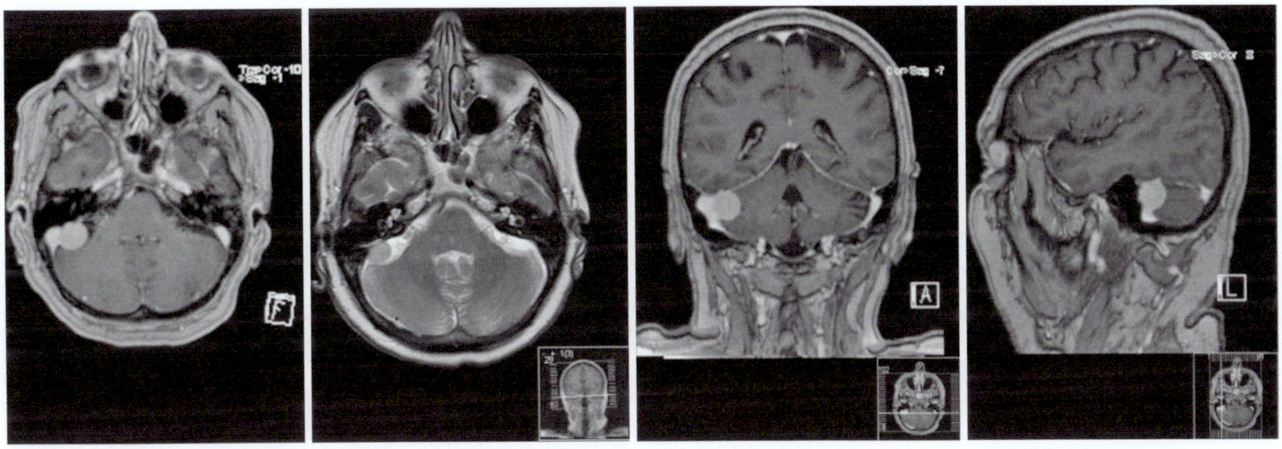

Fig. 8.35 Broad contact of the meningioma to the transverse sinus seen in axial, saggital and coronal view in the T1w sequence after Gd. Corresponding axial T2w dataset shows a moderate hypointensity (*second left image*)

Brain Metastases

Clinical History

Seventy-nine-year-old patient with metastatic SCLC; gamma-knife irradiation of a cerebellar metastasis 18 months ago; now rising CEA tumor marker values and unsuspicious extracranial staging.

Imaging Technique

PET measurement started 42 min after injection of 147 MBq FET. Simultaneous acquisition of MRI sequences (Dixon, T1, T2, CE T1 and T2 FLAIR).

Findings

Increased ring-shaped amino acid uptake in the left cerebellar hemisphere suggesting recurrent/viable metastasis with central necrosis. T1w image shows no relevant contrast enhancement. T2 FLAIR hyper intensity of the whole left cerebellar hemisphere may either be caused by peritumoral edema or post-radiogenic changes.

Teaching Points

FET-PET/MR for diagnosis of (recurrent) brain metastases is promising but must still be validated, due to the large heterogeneity of brain metastases.

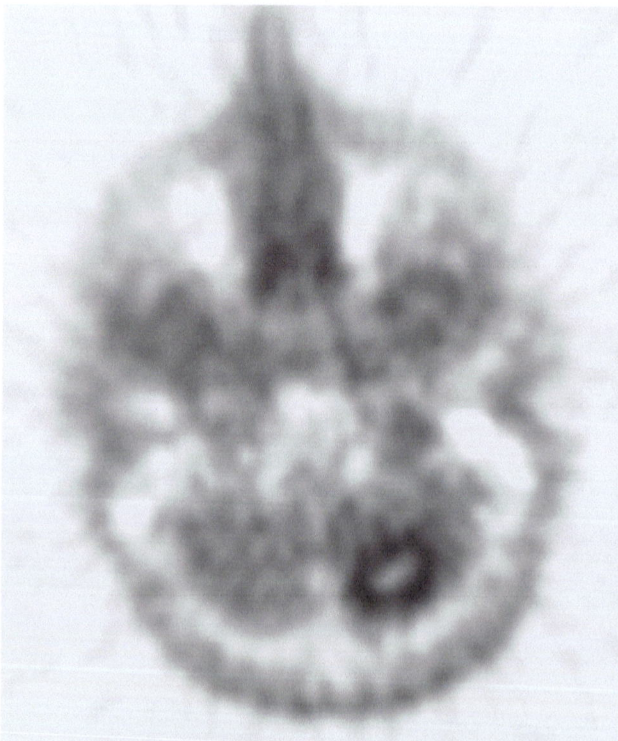

Fig. 8.36 Axial FET PET showing a left cerebellar circular tracer uptake with central defect compatible with local metastasis and a central necrosis

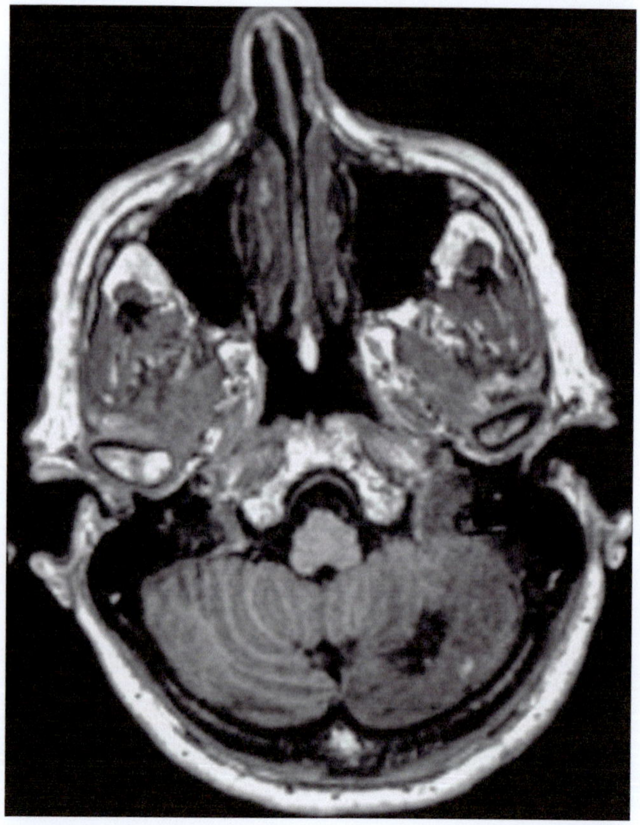

Fig. 8.37 Left cerebellar metastasis showing as low intensity lesion on T1 weighted (CE) MRI images

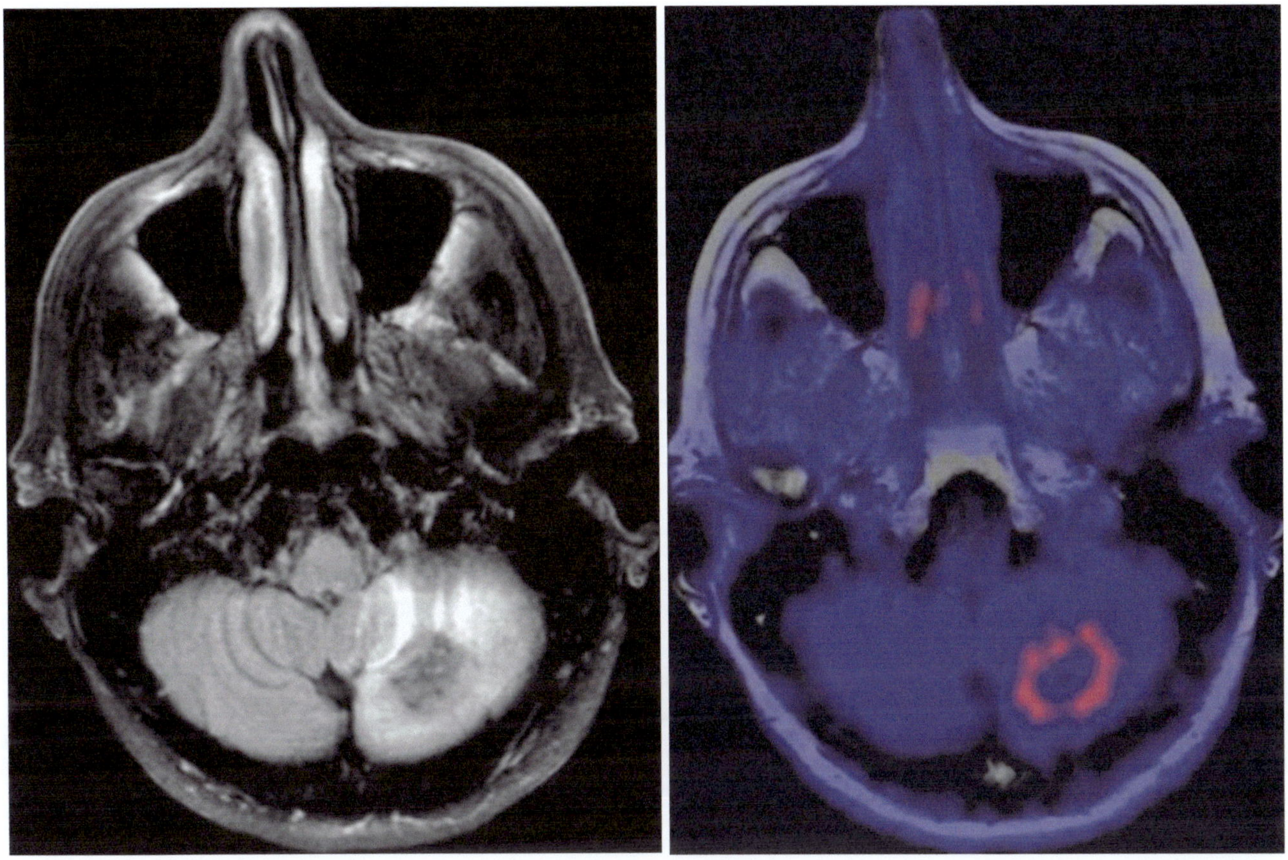

Fig. 8.38 T2 weighted Flair MRI image showing diffuse hyperintensity surrounding left cerebellar metastasis and the fused PET/MR image at the same level showing the hypermetabolic left cerebellar metastasis of a SCLC

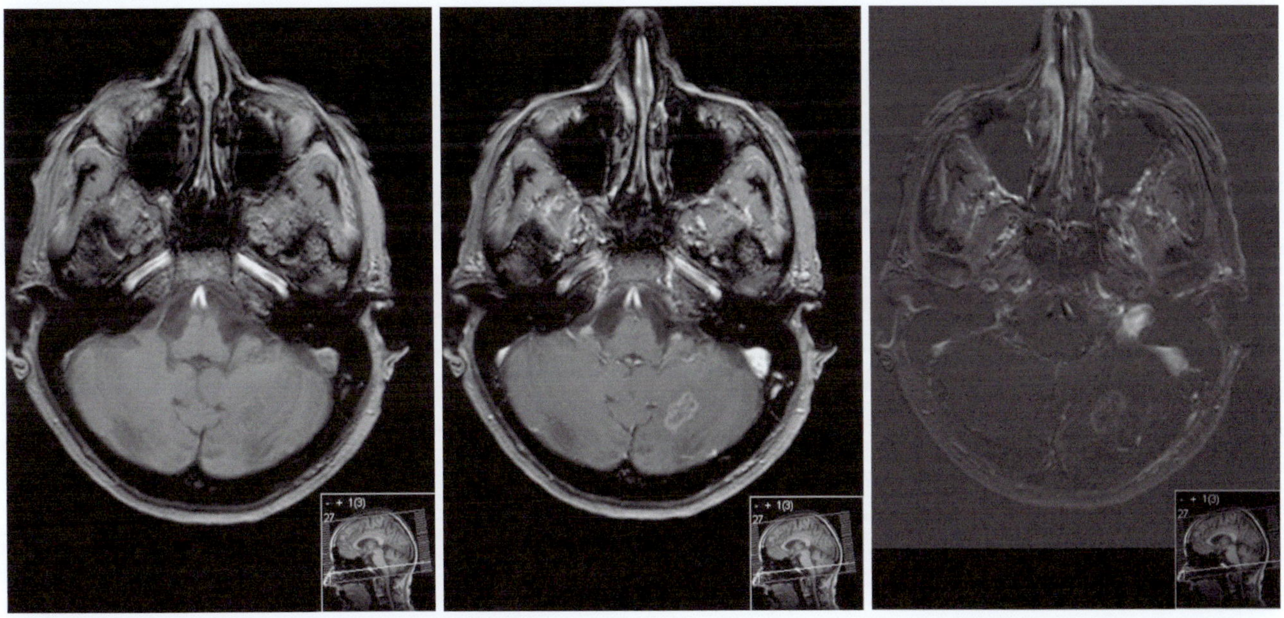

Fig. 8.39 Pre-therapeutic axial T1w images before (*left*) and after (*middle*) Gd injection as well as subtraction image (*right*) show initial circular contrast enhancement of the left cerebellar metastasis

Further Reading

Boss A, Bisdas S, Kolb A et al (2010) Hybrid PET/MRI of intracranial masses: initial experiences and comparison to PET/CT. J Nucl Med 51:1198–1205

Catana C, Drzezga A, Heiss WD, Rosen BR (2012) PET/MRI for neurologic applications. J Nucl Med 53:1916–1925

Garibotto V, Forster S, Haller S, Vargas MI, Drzezga A (2013) Molecular neuroimaging with PET/MRI. Clinical and Translational Imaging 1:53–63

Garibotto V, Heinzer S, Vulliemoz S et al (2013) Clinical applications of hybrid PET/MRI in neuroimaging. Clin Nucl Med 38:e13–e18

Herzog H, Langen KJ, Weirich C et al (2011) High resolution brainPET combined with simultaneous MRI. Nuklearmedizin 50:74–82

Khayal IS, McKnight TR, McGue C et al (2009) Apparent diffusion coefficient and fractional anisotropy of newly diagnosed grade II gliomas. NMR Biomed 22:449–455

Neuner I, Kaffanke JB, Langen KJ et al (2012) Multimodal imaging utilising integrated MR-PET for human brain tumour assessment. Eur Radiol 22(12):2568–2580

Noguchi T, Yoshiura T, Hiwatashi A et al (2008) Perfusion imaging of brain tumors using arterial spin-labeling: correlation with histopathologic vascular density. AJNR Am J Neuroradiol 29: 688–693

Popperl G, Gotz C, Rachinger W et al (2004) Value of O-(2-[18F]fluoroethyl)-L-tyrosine PET for the diagnosis of recurrent glioma. Eur J Nucl Med Mol Imaging 31:1464–1470

Schwenzer NF, Stegger L, Bisdas S et al (2012) Simultaneous PET/MR imaging in a human brain PET/MR system in 50 patients-Current state of image quality. Eur J Radiol 81(11):3472–3478

Terakawa Y, Tsuyuguchi N, Iwai Y et al (2008) Diagnostic accuracy of 11C-methionine PET for differentiation of recurrent brain tumors from radiation necrosis after radiotherapy. J Nucl Med 49: 694–699

Thorwarth D, Henke G, Muller AC et al (2011) Simultaneous 68Ga-DOTATOC-PET/MRI for IMRT treatment planning for meningioma: first experience. Int J Radiat Oncol Biol Phys 81:277–283

Vander Borght T, Asenbaum S, Bartenstein P et al (2006) EANM procedure guidelines for brain tumour imaging using labelled amino acid analogues. Eur J Nucl Med Mol Imaging 33:1374–1380

9 Pediatric Oncology

M. Eiber, L. Merlini, O. Ratib, K. Scheidhauer, M. Souvatzoglou, C. Tabouret-Viaud, and T. Zand

Contents

M. Eiber (✉)
Department of Radiology, Klinikum Rechts der Isar, Technische Universität München, Munich, Germany
e-mail: matthias.eiber@tum.de

L. Merlini
Division of Pediatric Radiology, Department of Medical Imaging, Geneva University Hospitals, Geneva, Switzerland

O. Ratib
Division of Nuclear Medicine and Molecular Imaging, Department of Medical Imaging, Geneva University Hospitals, Geneva, Switzerland

K. Scheidhauer • M. Souvatzoglou
Department of Nuclear Medicine, Technische Universität München, Munich, Germany

C. Tabouret-Viaud
Division of Nuclear Medicine and Molecular Imaging, Department of Medical Imaging, Geneva University and Geneva University Hospitals, Geneva, Switzerland

T. Zand
Division of Pediatric Radiology, Department of Medical Imaging, Geneva University and Geneva University Hospitals, Geneva, Switzerland

Pediatric Oncology

In pediatric oncology ^{18}F-FDG PET/CT imaging is used mainly for staging and restaging of lymphoma and soft tissue and bone tumors. In this special patient collective minimizing the radiation dose is one of the major goals. With the introduction of PET/MR, the CT exposure component previously produced in PET/CT studies potentially can be eliminated [1]. Preliminary reports state that compared to PET/CT the radiation exposure from a single hybrid imaging PET/MR-scan is reduced by around 80 %, to only one effective dose of 4.6 mSv [2, 3]. In addition, especially in bone tumors (e.g. Ewing-sarcoma, multifocal osteosarcoma) patient require both whole-body MR and ^{18}F-FDG PET and, therefore, the combination of both examinations in one single session has also substantial logistical advantages (e.g. only one anesthesia).

Furthermore, compared to PET/CT this technique also enables whole-body diffusion-weighted imaging (DWI) providing additional information about cellularity and nuclear/cytoplasmic ratio of tumors. Recent studies in pediatric patients with lymphoma demonstrated high sensitivity for the detection of lesions and allows quantitative assessment of diffusion that may aid in the evaluation of malignant lymphomas [4]. For soft-tissue and bone tumors the advantage of PET/MR compared to PET/CT also lies in its high soft-tissue contrast [5]. ^{18}F-FDG PET/CT does not provide exact information as MRI for T-staging in sarcomas, however it can give additional prognostic information [6, 7]. e.g. in one study assessing therapy response in pediatric osteosarcomas ^{18}F-FDG PET could discriminate responders from nonresponders [8]. In regards of the advantages of both modalities integrated PET/MRI can replace PET/CT for these indications with a focus of the ^{18}F-FDG PET component for prognostic questions and assessment of N-stage and M-stage and the MR-examination on local staging.

O. Ratib et al. (eds.), *Atlas of PET/MR Imaging in Oncology*,
DOI 10.1007/978-3-642-31292-2_9, © Springer-Verlag Berlin Heidelberg 2013

Follow-up of Intestinal Adenocarcinoma

Clinical History

Seventeen-year-old patient after surgery and chemotherapy of a mucinous intestinal adenocarcinoma with complete remission 21 months after seven cycles of chemotherapy. Follow up study for staging of possible recurrence of an abdominal mass.

Imaging Technique

PET: Whole-body PET acquired 60 min after injection of 369 MBq of ^{18}F-FDG, 57 kg/157 cm patient, with 5.2 mmol/L of fasting glycemia.

MRI: Whole body atMR (T1 weighted), supine position. 3D Dixon, T2 weighted and STIR whole-body MRI.

Findings

PET/MR images confirmed the recurrence of tumoral tissue in a polymorphic mass in the pre-sacral area with combined solid and cystic components and increased FDG uptake in the sold parts of the tumor.

Teaching Points

While MR may sometimes be limited for evaluation of abdominal masses, PET/MR may provide adequate evaluation of solid masses in follow up of young patients avoiding unnecessary radiation from multiple PET/CT studies.

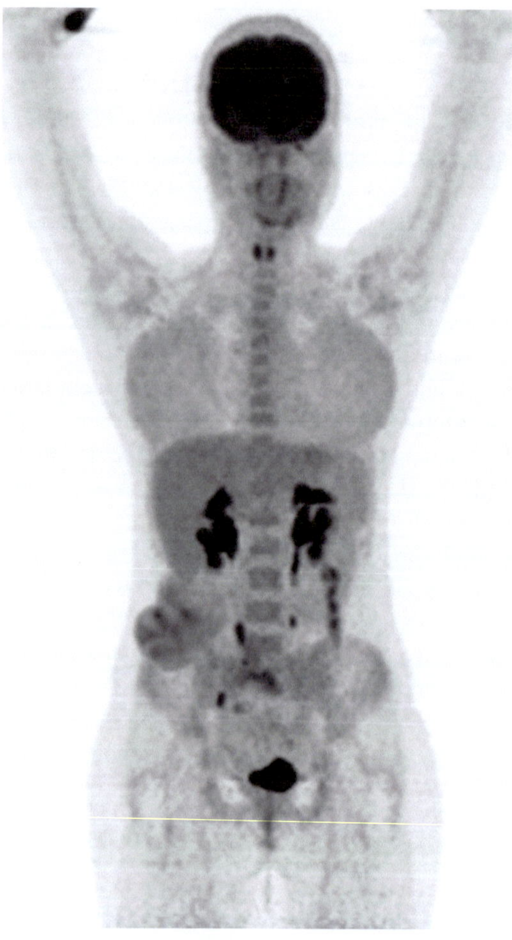

Fig. 9.1 Coronal MIP reconstruction of PET images shows multiple focal areas of FDG uptake in the abdomen and mild diffuse uptake in the colostomy located on the right

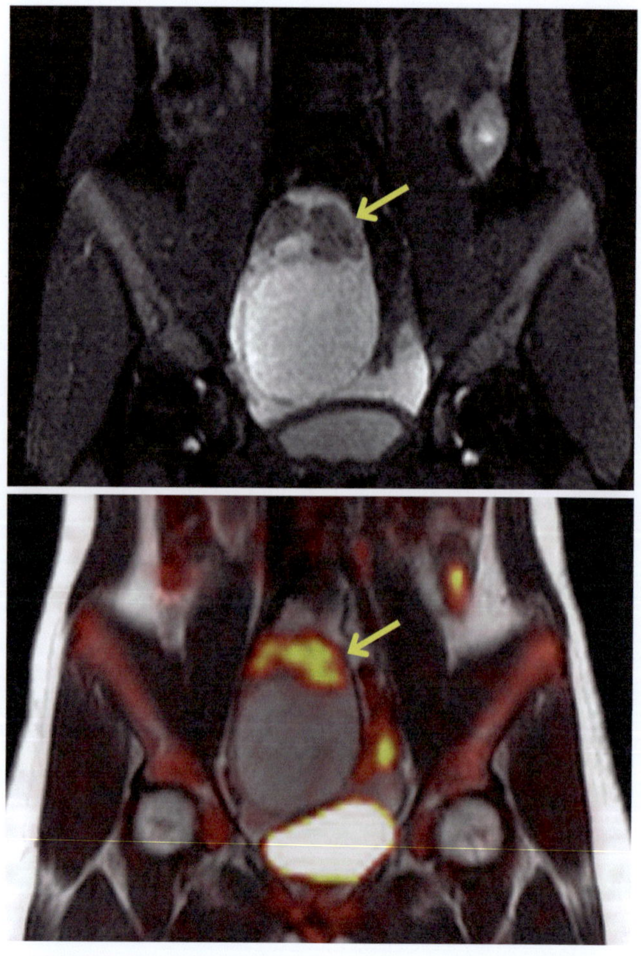

Fig. 9.2 Coronal STIR MR (*top*) and T2 weighted TSE PET/MR (*bottom*) images of the retro-peritoneal mass (*arrow*) with cystic and solid components with increased focal uptake of FDG

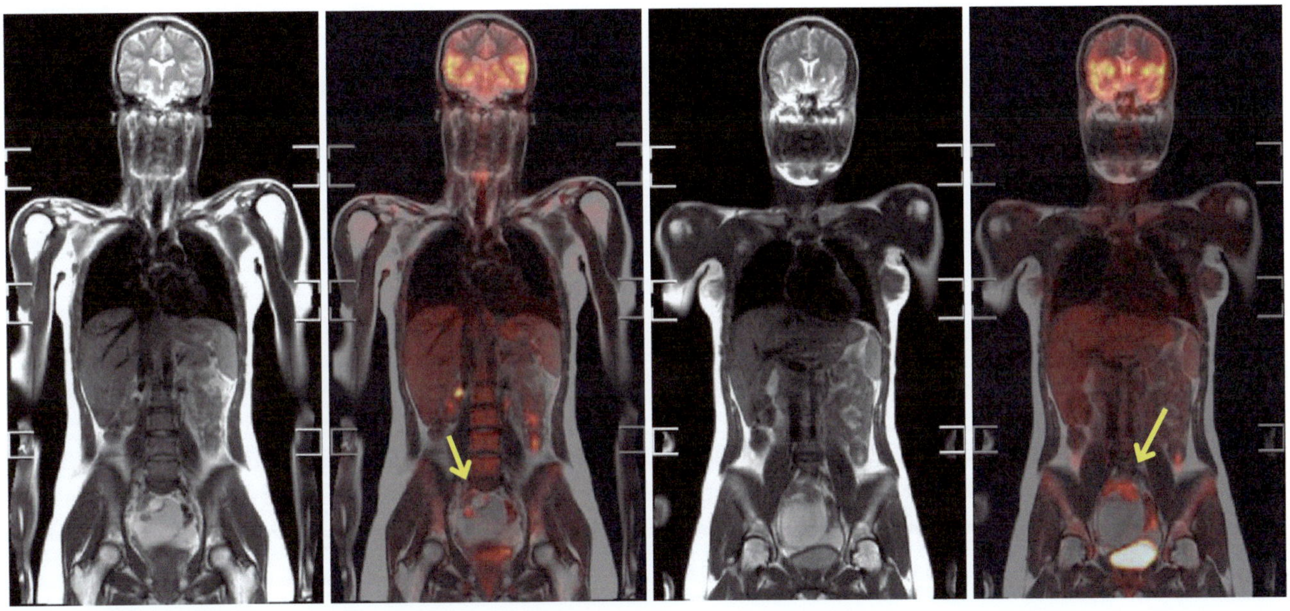

Fig. 9.3 Whole-body coronal T2 weighted TSE MR images fused with corresponding PET images showing the localization of the retro-peritoneal mass (*arrow*)

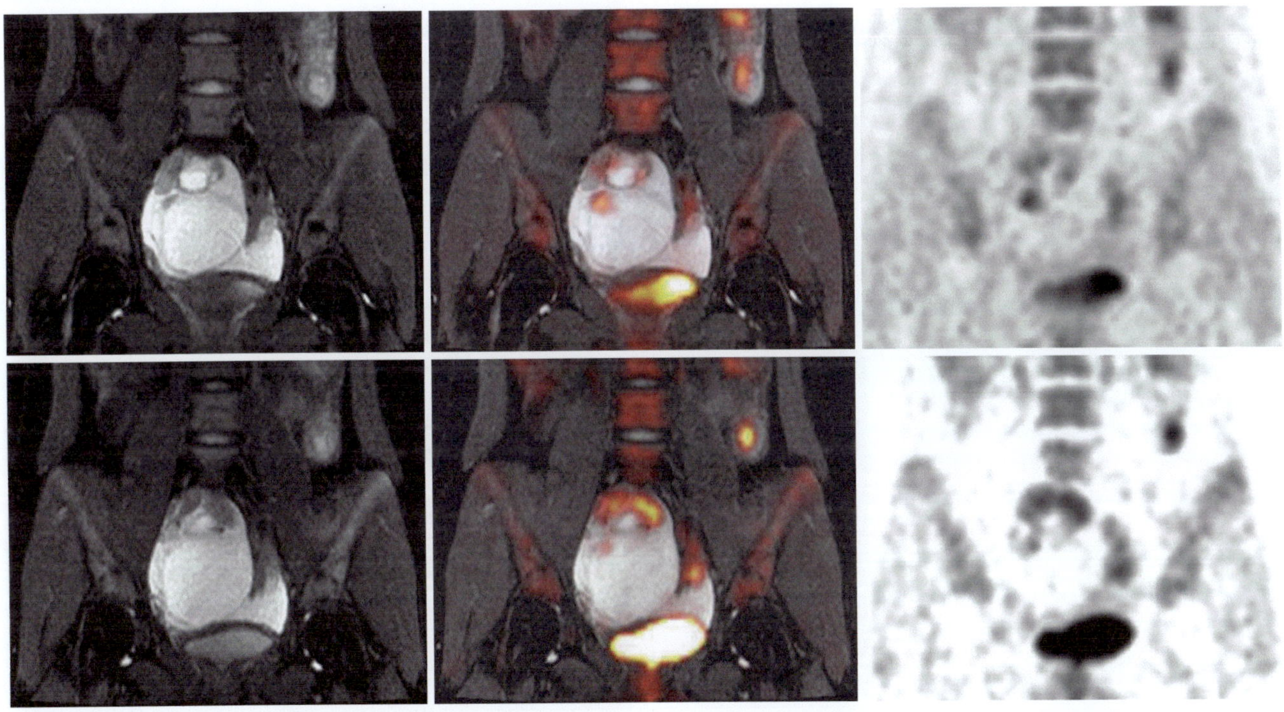

Fig. 9.4 Two adjacent coronal planes of STIR MR sequences fused with PET images of the same location showing the heterogeneous composition of the pelvic mass with a large cystic component

Follow-up of Renal Cyst

Clinical History

Sixteen-year-old patient followed for a left renal cyst since 2001 with a recent change in morphology that could suggest malignant transformation.

Imaging Technique

PET: Whole-body PET acquired 60 min after injection of 370 MBq of ^{18}F-FDG.

MRI: Whole body atMR (T1 weighted), supine position. 3D Dixon and T2 weighted whole-body MRI . Followed by diagnostic MRI, with HASTE diffusion and eThrive sequences.

Findings

PET/MR showed a normal study without evidence of abnormal tracer uptake at the level of the cyst or in any other distant lymph nodes.

Teaching Points

PET/MR could replace PET/CT in pediatric cases where exclusion of malignant tumors is required with the added value of combining of PET's negative predictive value and the ability of MRI for tissue and lesion characterization.

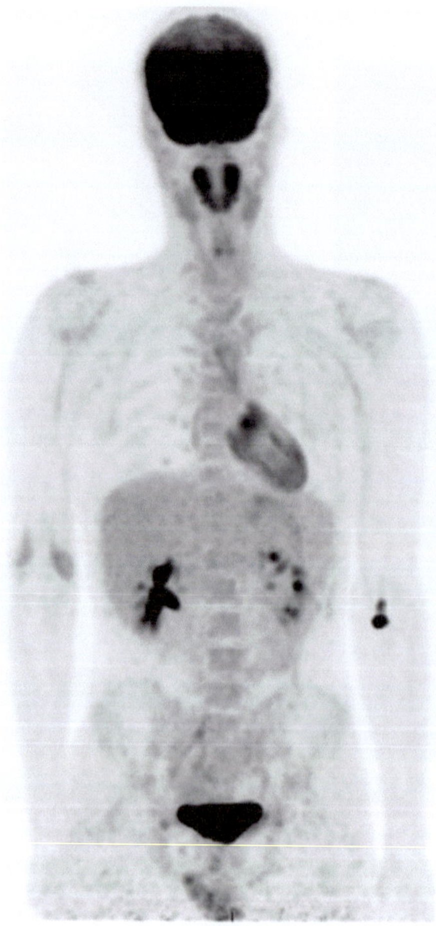

Fig. 9.5 Coronal MIP reconstruction of PET images with no evidence of abnormal PET uptake in the kidney or abdomen

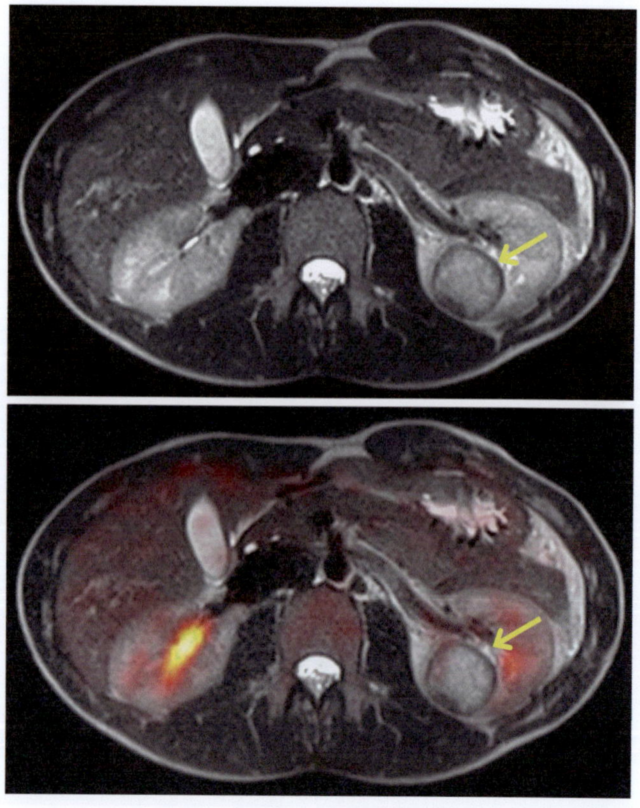

Fig. 9.6 Axial respiratory gated T2 weighted HASTE (*top*) and fusion with corresponding PET image (*bottom*) with no abnormal tracer uptake around the renal cyst (*arrow*)

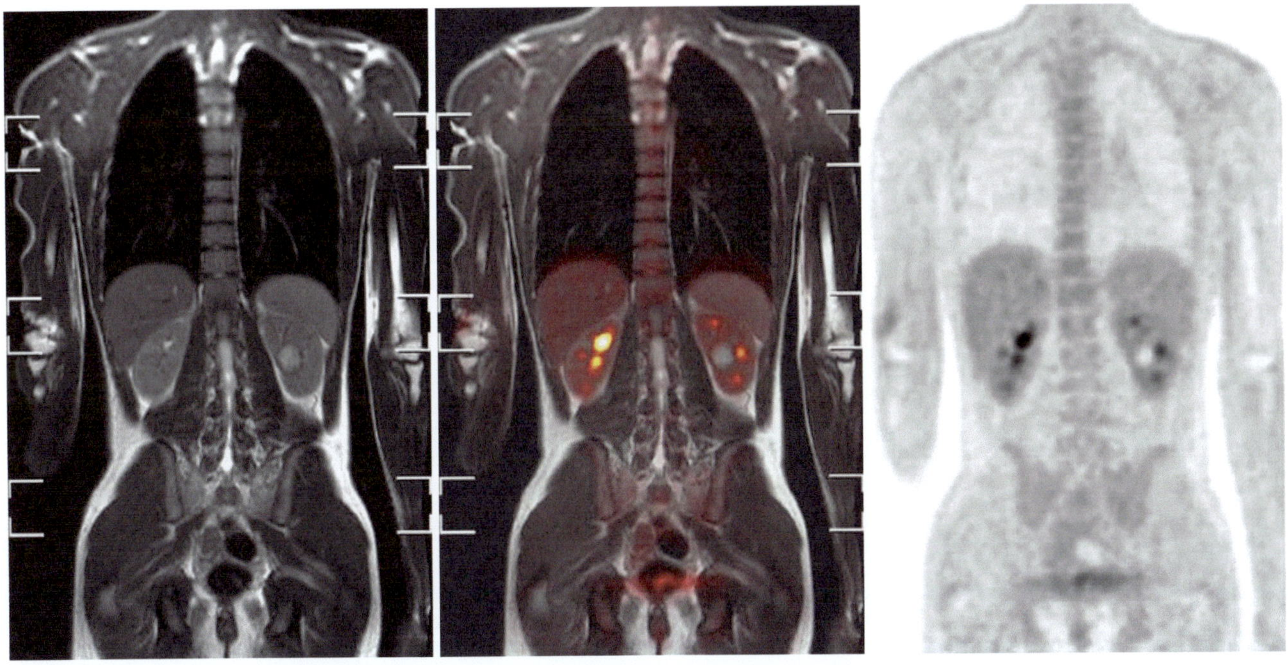

Fig. 9.7 Coronal reformatted images from whole-body T2 weighted TSE images fused with corresponding PET images showing no abnormal tracer uptake

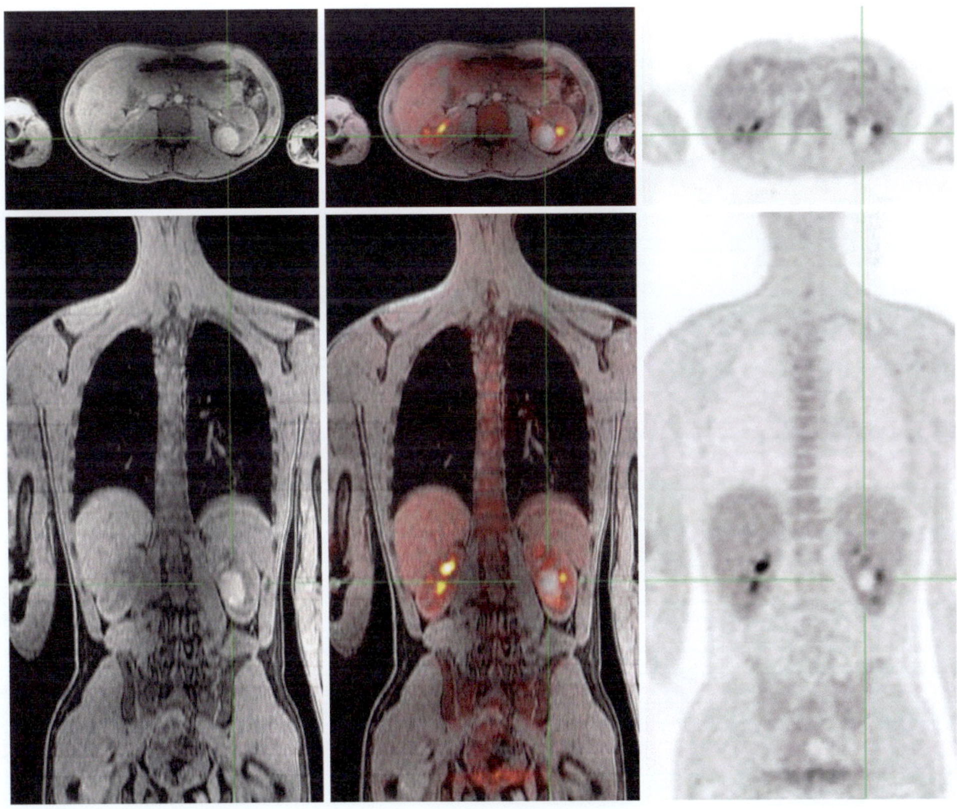

Fig. 9.8 Multiplanar reformatting of whole-body 3D Dixon sequence at the level of the renal cyst

Follow-up Post Treatment of Hodgkin Disease

Clinical History

Sixteen-year-old patient after treatment by chemotherapy for Hodgkin disease. Assessment of end of treatment.

Imaging Technique

PET: Whole-body PET acquired 60 min after injection of 370 MBq of ^{18}F-FDG.

MRI: Whole body atMR (T1 weighted), supine position. 3D Dixon, DWIBS and T2 weighted whole-body MRI sequences.

Findings

PET/MR showed a normal study with complete regression of mediastinal mass seen on the PET/CT study performed prior to initiating chemotherapy treatment.

Teaching Points

PET/MR could replace PET/CT in pediatric follow up studies for assessment of the efficacy of oncological treatments.

PET/MR fusion allows better differentiation of lymph node tracer uptake and brown fat uptake of FDG.

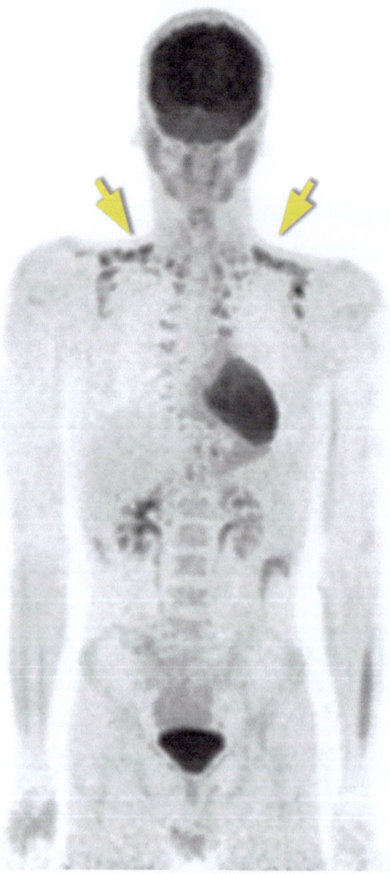

Fig. 9.9 Coronal MIP reconstruction of PET images with no evidence of abnormal tracer uptake. Note the diffuse heterogeneous uptake in brown fat (*arrows*)

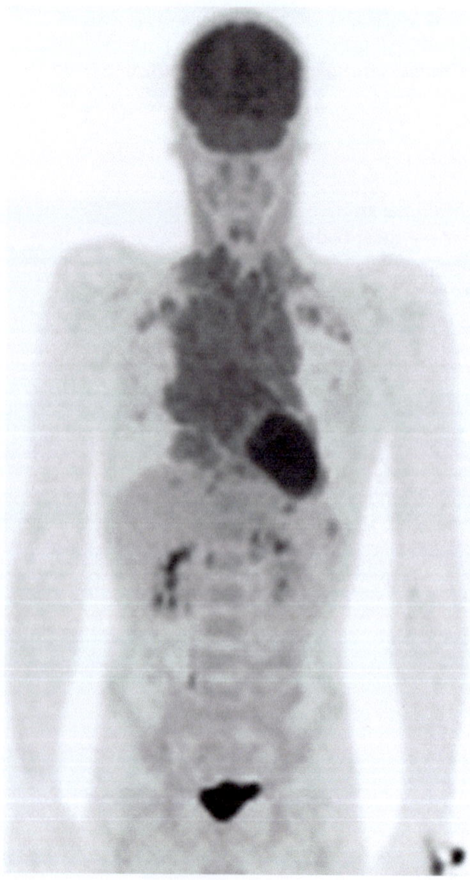

Fig. 9.10 Comparative whole body PET study prior to chemotherapy showing the large mediastinal mass of Hodgkin lymphoma

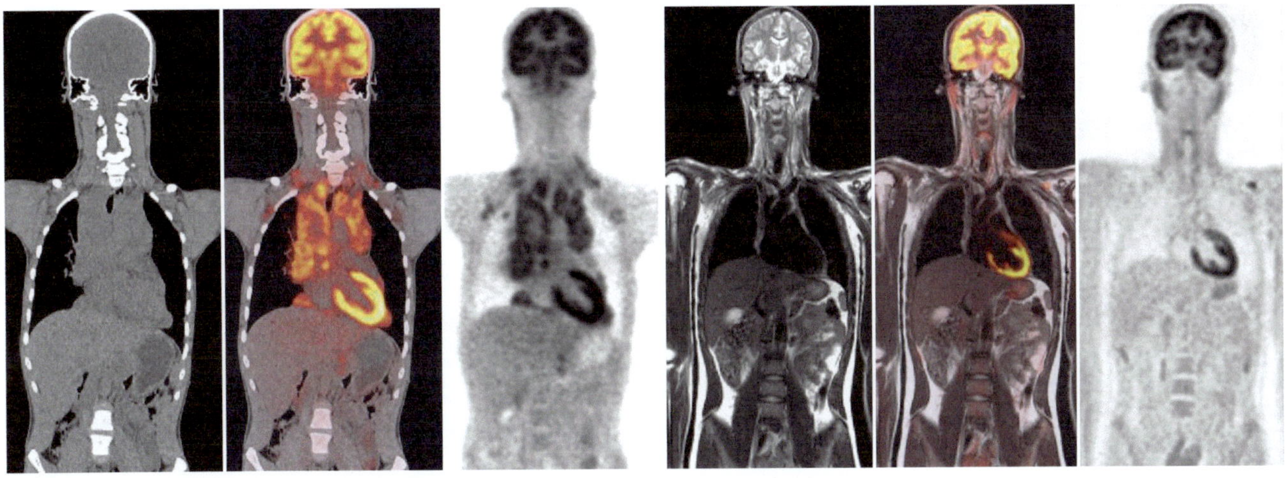

Fig. 9.11 Comparison of pre-treatment PET/CT study (*left*) and post chemotherapy PET/MR study (*right*) showing complete response to therapy with disappearance of all mediastinal masses

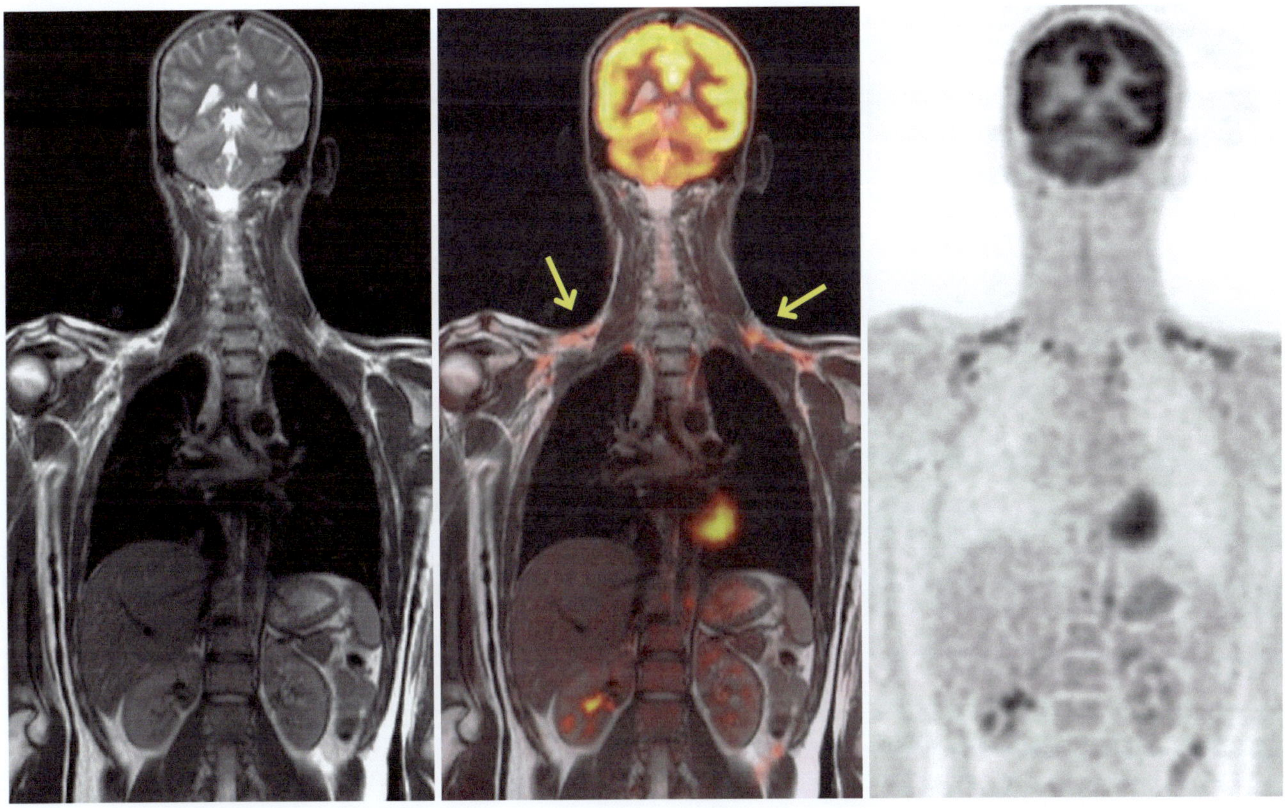

Fig. 9.12 Coronal fused images of PET/MR showing the localization of brown fat uptake (*arrows*)

Long-Term Follow-up of Hodgkin Disease

Clinical History

Fifteen-year-old patient referred for follow-up 2 years after treatment by chemotherapy and radiotherapy for Hodgkin disease.

Imaging Technique

The acquisition was performed on a Philips whole-body hybrid Ingenuity TF PET/MR scanner.

PET: Whole-body PET acquired 60 min after injection of 370 MBq of ^{18}F-FDG.

MRI: Whole body atMR (T1 weighted), supine position. 3D Dixon, STIR and T2 weighted whole-body MRI sequences.

Findings

PET/MR showed a normal study with complete regression of thoracic enlarged lymph nodes seen on the PET/CT study performed prior to initiating treatment.

> **Teaching Points**
>
> PET MR could replace PET/CT in pediatric follow up studies for assessment of the efficacy of oncological treatments particularly in lymphoma patients.
>
> PET/MR fusion allows better differentiation of lymph node tracer uptake and brown fat uptake of FDG.

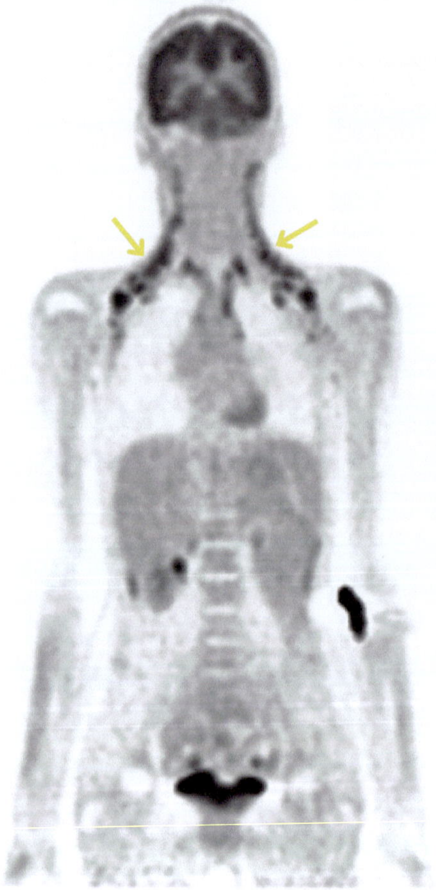

Fig. 9.13 Coronal MIP of PET images with no evidence of abnormal tracer uptake, except physiological uptake in brown fat (*arrows*)

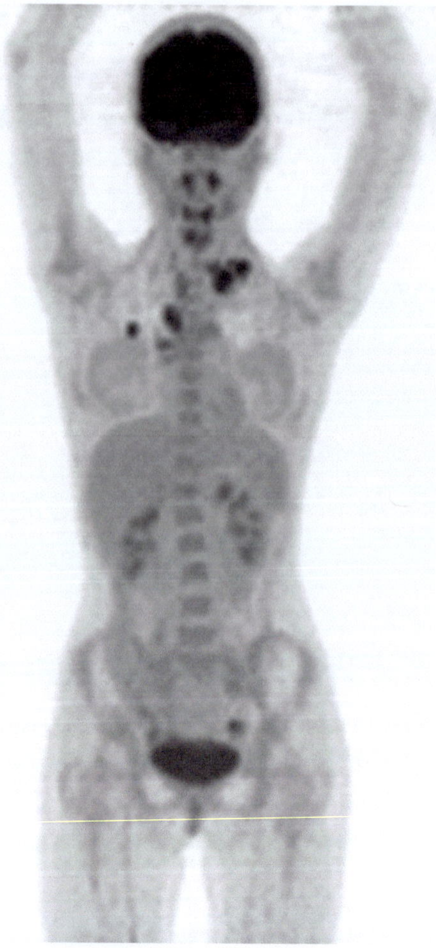

Fig. 9.14 Comparative whole body PET study performed 2 years earlier prior to treatment showing multiple hypermetabolic lymph nodes of Hodgkin lymphoma

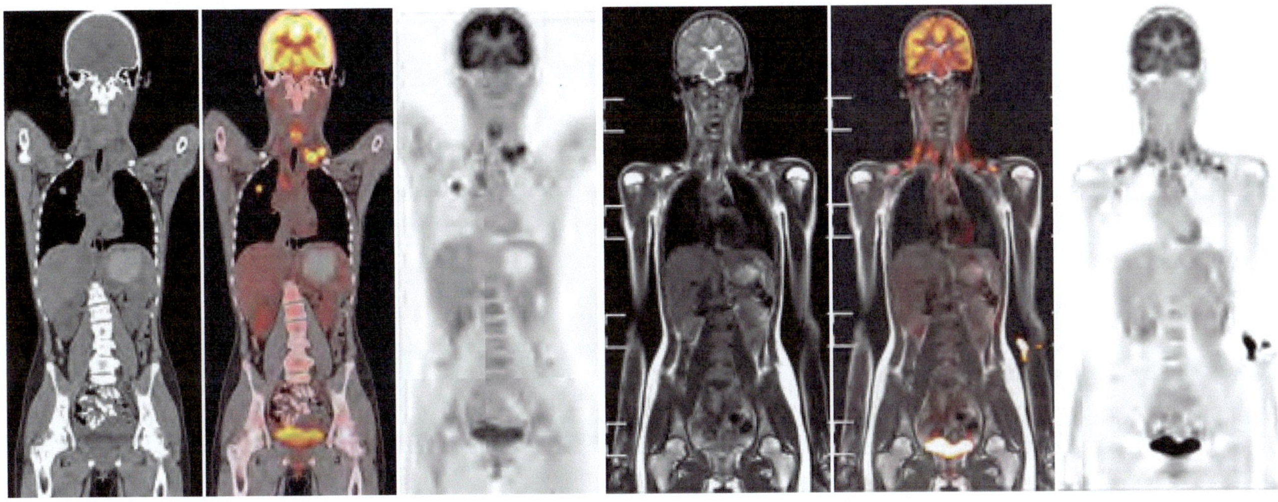

Fig. 9.15 Comparison of pre-treatment PET/CT study (*left*) and 2 years follow-up post treatment PET/MR study (*right*) showing complete response to therapy. Focal FDG uptake bilaterally correspond to physiological brown fat uptake

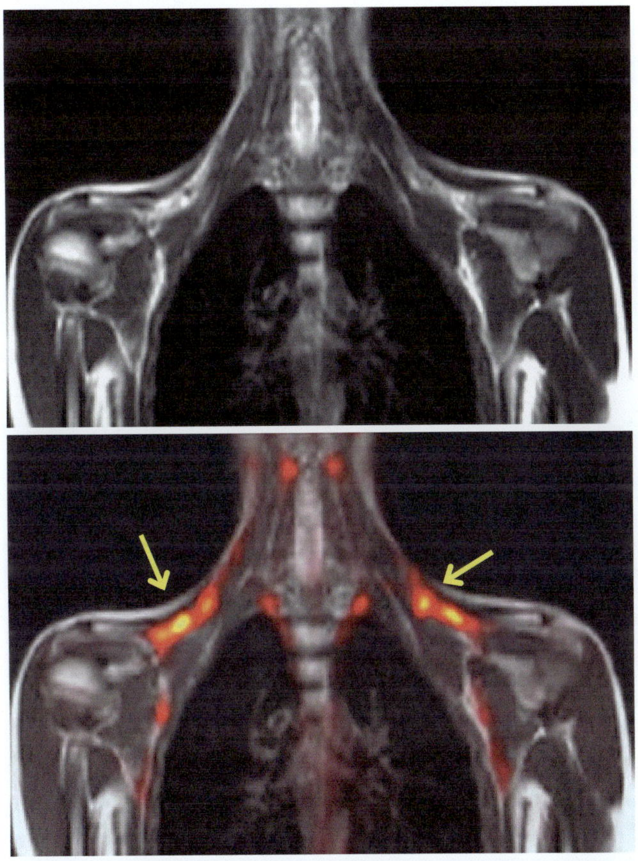

Fig. 9.16 Coronal fused images of PET/MR showing the localization of brown fat uptake (*arrows*)

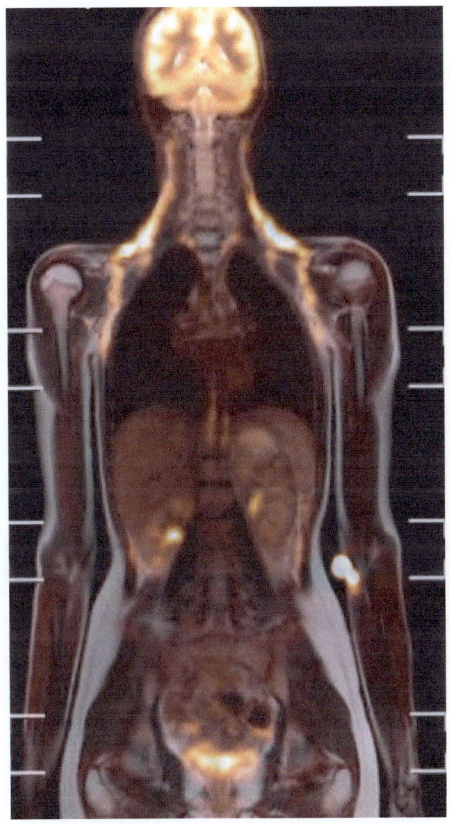

Fig. 9.17 Coronal fused whole-body images showing no abnormal focal uptake except brown fat uptake

PET/MR in Langerhans Cell Histiocytosis

Clinical History

A 12-year-old patient presents with pain in the left hip since several weeks. A prior X-ray revealed an osteolytic lesion in the left ileal bone suspicious for Langerhans cell histiocytosis.

Imaging Technique

Whole body PET/MR images acquired 135 min after iv injection 335 MBq 18F-FDG, 58 kg.

8 beds × 3 min together with whole body cor T2w STIR. 1 bed (pelvis) a 15 min together with cor T1w TSE before and after Gadolinium, ax T2w TSE and ax T1w fs TSE after Gadolinium. Additional sequences for the brain: ax T2w flair and MPRage after Gadolinium. Head/neck and four body coils.

Findings

Besides extensive activity due to brown fat a PET/positive lesion with intense contrast enhancement is demonstrated in the left ileal bone. No other suspicious lesions could be visualized both in MRI and PET.

> **Teaching Points**
>
> The combination of whole-body PET and MR can aid in excluding or confirming the presence of multiple lesions in Langerhans cell histiocytosis. This is essential information for the clinician in the further treatment of those patients.

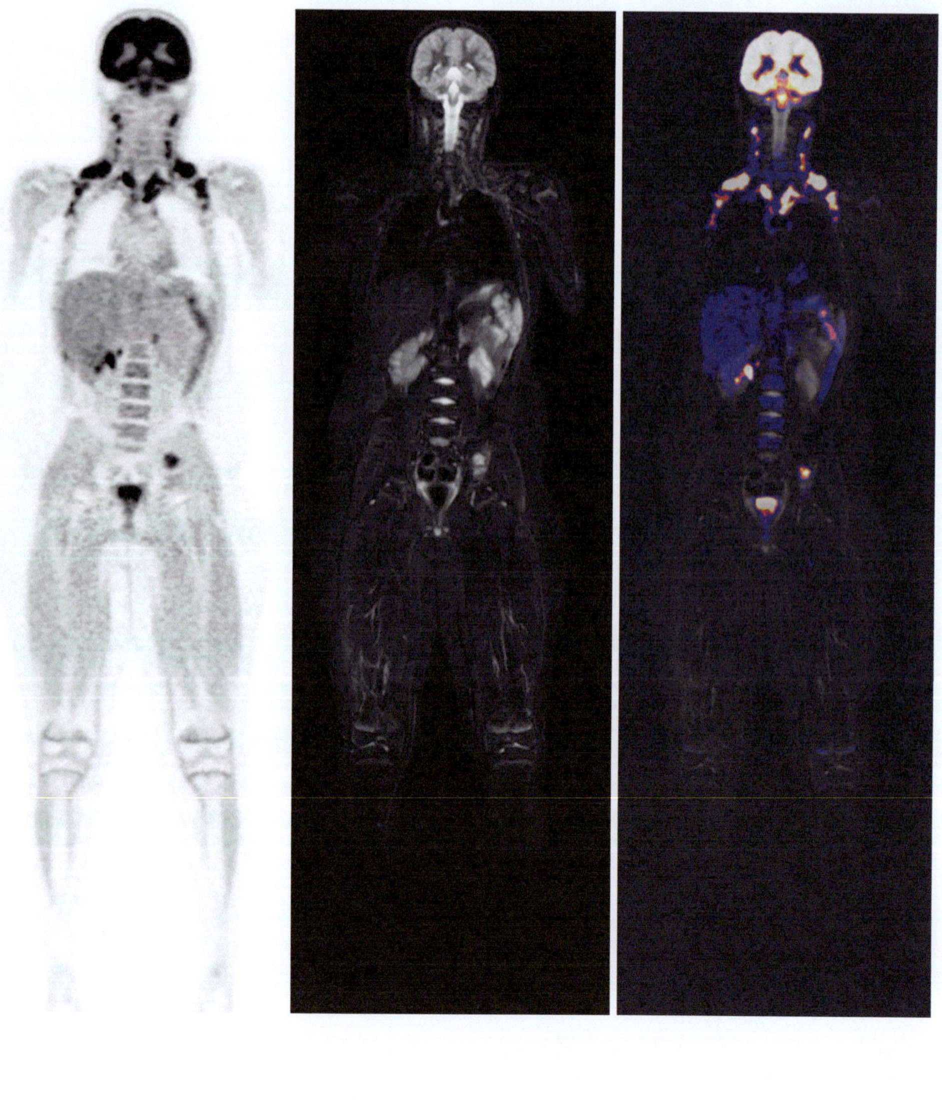

Fig. 9.18 Coronal whole body PET demonstrates intense FDG-accumulation due to brown fat. In addition a focal moderate uptake could be found in the left ileal bone (*left*). In the whole body coronal T2w STIR sequence only one lesion is confirmed by a hyperintense signal (*middle*). Additional fusion between coronal T2w stir and PET shows a good correlation between the single lesion in PET and MRI (*right*)

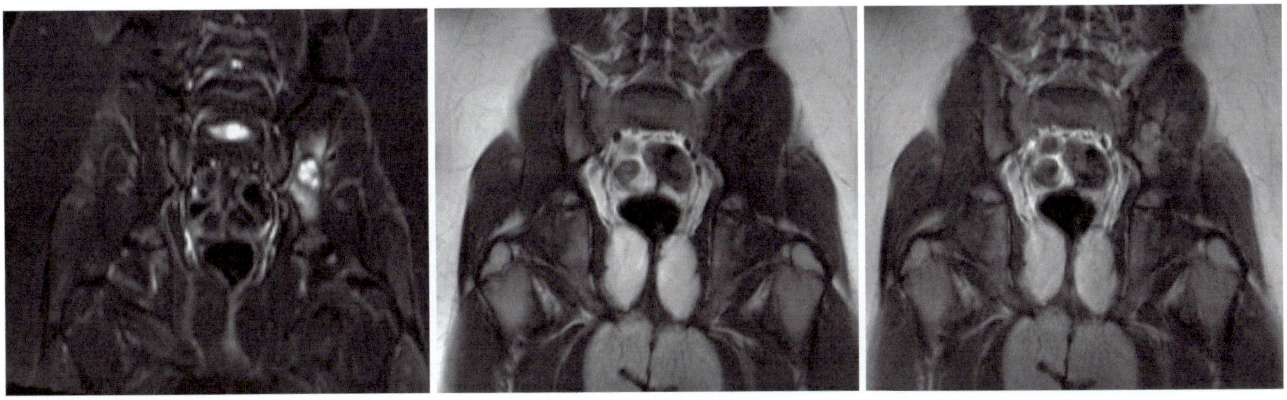

Fig. 9.19 Coronal T2w STIR reveals a hyperintense lesion in the right ileal bone with surrounding edema (*left*). Corresponding coronal T1w TSE demonstrate moderate to intense contrast enhancement of the lesion (*middle* and *right*)

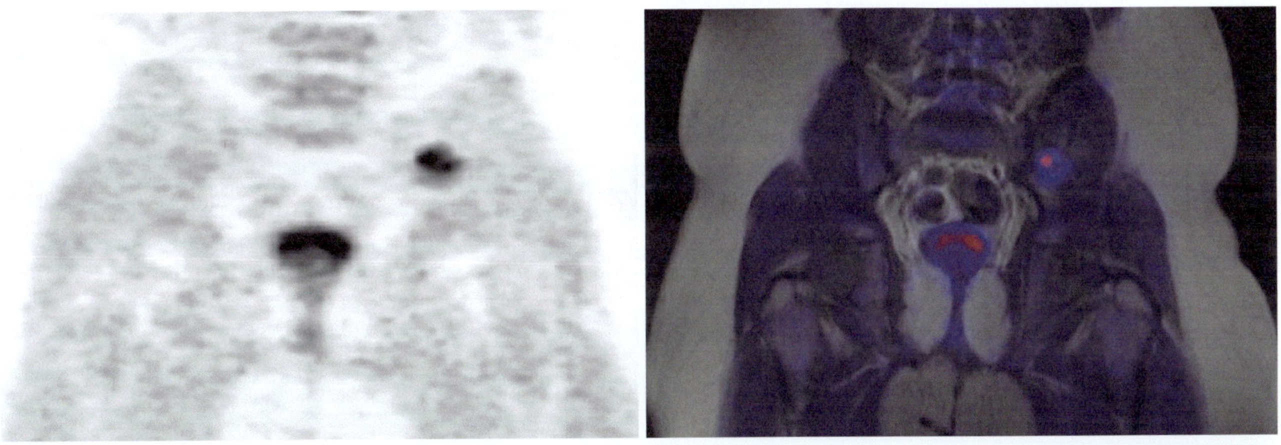

Fig. 9.20 Coronal PET (*left*) and fused images (*right*) show a good anatomical correlation between the moderate increased focal FDG-metabolism and the abnormality in MRI

Fig. 9.21 No involvement of the brain espc. the hypophyseal stalk can be found in the sagittal reformatted MPR age after Gadolinium (*top left*). The anatomical extent of the lesion in the left ileal bone is outlined in the axial T1w TSE fs after Gadolinium sequences (*top right*). Axial PET and fused images demonstrate the highest uptake in PET in the region of the most intense contrast enhancement (*lower row*)

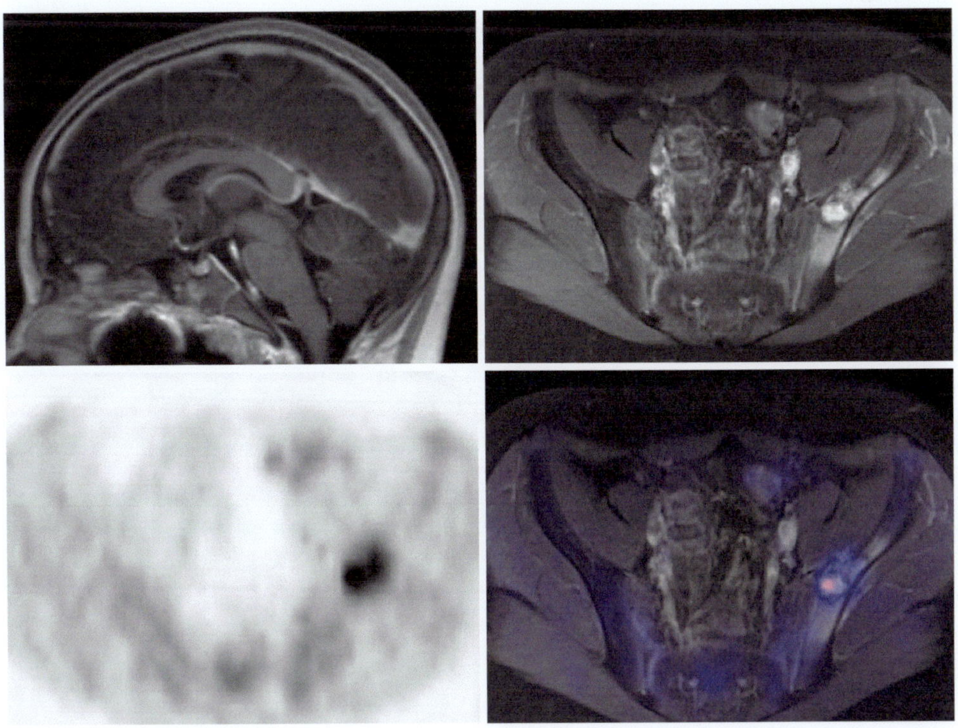

Ewing Sarcoma

Clinical History

Eleven year old boy with a large symptomatic tumor of the left pelvis, a histologically proven Ewing sarcoma of the left os ilium.

Imaging Technique

Whole body PET/MR images acquired pre- and post-therapy 135 min (Fig. 9.22), resp. 140 min (Fig. 9.23) after i.v injection of 198 MBq, resp. 123 MBq 18F-FDG, 27 kg.

7 beds × 3 min together with coronal T2 STIR and coronal T1 TSE. T1 VIBE Dixon for attenuation correction.

Findings

High FDG-uptake of the primary Ewing sarcoma of the left os ilium, corresponding to the T1-hypointense tumor lesion shown in Fig. 9.22.

Images acquired 8 month later after RCTx show no more tracer uptake in the lesion. MRT shows residual tumor lesion in the left os ilium exhibiting hypointense signal in the T1-sequence.

Teaching Points

FDG-PET is able to demonstrate good therapeutic response of the treatment indicating no active tumor. MRT shows the large decrease of the lesion size. Combination of PET and MR could be a valuable tool assessing the response to therapy of bone tumors. Images also show the conversion to fatty bone marrow in the lumbar spine after RCTX, in contrast to the thoracic spine.

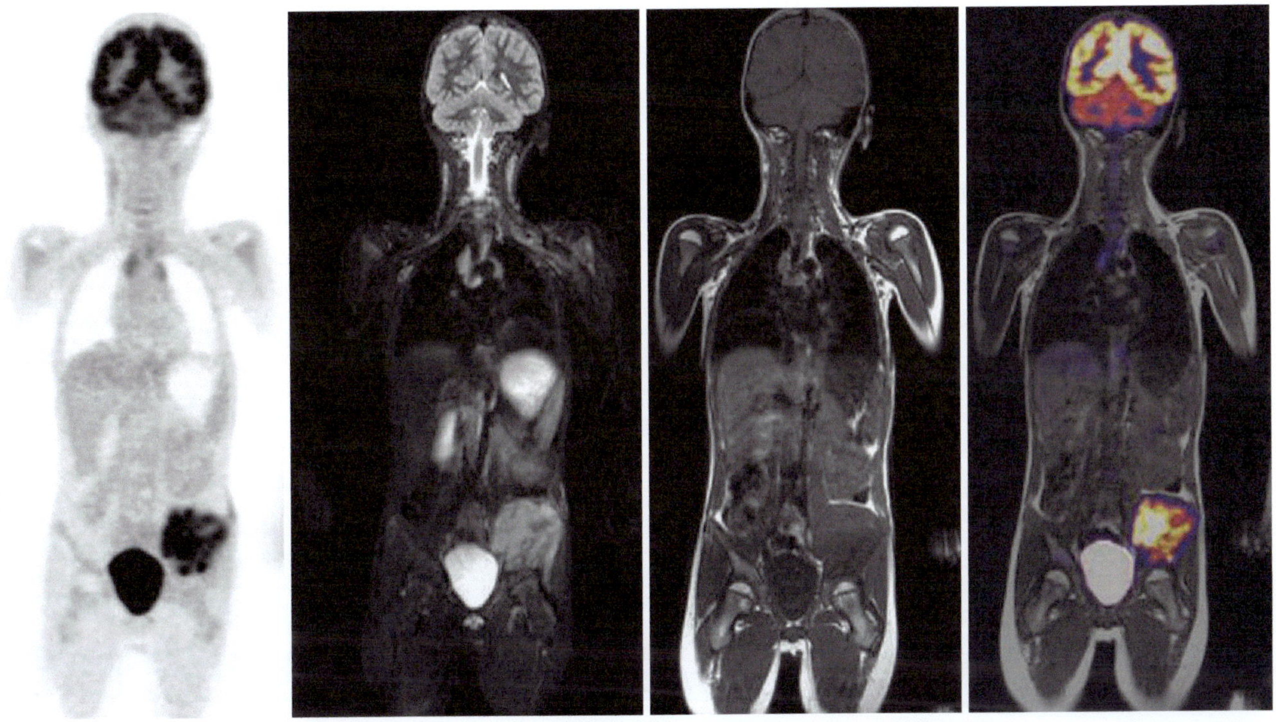

Fig. 9.22 Coronal T1 TSE whole body shows a hypointense homogenous lesion of the left os ilium, infiltrating the soft tissue structures of the pelvis. The space occupying lesion is hyperintense in the T2 STIR. PET shows an intensive glucose utilization of the whole tumor, no other lesions

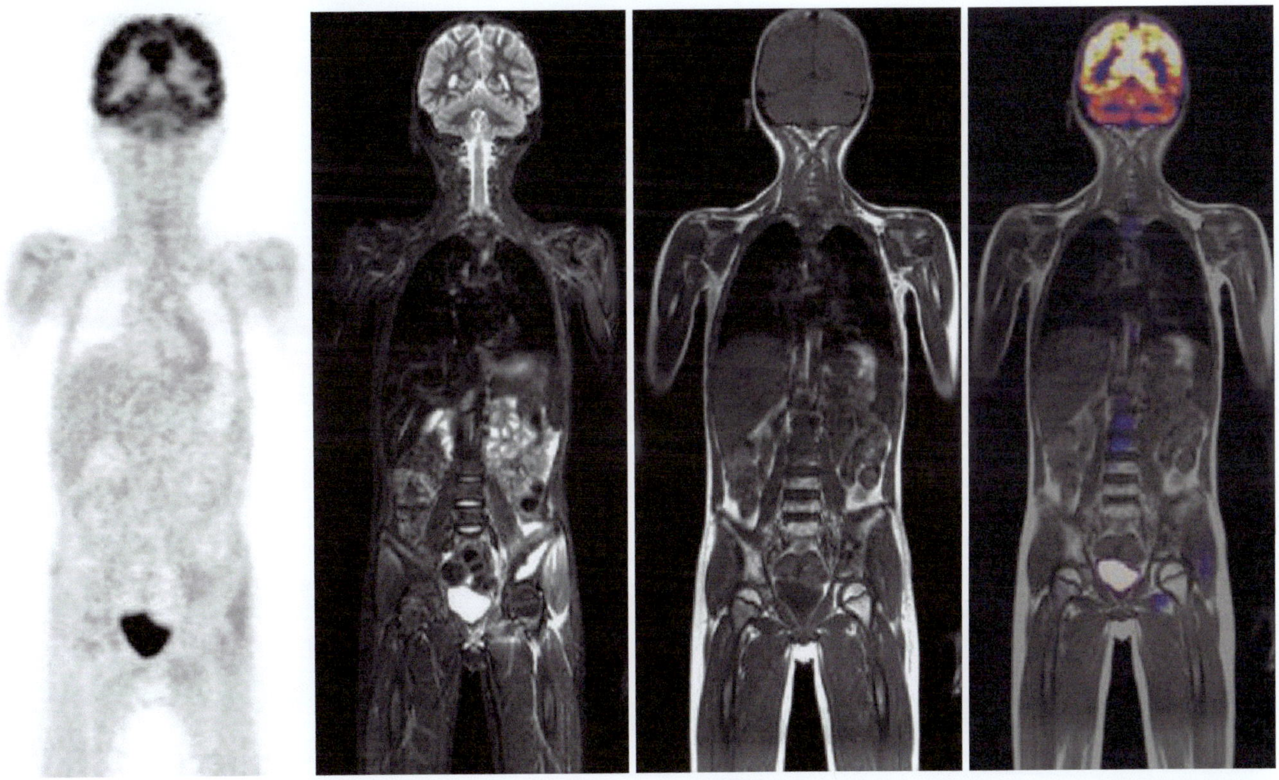

Fig. 9.23 After RCTx – 8 months later – tumor shrinkage is demonstrated in the MR component of the scan. However, a residual T1 hypointense/T2 hyperintense lesion is detected exhibiting no increased glucose utilization, indicating no active tumor. Further, a T2 hyperintense signal alteration is observed in the soft tissue surrounding the lesion indicating most probably an unspecific postactinic reaction

Recurrent Ewing's Sarcoma

Clinical History

Eight years old boy after RTx (12/2011) of a Ewing's Sarcoma of the cervical spine exhibiting intraspinal involvement. First scan (09/2012) was performed for restaging to exclude local or systemic recurrence. Consecutively patient received surgical treatment to resect the finding of the scan. Second scan (01/2013) was performed in the frame of follow up.

Imaging Technique

PET/MR 171 min and 153 min p.i. of 100 and 107 MBq 18F-FDG, 23 kg, 7 bed positions 3 min per bed position T1 VIBE Dixon for attenuation correction.

MR component first scan: cor T1 TSE, cor T2 STIR, sag T1 TSE post GD, cor T1 SPIR post GD; second scan: cor T1 TSE, cor T2 STIR.

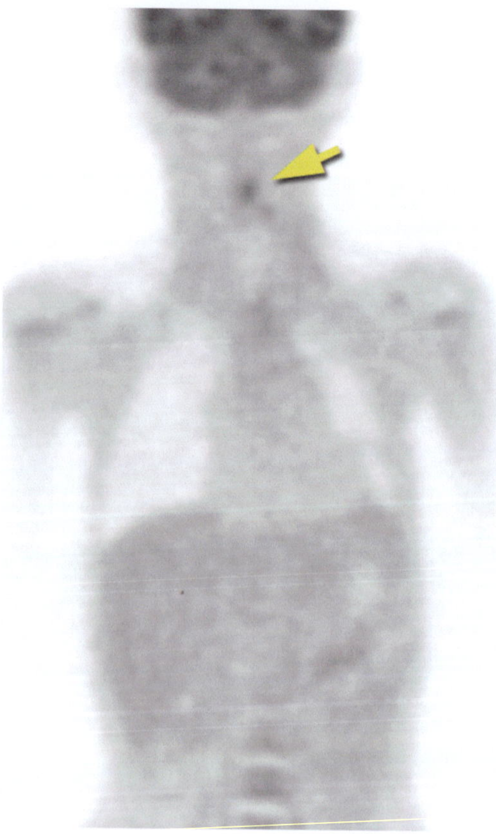

Fig. 9.24 Coronal PET shows the lesion exhibiting a moderate focal 18F-FDG uptake (*arrow*) giving evidence of disease recurrence

Findings

There is focally increased glucose uptake in the cervical spine, corresponding to an intraspinal space occupying lesion also visible on the MR component of the scan (Fig. 9.24). The lesion is contrast agent enhancing (Fig. 9.25). The PET/MR fused image demonstrates the lesion exhibiting a moderate 18F-FDG uptake, suspect of recurrence of Ewing Sarcoma (Fig. 9.24). Surgical resection confirmed recurrent disease. The second scan performed after surgery showed no evidence of recurrent disease. The increased uptake shown on the fused images cervicaly and periclavicularly (Fig. 9.26) corresponds to fat tissue in the MR and corresponds unspecific uptake in brown fat.

Teaching Points

MRI is the method of choice to assess intraspinal involvement in disease. Simultaneous PET/MR imaging increased localization certainty of the hypermetabolic lesion shown in PET. Additionally it increased confidence in characterizing the space occupying lesion demonstrated in the MR component of the scan. The good distinction of fat tissue in the MR from other tissue (e.g. lymph nodes) helps in the evaluation of patients exhibiting increased glucose utilization in brown fat.

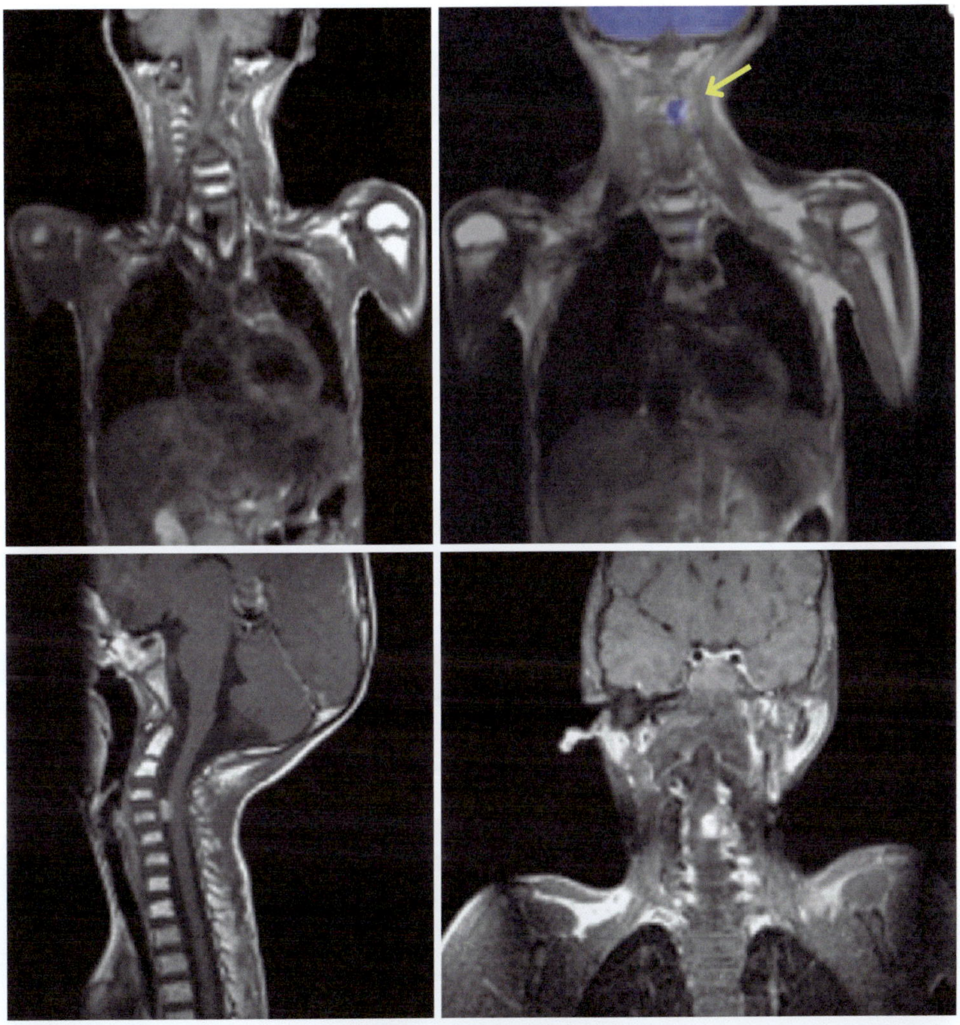

Fig. 9.25 Intraspinal lesion enhancing contrast shown most clearly in the sag T1 TSE post GD and in the cor T1 SPIR post GD (*both images in bottom row*). Coronal fused PET/MR images (*top right*) demonstrate the lesion exhibiting a moderate focal 18F-FDG uptake (*arrow*) giving evidence of disease recurrence

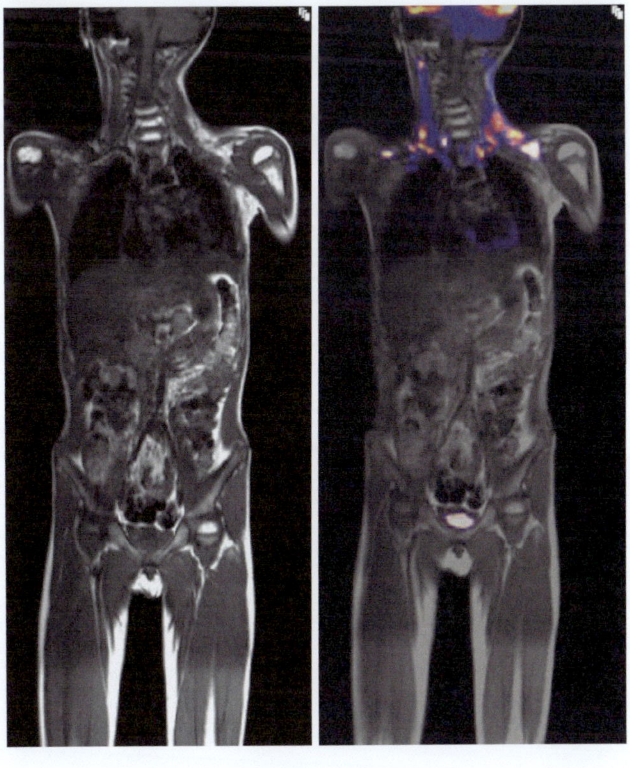

Fig. 9.26 Follow up PET/MR. The former lesion is not visible any more in condition after surgical excision. No new suspicious lesion was observed. Note the accurate correspondence of the increased glucose utilization cervical and periclavicular to fat tissue as shown in the MR component of the scan, indicating unspecific activity in brown fat

Multifocal Ewing Sarcoma

Clinical History

Fifteen years old patient treated with radiotherapy and chemotherapy for Ewing Sarcoma in the right humerus (until 09/2011). He was referred for restaging in the frame of follow up (03/2012).

Imaging Technique

PET/MR 136 min p.i. of 283 MBq 18F-FDG, 41 kg, 7 bed positions 3 min per bed position, T1 VIBE Dixon for attenuation correction.

MR component: cor T1 TSE, cor T2 STIR, sag T1 TSE, sag T2 STIR.

Findings

PET/MR raises suspicion of a multifocal recurrence of Ewing Sarcoma with hypermetabolic foci in multiple sites (Fig. 9.27). In all cases a typical T1 hypointense/T2 hyperintense signal alterations can be observed (Fig. 9.28).

Teaching Points

PET/MR is a valuable whole body imaging method for diseases which can involve multiple sites. The high sensitivity of MR in assessing bone marrow involvement adds in the high sensitivity of PET in restaging of Ewing Sarcoma. Furthermore the radiation exposure of PET/MR for pediatric patients is lower compared to PET/CT.

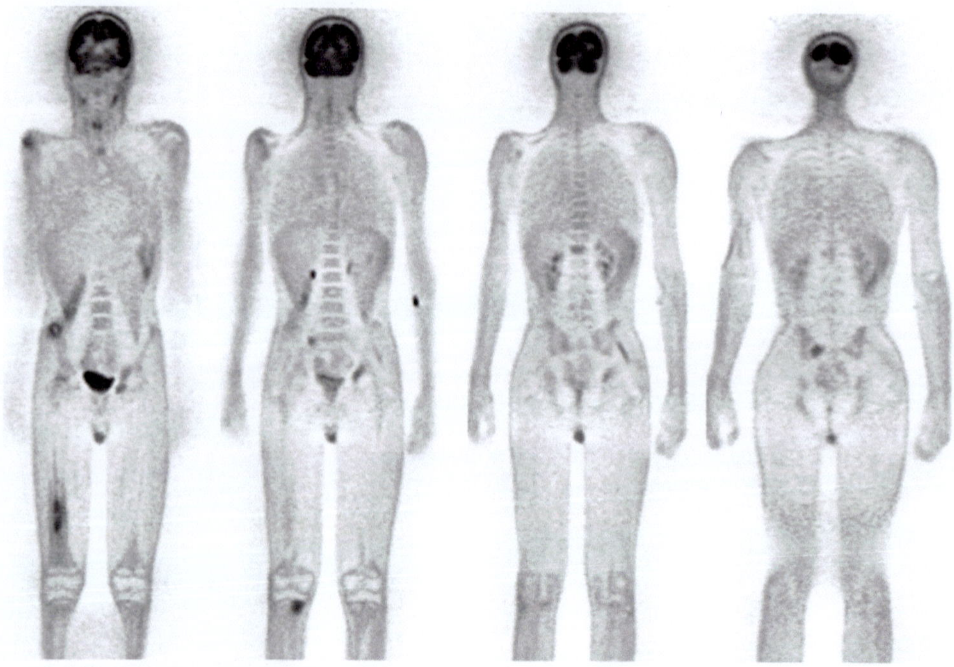

Fig. 9.27 Coronal PET/MR images at different levels showing hypermetabolic foci in the right femur, in both iliac bones, in the right medial tibia condyles, in the 12th thoracic vertebral bone and in the right sacral bone

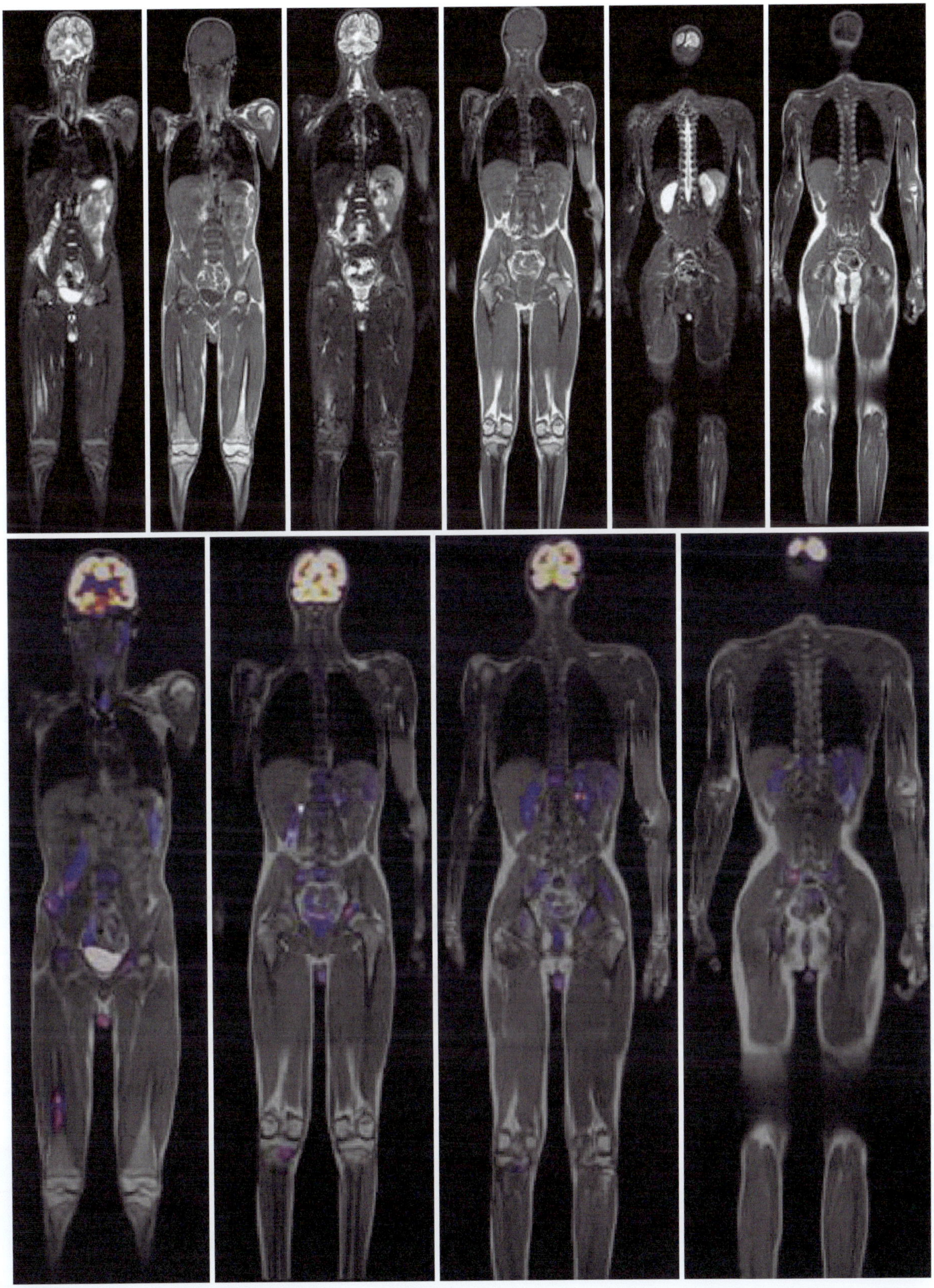

Fig. 9.28 cor T1 TSE, cor T2 STIR (*top*) and PET/MR fused images (*bottom*) of the sites suspected to be involved in the disease. All the hypermetabolic foci present with a T1 hypointense/T2 hyperintense signal alteration in MR suggesting bone marrow manifestations of Ewing Sarcoma. Additionally MRI provides detailed anatomical and diagnostic information. Note the T2 hyperintense signal alteration in the periost surrounding the manifestation in the right femoral bone suggesting periostal reaction

Treatment Follow-up of Lymphoma

Clinical History

Sixteen years old patient with Hodgkin lymphoma diagnosed after biopsy of a cervical lymph node referred for staging and follow up after two cycles of chemotherapy.

Imaging Technique

PET/MR 162 and 127 min p.i. of 327 and 387 MBq 18F-FDG, 60 kg, 5 bed positions 4 min per bed position T1 VIBE Dixon for attenuation correction.

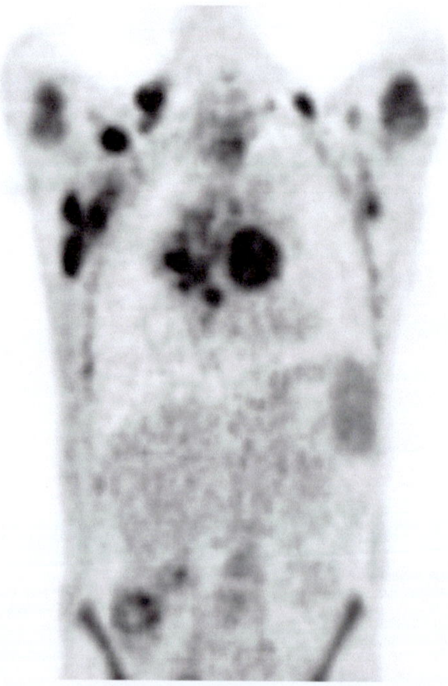

Fig. 9.29 Coronal PET demonstrates extensive FDG-uptake in cervical, axiallary and mediastinal lymph nodes

MR sequences in both scans: cor T2 STIR, ax VIBE fs post GD, thorax cor T2 haste fs.

Findings

In the pretherapeutic scan there are multiple foci of increased glucose utilization/enlarged lymph nodes in the cervical, axillary and mediastinal lymph node stations with infiltration of the sternum (Figs. 9.29, 9.31). Additionally in the MR component pleural effusion is observed. Further, increased homogenous uptake in the bone marrow can be noted indicating probably bone marrow activation, however bone marrow involvement can not be excluded.

In the scan after two cycles of CTx enlarged lymph nodes are demonstrated in the axilla in the MR component, however there is a decrease in number and size observed (Figs. 9.30 and 9.32). The lymph nodes exhibit tracer accumulation in the same range as that of blood pool (Fig. 9.30). The scan indicates a good response to chemotherapy.

> **Teaching Points**
>
> MRI has an equal performance to CT in imaging lymph node involvement in lymphoma. PET is a valuable staging and restaging method for FDG avid lymphomas. As the overall life expectancy of children with lymphoma can be long and in many cases not reduced compared to that of healthy population, it is important to keep radiation exposure as low as possible. Therefore, combining the anatomical MRI-information and the high accuracy of PET in detecting viable lymphoma tissue, could become the preferred choice compared to PET/CT when evaluating lymphoma in children.

Fig. 9.30 Coronal PET slices in different levels of the PET/MR after two cycles of CTx

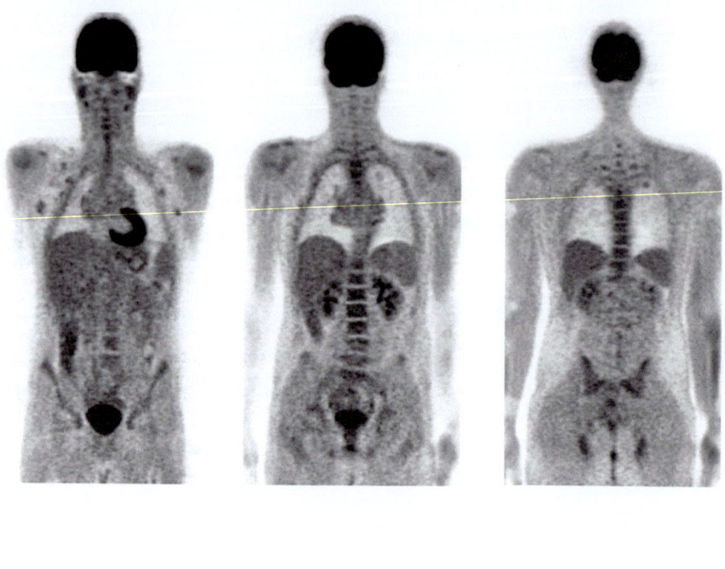

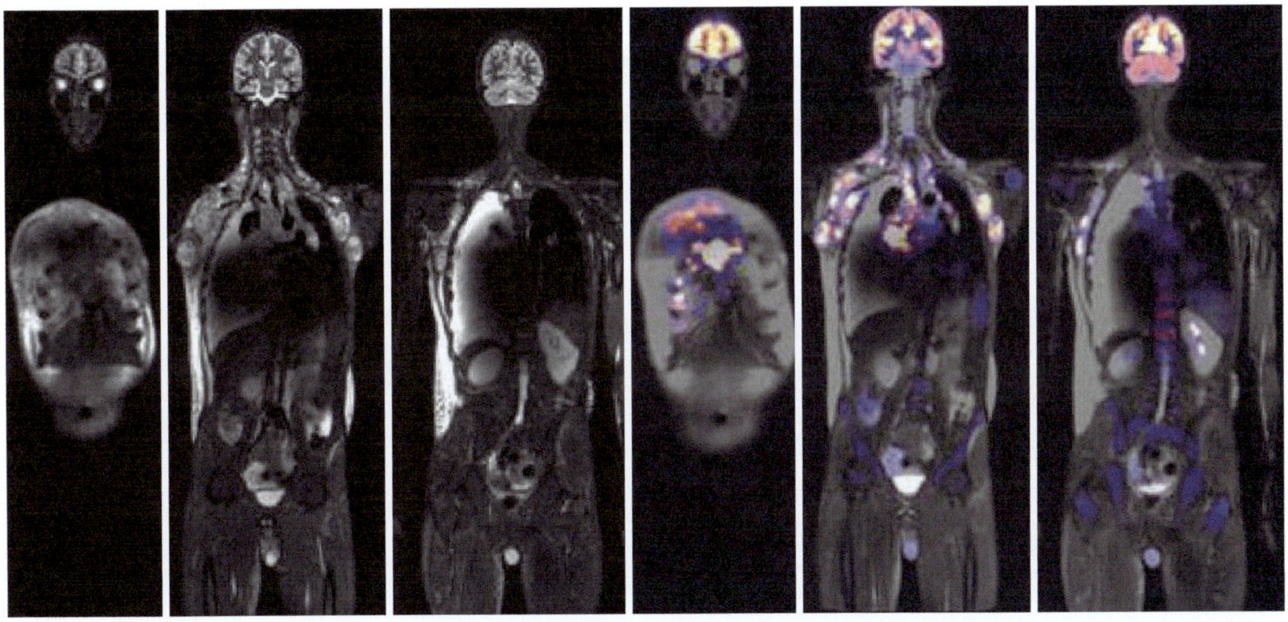

Fig. 9.31 Slices in different levels of the cor T2 STIR and PET/MR fused images. The enlarged lymph nodes are presenting as T2 hyperintense signal alterations in the MR component. Note the pleural effusion imaged in the MR component and the lymphoma manifestation destructing the sternum best seen in the fused images

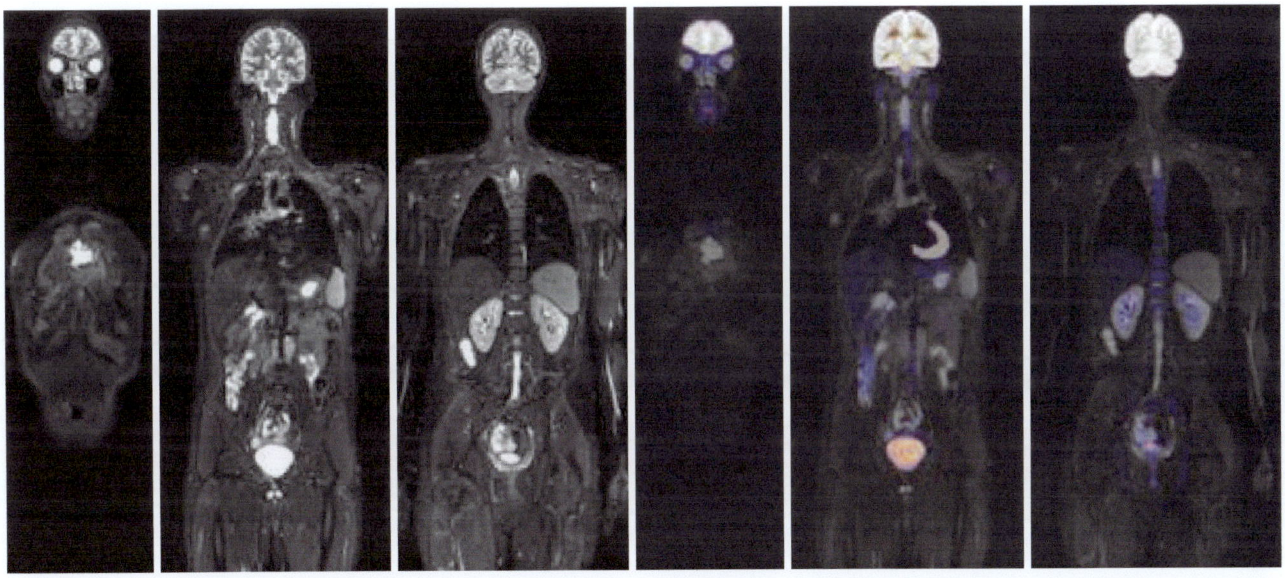

Fig. 9.32 PET/MR after two cycles of chemotherapy. Enlarged, T2 hyperintense lymph nodes in the axilla can be observed, however compared to the pretherapeutic scan they are reduced in number and size. The pleural effusion is resolved. Overall a good response to treatment can be reported

References

1. Pichler BJ, Kolb A, Nägele T, Schlemmer H-P (2010) PET/MRI: paving the way for the next generation of clinical multimodality imaging applications. J Nucl Med 51(3):333–336
2. Hirsch FW, Sattler B, Sorge I, Kurch L, Viehweger A, Ritter L et al (2013) PET/MR in children. Initial clinical experience in paediatric oncology using an integrated PET/MR scanner. Pediatr Radiol (in press)
3. Chawla SC, Federman N, Zhang D, Nagata K, Nuthakki S, McNitt-Gray M et al (2010) Estimated cumulative radiation dose from PET/CT in children with malignancies: a 5-year retrospective review. Pediatr Radiol 40(5):681–686
4. Kwee TC, Takahara T, Vermoolen MA, Bierings MB, Mali WP, Nievelstein RAJ (2010) Whole-body diffusion-weighted imaging for staging malignant lymphoma in children. Pediatr Radiol 40(10):1592–1602; quiz 1720–1721
5. Sinha S, Peach AHS (2010) Diagnosis and management of soft tissue sarcoma. BMJ 341(1):c7170–c7170
6. Tateishi U, Hosono A, Makimoto A, Nakamoto Y, Kaneta T, Fukuda H et al (2009) Comparative study of FDG PET/CT and conventional imaging in the staging of rhabdomyosarcoma. Ann Nucl Med 23(2):155–161
7. Baum SH, Frühwald M, Rahbar K, Wessling J, Schober O, Weckesser M (2011) Contribution of PET/CT to prediction of outcome in children and young adults with rhabdomyosarcoma. J Nucl Med 52(10):1535–1540
8. Denecke T, Hundsdörfer P, Misch D, Steffen IG, Schönberger S, Furth C et al (2010) Assessment of histological response of paediatric bone sarcomas using FDG PET in comparison to morphological volume measurement and standardized MRI parameters. Eur J Nucl Med Mol Imaging 37(10):1842–1853

Lymphoma, Lung and other Tumors

10

M. Eiber, A. Baskin, M. Essler, K. Holzapfel,
O. Ratib, K. Scheidbauer, and J.-P. Willi

Contents

M. Eiber (✉) • K. Holzapfel
Department of Radiology,
Technische Universität München,
Munich, Germany
e-mail: matthias.eiber@tum.de

A. Baskin • O. Ratib • J.-P. Willi
Department of Medical Imaging,
Division of Nuclear Medicine and Molecular Imaging,
Geneva University and Geneva University Hospitals,
Geneva, Switzerland

M. Essler • K. Scheidbauer
Department of Nuclear Medicine,
Technische Universität München,
Munich, Germany

Lymphoma, Lung and Other Tumors

In both Hodgkin disease and non-Hodgkin lymphoma, imaging plays an important role for primary diagnosis and staging [1]. Except for cerebral lymphoma, whole-body MRI is of high research interest but not clinical routine in the staging algorithm of lymphoma patients. This situation could change quickly, and whole-body MRI might become a good alternative to CT [2]. Especially when combining with whole-body diffusion-weighted MRI, with a its high sensitivity could improve the diagnostic accuracy for the staging of Hodgkin disease and non-Hodgkin lymphoma [3, 4]. Alternatively, combing MR and 18F-FDG PET might further increase diagnostic accuracy and play an important role as research tool in evaluating the strengths and draw-backs of both modalities directly against each other. This might also give additional data on the view of some authors who argue that ^{18}F-FDG PET/CT might even eliminate the need for bone marrow biopsy in the primary staging of Hodgkin disease because ^{18}F-FDG PET/CT is highly sensitive and specific for bone marrow involvement in this disease, at 92 % and 90 % respectively [5]. Additional information using PET/MR could be specifically gained from diffusion-weighted sequences in the case of indolent lymphomas [6]. Finally due the lack of radiation exposure of MRI, compared with CT, PET/MRI may get an alternative to PET/CT especially in young patients with good prognosis.

MR in general is considered to be inferior to CT for staging of lung cancer and detection of pulmonary metastases [7, 8]. However MRI, including DWI sequences, has been shown to detect 100 % of lung metastases larger than 7 mm found on CT and the presence of small metastases is often no therapeutically relevant [9, 10]. Hereby first preliminary data indicate an equivalent accuracy of PET/MR and PET/CT for lung lesions [11]. In addition, new developments like half-Fourier, single-shot, turbo spin echo sequences have substantially improved the lung-tissue contrast of MRI in the recent years [8]. With regard to local tumor infiltration into adjacent structures MRI might improve T-staging when compared to CT.

O. Ratib et al. (eds.), *Atlas of PET/MR Imaging in Oncology*,
DOI 10.1007/978-3-642-31292-2_10, © Springer-Verlag Berlin Heidelberg 2013

Diffuse Large B-Cell Lymphoma

Clinical History

Thirty-eight-year-old patient with diffuse large B-cell lymphoma (originally as gastric MALT). Follow-up study acquired after two cycles of chemotherapy. Status post renal transplant at age of 19.

Imaging Technique

PET: Whole-body PET acquired 60 min after injection of 369 MBq of ^{18}F-FDG, 57 kg/157 cm patient, with 5.2 mmol/L of fasting glycemia.

MRI: Whole body atMR (T1 weighted), supine position. 3D FFE T1 weighted (eThrive) whole-body MRI.

Findings

Initial staging study prior to treatment showed multiple hypermetabolic lymph nodes in the coeliac and retroperitoneal areas. Super diaphragmatic extension showed a single positive supraclavicular lymph node. Follow-up study after two cycles of chemotherapy show complete normalization of lymph nodes metabolic activity.

Teaching Points

Although whole-body MR images may not provide similar diagnostic anatomical resolution as PET/CT, PET/MR may be a valuable alternative technique for assessment of the extent of the disease and response to chemotherapy particularly in patients with limited renal function that may be at risk of renal toxicity from CT contrast media.

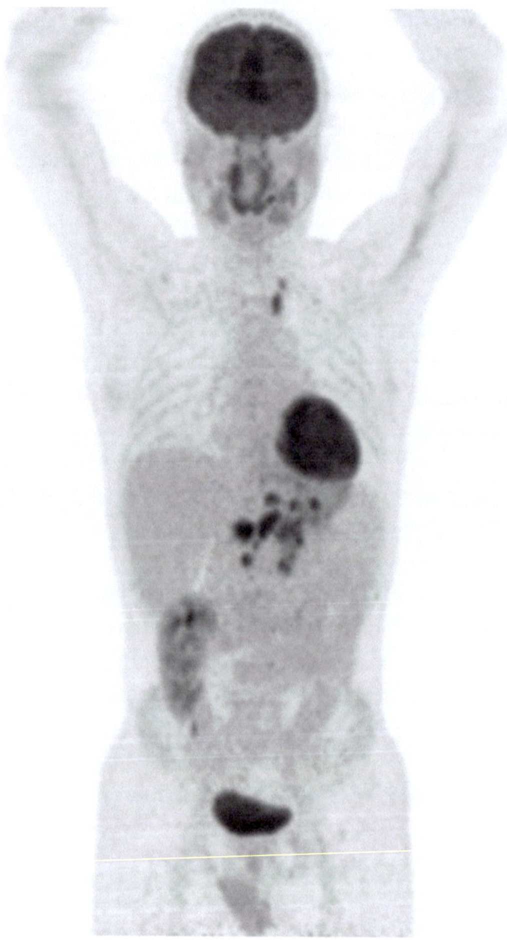

Fig. 10.1 Coronal MIP reconstruction of PET images acquired at the time of the diagnosis showing diffuse hyper-metabolic lymph nodes in the coeliac and retroperitoneal area and in the upper left clavicular area

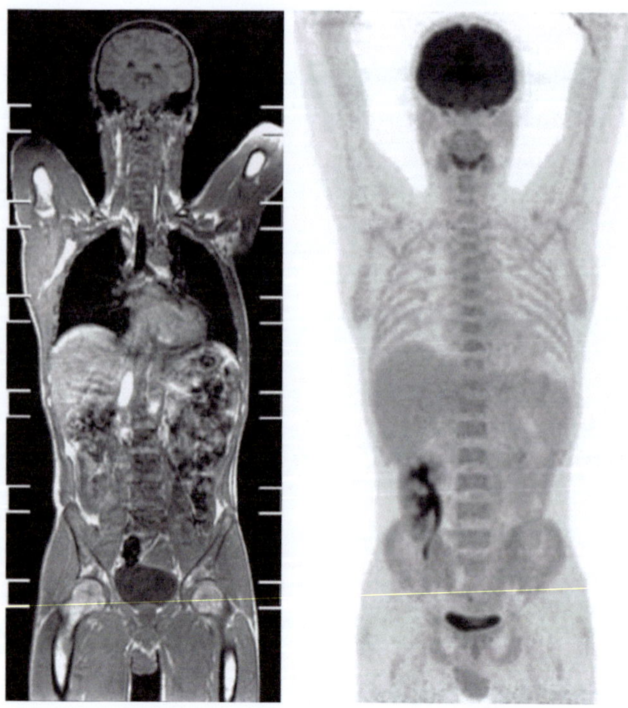

Fig. 10.2 Whole body coronal MR and PET images showing complete resolution of the hyper metabolic lymph nodes 2 month later after two cycles of chemotherapy

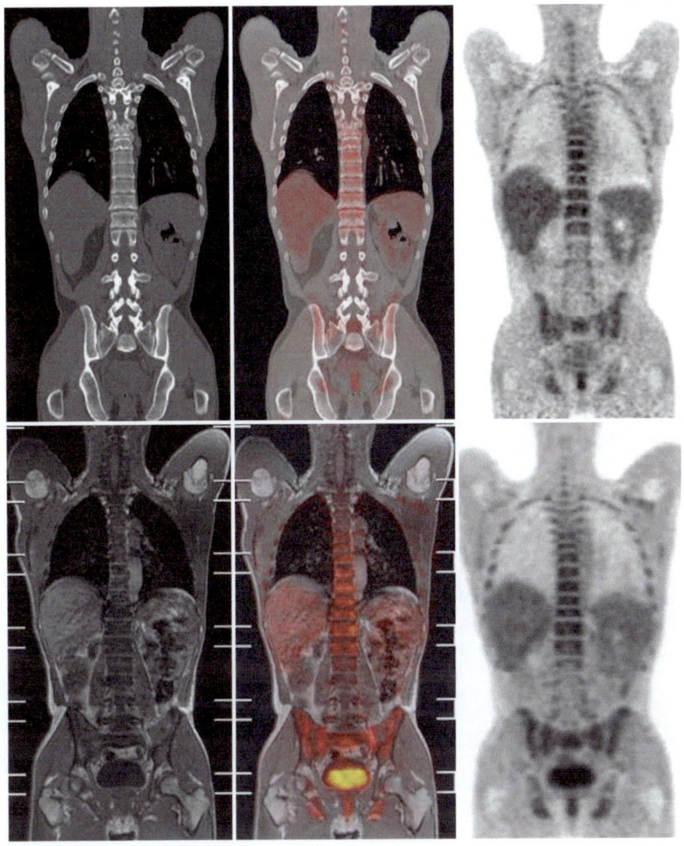

Fig. 10.3 Comparison of coronal PET/CT (*top*) and PET/MR (*bottom*) images acquired after chemotherapy showing complete resolution of abdominal and thoracic metabolic lymph nodes. Note the medullar hyper-metabolism post chemotherapy

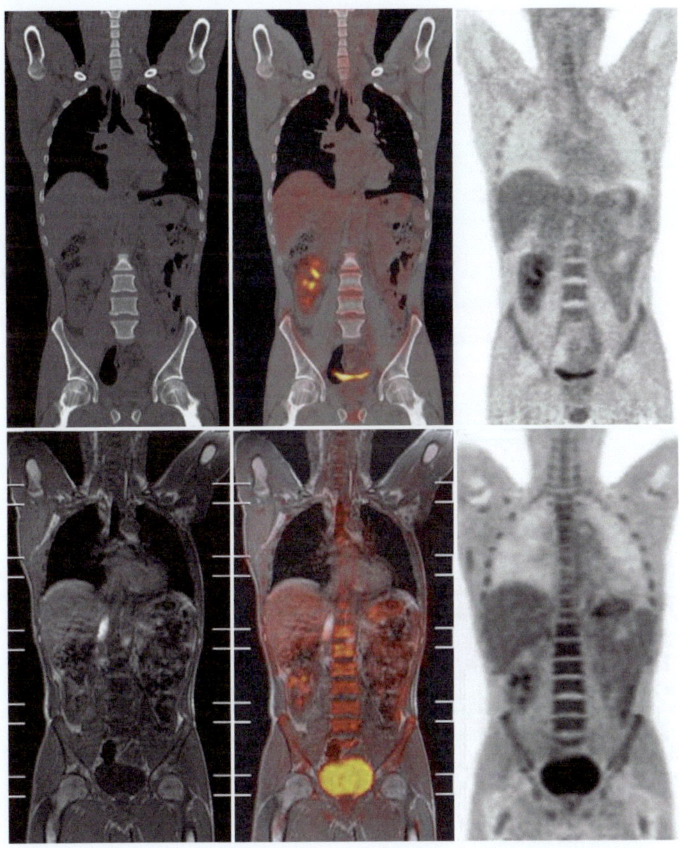

Fig. 10.4 Coronal images of PET/CT (*top*) and PET/MR (*bottom*) studies located more posteriorly. Notice the right transplanted kidney

Recurrence of Chondrosarcoma

Clinical History

Thirty-five-year-old patient with a history of surgical removal of a mixoide chondrosarcoma of the left thigh followed by radio- and chemo-therapy 2 years ago. Current study requested for investigation of recurrence of extra-articular multi-metastatic extension of the original tumor.

Imaging Technique

PET: Whole-body PET acquired 60 min after injection of 369 MBq of ^{18}F-FDG, 57 kg/157 cm patient, with 5.2 mmol/L of fasting glycemia.

MRI: Whole body atMR (T1 weighted), supine position followed by a whole body 3D FFE T1 weighted (eThrive) MRI.

Findings

Current study shows recurrence of soft tissue lesion of the left thigh with focal increase in FDG uptake with remote metastatic extension of hepermetabolic lesions in the iliac and peritoneal area of the left abdomen and pelvic area.

Teaching Points

For soft tissue tumors, high-resolution MR images can provide more adequate soft tissue differentiation and anatomical localization than CT images

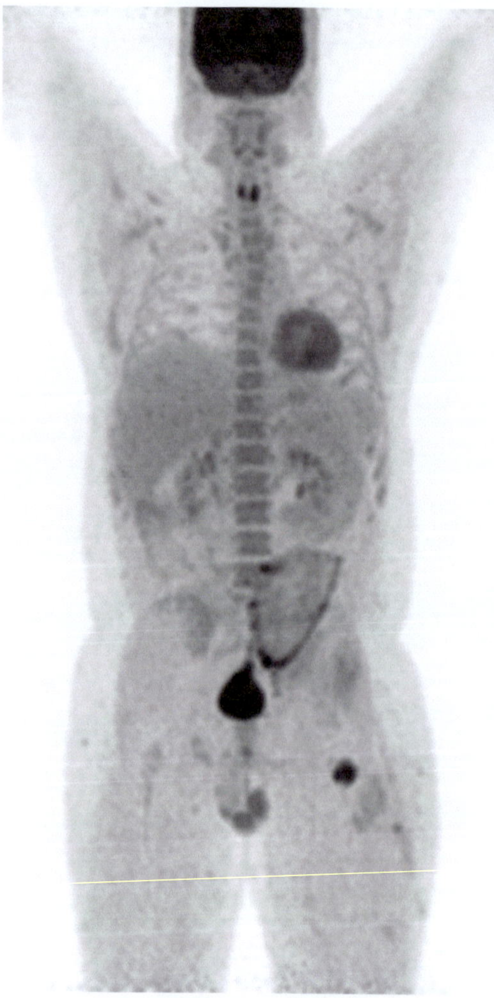

Fig. 10.5 Whole body volume MIP rendering of PET images showing focal uptake in the tumor region of the left thigh and distant focal uptake lesions in the abdomen

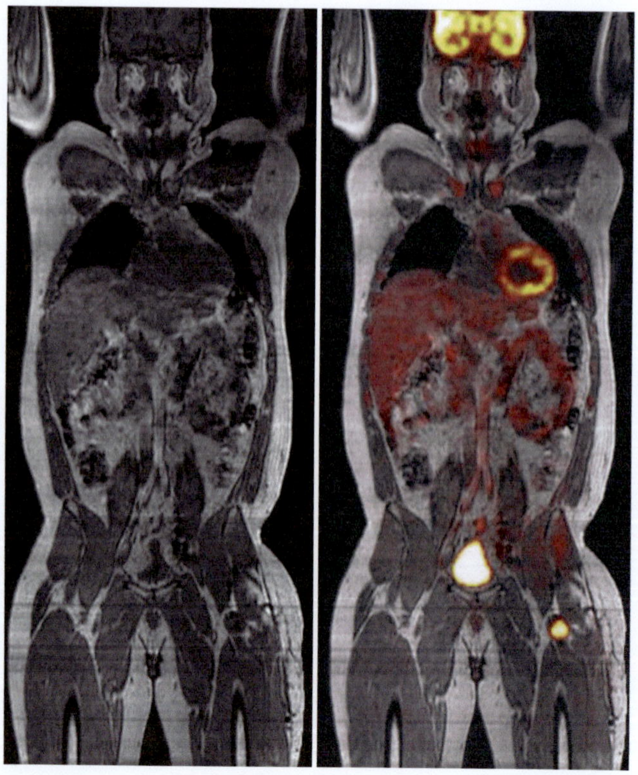

Fig. 10.6 Coronal MPR of whole-body eThrive MRI images (*left*) and fusion with PET images (*right*)

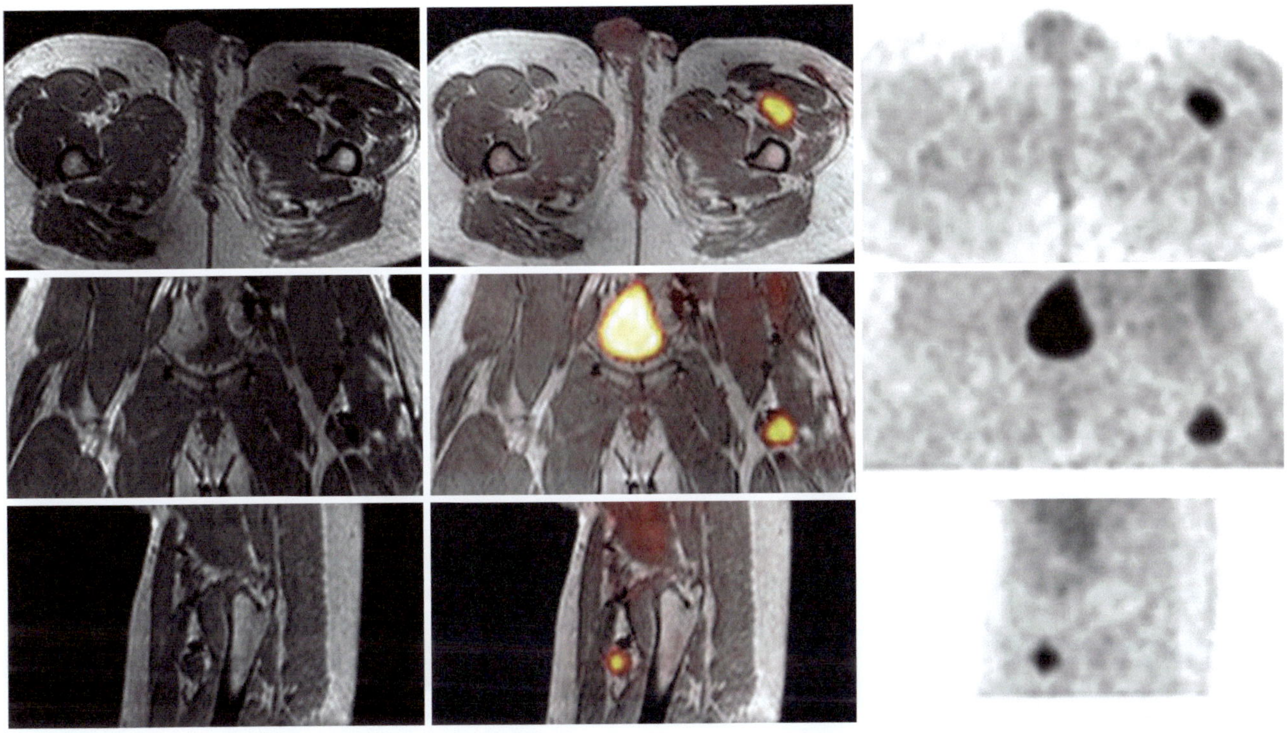

Fig. 10.7 Multi-planar reformatted (MPR) images of high resolution TSE T2 weighted (eThrive) MRI images fused with PET images at the level of the muscular lesion in the left thigh

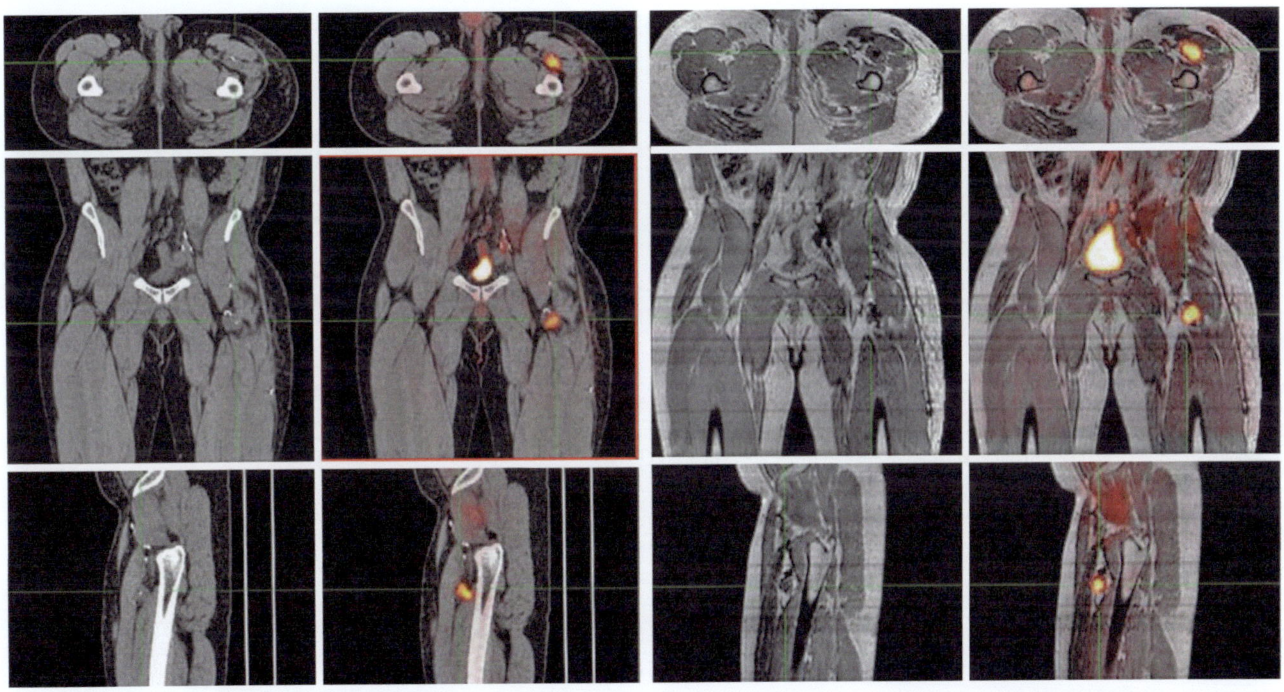

Fig. 10.8 Comparison of PET/CT (*left*) and PET/MR (*right*) multi-planar (MPR) reformatted images of the pelvis and mid thigh region obtained from whole-body 3D images

Metastatic Pulmonary Cancer (NSCLC)

Clinical History

Seventy-year-old patient diagnosed with non-small cell lung cancer (NSCLC) with liver metastases. Follow-up study requested 3 months after chemotherapy.

Imaging Technique

PET: Whole-body PET acquired 60 min after injection of 370 MBq of ^{18}F-FDG.

MRI: Whole body atMR (T1 weighted), supine position. 3D FFE T1 weighted (eThrive) MRI followed by coronal high-resolution breath-hold HASTE images of the upper abdomen.

Findings

PET/MR shows left lower lobe lung cancer with metastatic mediastinal lymph node and heterogeneous tracer uptake in large lesion (7 × 9 cm) in right liver segments VI/VII corresponding to metastatic disease.

Teaching Points

For liver metastases, high-resolution breath-hold MR images can provide better definition and tissue characterization than contrast-enhanced CT images.

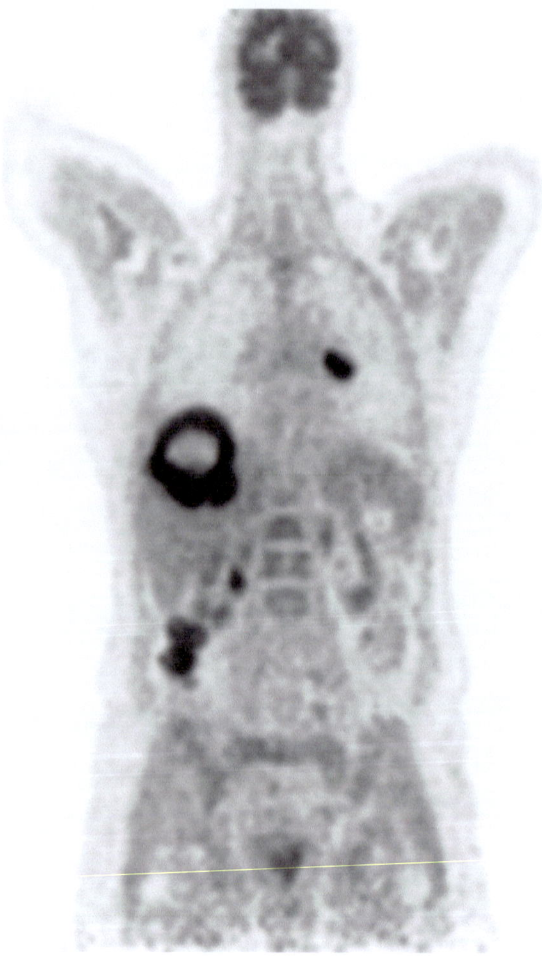

Fig. 10.9 Coronal view of volume rendered MIP of PET images showing focal FDG uptake in the left para-hillar region and a large metastatic lesion of the liver with central hypometabolism corresponding to necrotic tissue

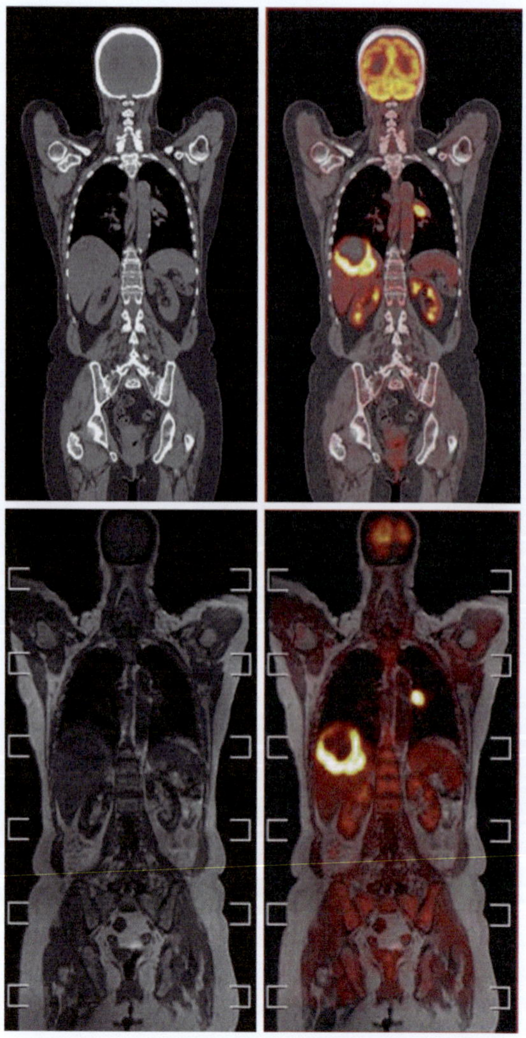

Fig. 10.10 Comparison of coronal views of whole body PET/CT (*top*) and low resolution whole-body PET/MR (*bottom*)

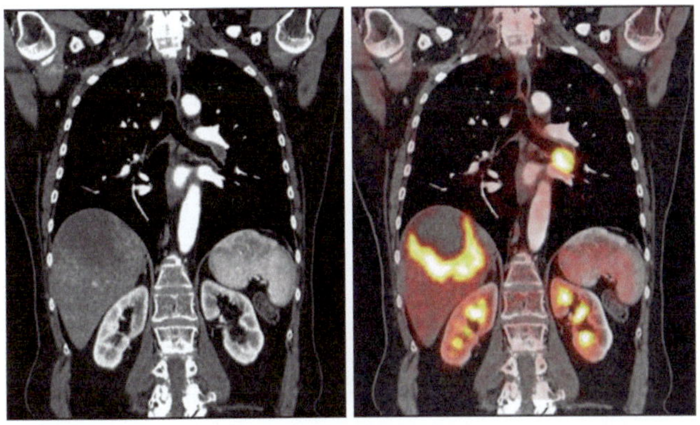

Fig. 10.11 High-resolution contrast-enhanced CT (*left*) and fusion (*right*) of PET/CT images of the thorax and upper abdomen

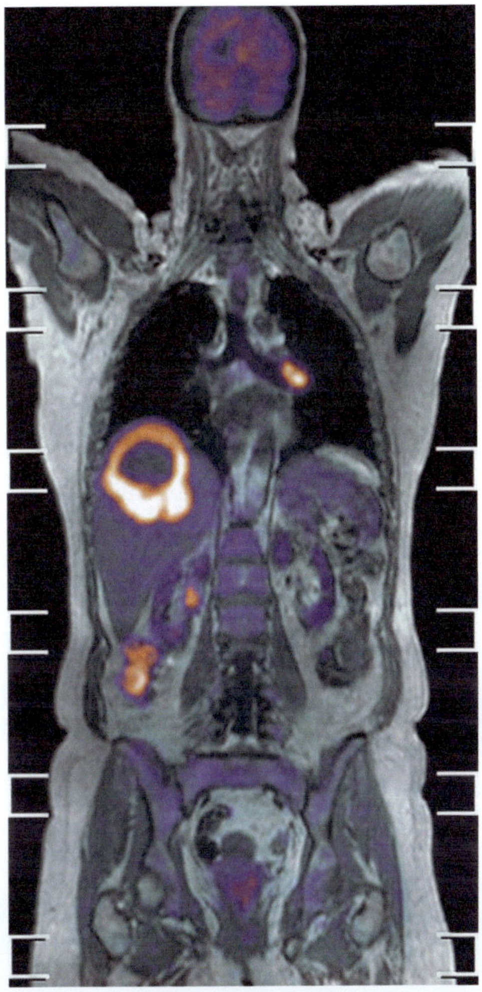

Fig. 10.12 Coronal view of low-resolution whole-body MR fused with corresponding PET image

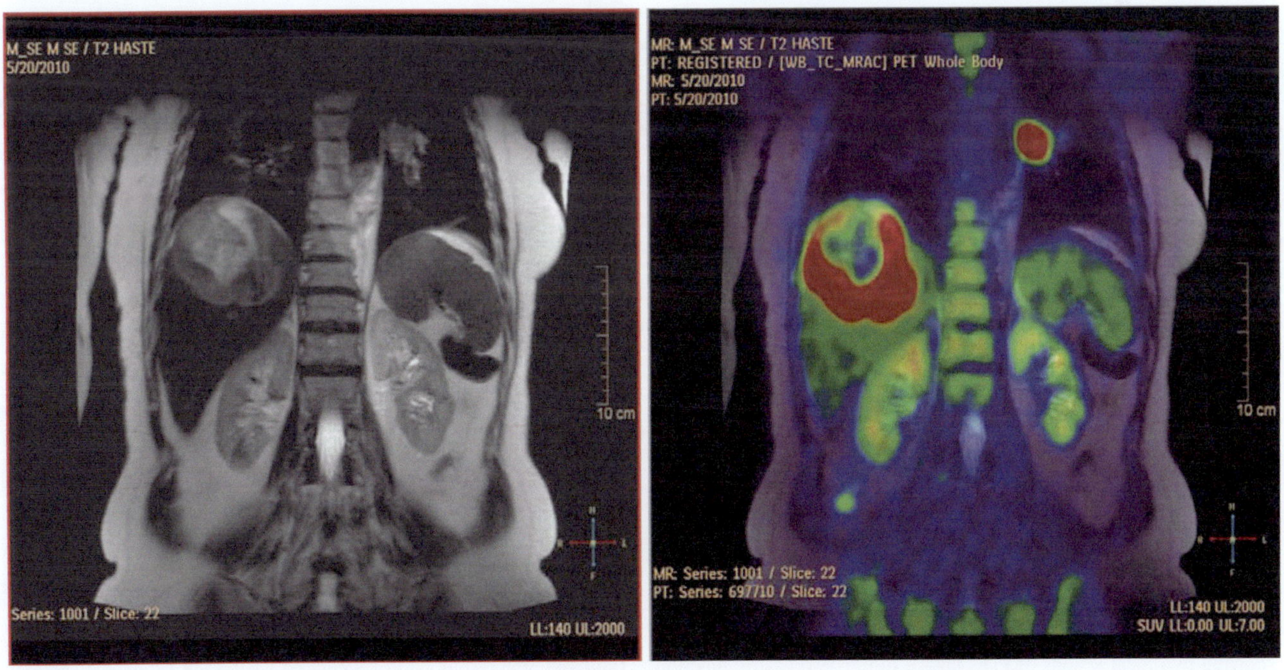

Fig. 10.13 High-resolution breath-hold coronal HASTE MR image (*left*) with corresponding PET/MR image (*right*)

Esophageal Cancer with Liver Metastases

Clinical History

Sixty-year-old patient investigated for staging of a distal esophageal adenocarcinoma of the oeso-gastric junction. Status post chemotherapy.

Imaging Technique

PET: Whole-body PET acquired 60 min after injection of 370 MBq of ^{18}F-FDG.

MRI: Whole body atMR (T1 weighted), supine position. Followed by a complementary diagnostic MRI study acquired on a Siemens Espree including a T2 HASTE MRI sequences in coronal. 3D FFE T1 weighted (eThrive) sequence with contrast injection.

Findings

PET/MR shows the hypermetabolic tumor lesion of the oeso-gastric junction, and a focal metastatic lesion of the liver with high FDG uptake. Incidental finding of a benign hepatic lesion without tracer uptake, most likely an hemangioma.

Teaching Points

Combination of diagnostic MR sequences and PET images allow to better differentiate malignant from benign lesions of the liver.

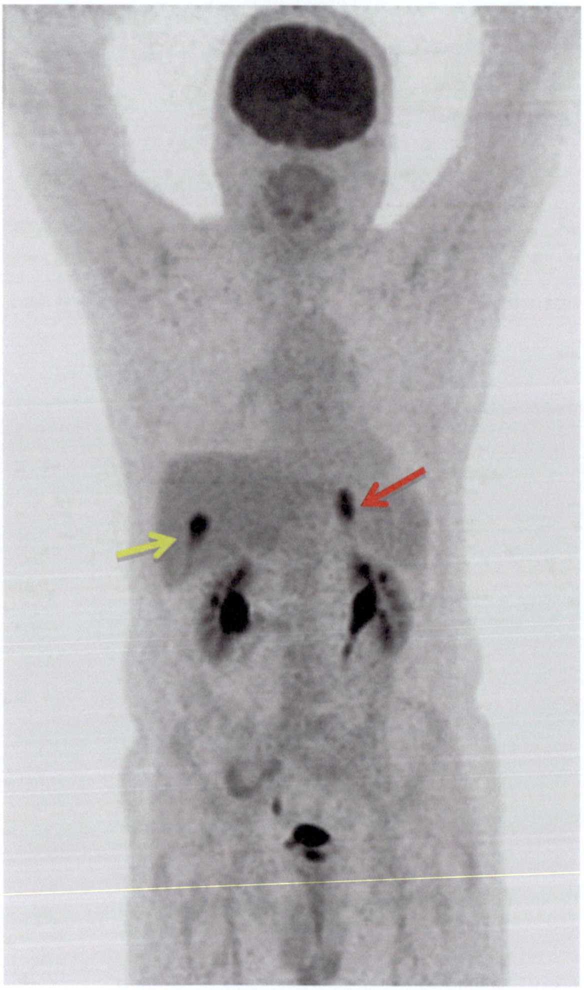

Fig. 10.14 Coronal view of volume rendered MIP of PET images showing two focal lesions of FDG uptake in the oeso-gastric junction (*red arrow*) and in a liver metastasis (*yellow arrow*)

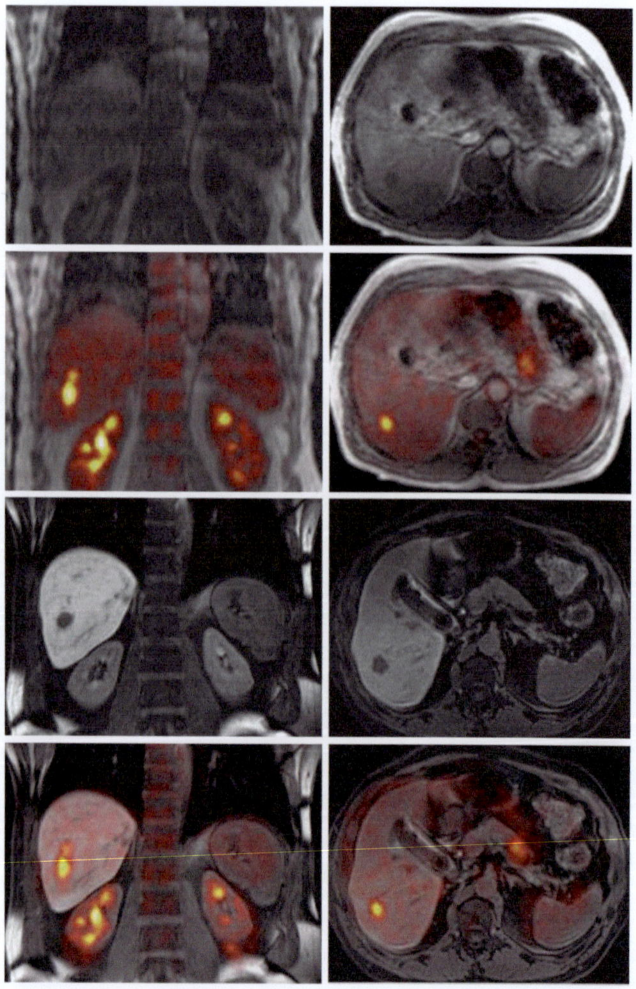

Fig. 10.15 Comparison of low-resolution whole-body MRI images (*top*) and high resolution (T1 weighted VIBE) MR sequences (*bottom*) fused with corresponding PET images

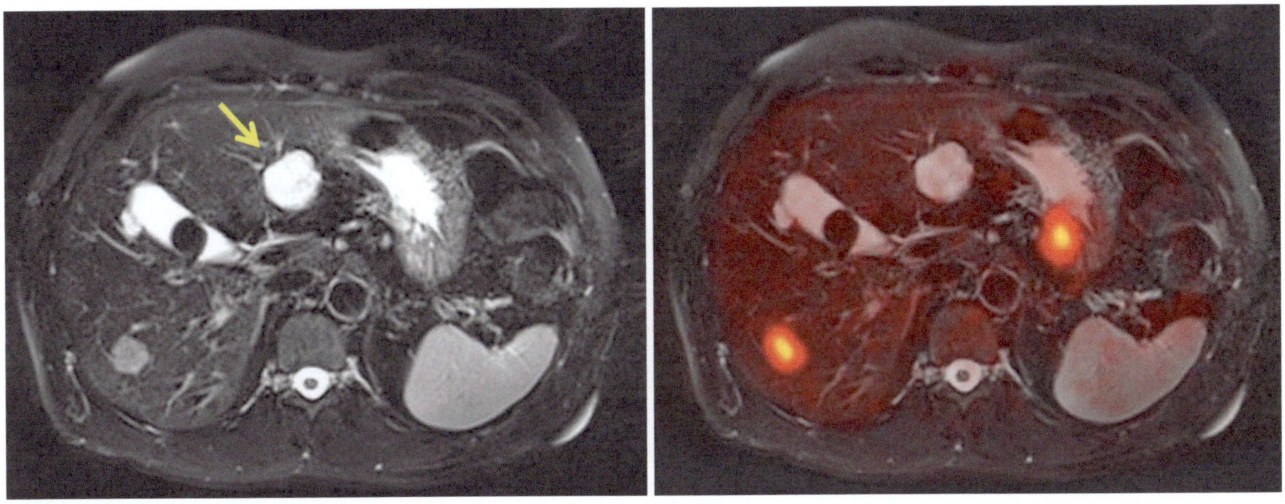

Fig. 10.16 High-resolution 2D fat-saturated "BLADE" MR images (*left*) fused with corresponding PET image (*right*) showing a benign lesion (*arrow*) with absence of FDG uptake on PET

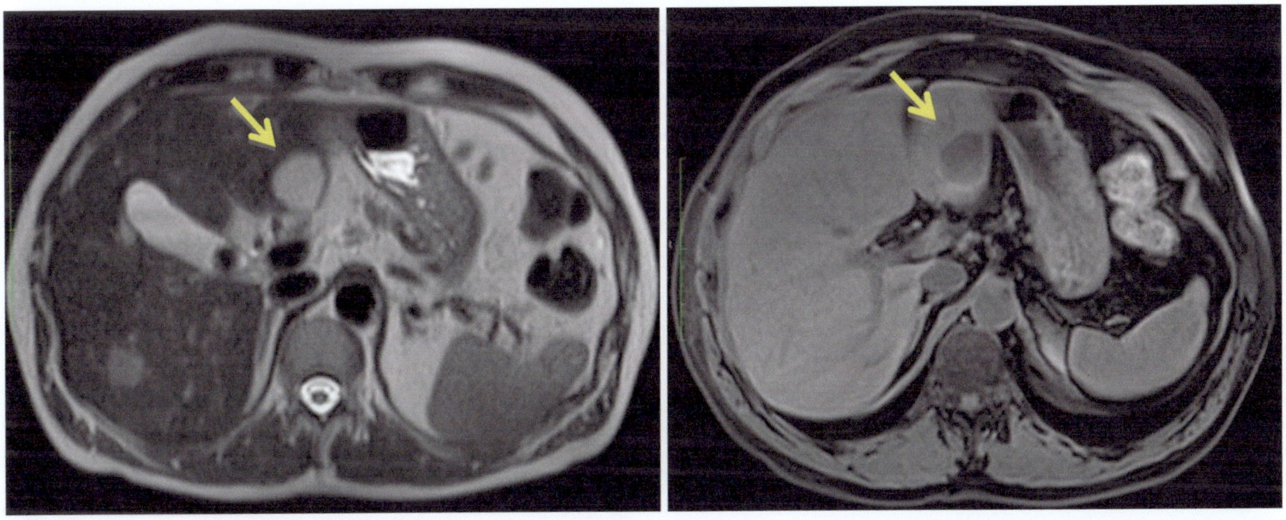

Fig. 10.17 Two different MR sequences of the liver T2 weighted HASTE (*left*) and T1 weighted eThrive (*right*) allowing to better characterize benign lesion (*arrow*) from metastatic lesions

Multi-Focal Lung Tumor

Clinical History

Seventy-year-old patient with history of smoking and incidental finding of a lung tumor on chest X-ray performed for investigation of resistant cough. Histology confirmed pulmonary carcinoma (cT2a cN3 cN0, stage IIB). Study requested for staging post chemotherapy.

Imaging Technique

PET: Whole-body PET acquired 60 min after injection of 370 MBq of ^{18}F-FDG.

MRI: Whole body atMR (T1 weighted), supine position. 3D FFE T1 weighted (eThrive) MRI followed by respiratory-gated T2 weighted HASTE images acquired in coronal and axial planes.

Findings

PET/MR shows a hypermetabolic lung lesion of the apical segment of the left lower pulmonary lobe. Identification of multiple metastatic lymph nodes with intense focal uptake of FDG in the paratracheal, hilar and subcarenal areas.

Teaching Points

While MR sequences are not optimal for examination of lung parenchyma that is best evaluated by CT, high resolution MR sequences can however provide sufficient anatomical details for identification and localization of lesions with high FDG uptake.

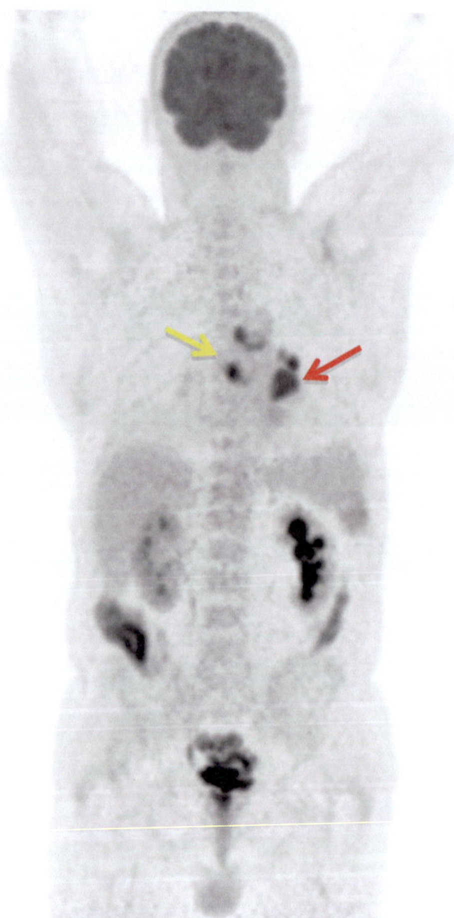

Fig. 10.18 Coronal vie of volume rendered MIP images of PET showing the lung tumor of the lower left lobe (*red arrow*) and dissemination on the mediastinal lymph nodes (*yellow arrow*)

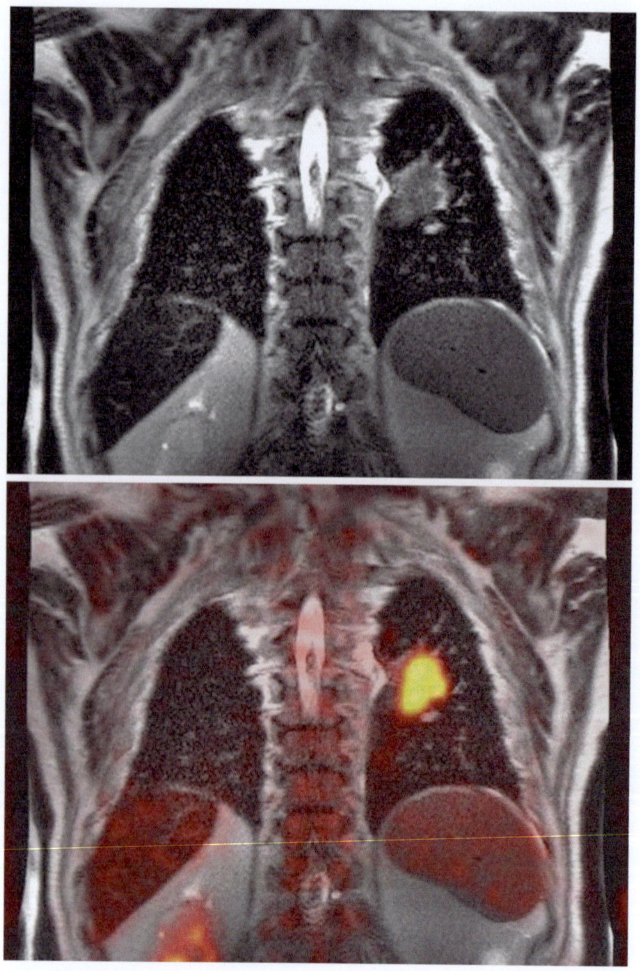

Fig. 10.19 Coronal respiratory-gated T2 weighted HASTE images (*top*) fused with corresponding PET image (*bottom*) showing high metabolic activity of the lung tumor

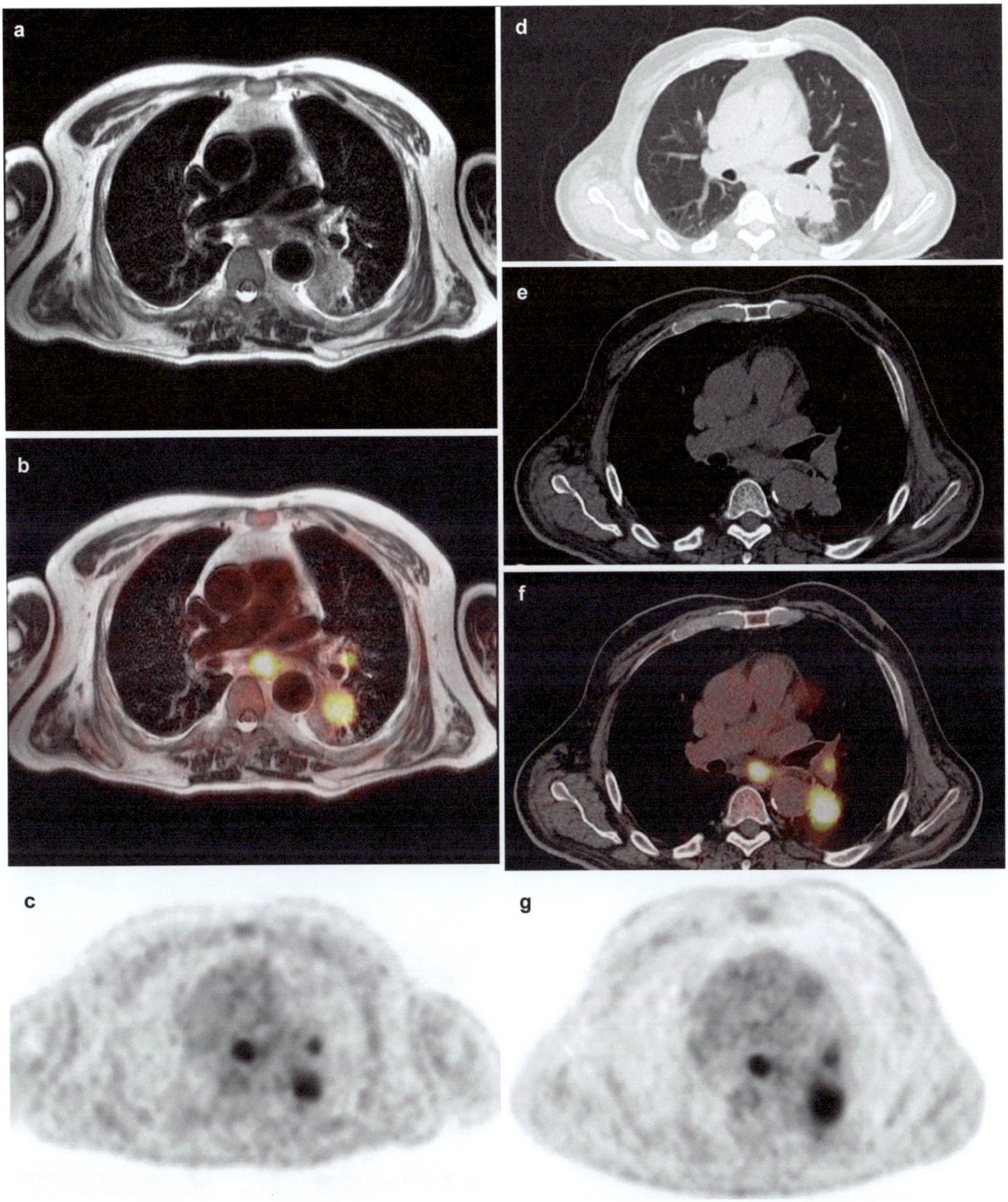

Fig. 10.20 Comparison of PET/MR (*left*) and PET/CT studies. Axial respiratory-gated T2 weighted HASTE images (**a**) fused with corresponding PET image (**b**), and axial CT with lung window setting (**d**) and soft tissue setting (**e**) fused with corresponding PET images (**f**). Both (**c**) and (**g**) show the PET images at the same level of the two studies

Brain Metastasis of Unknown Origin

Clinical History

Sixty-two-year-old patient discovered having a brain metastases in the left cerebellum on an MRI performed for investigating recurrent headaches. Current study requested for staging and identification of the original tumor. Patient also known for renal insufficiency and multiple renal cysts.

Imaging Technique

PET: Whole-body PET acquired 60 min after injection of 369 MBq of ^{18}F-FDG, 57 kg/157 cm patient, with 5.2 mmol/L of fasting glycemia.

MRI: Whole body atMR (T1 weighted), supine position. 3D FFE T1 weighted (eThrive) MRI followed by a complete diagnostic MRI study of the abdomen.

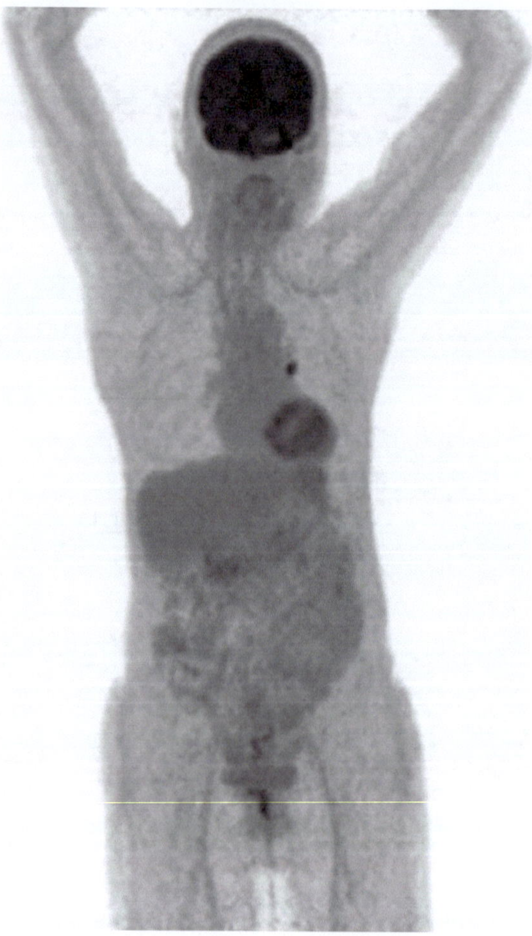

Fig. 10.21 Volume rendered MIP of whole-body PET showing a single focal uptake of a lesion in the hilar region of the left lung

Findings

PET/MR shows a focal hypermetabolic lesion of the hilum of the left lung. Standard whole-body MRI could not clearly characterize the lung lesion but complimentary PET/CT confirmed the suspicion of lung cancer. Additional high resolution MRI showed polycystic renal disease and incidental finding of an aortic dissection.

Teaching Points

For proper characterization of suspicious lung tumor, additional CT image are required. But PET/MR allows to properly stage the extent of remote metastatic lesions.

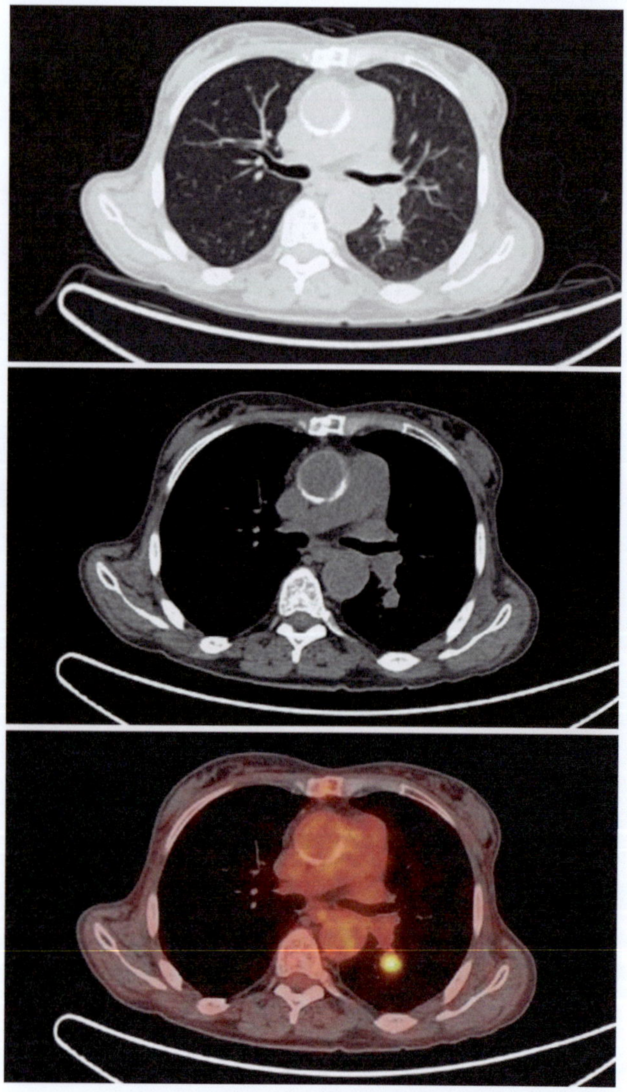

Fig. 10.22 Axial CT with lung window setting (*top*) and soft tissue setting (*middle*) fused with corresponding PET images (*bottom*)

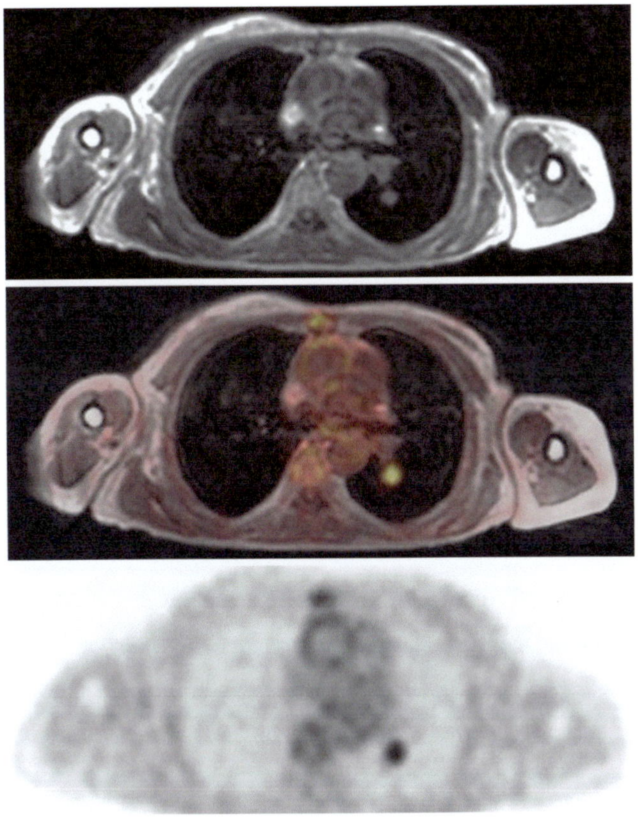

Fig. 10.23 Standard low-resolution whole body MRI sequences used for attenuation correction (*top*) have limited resolution for lung parenchyma

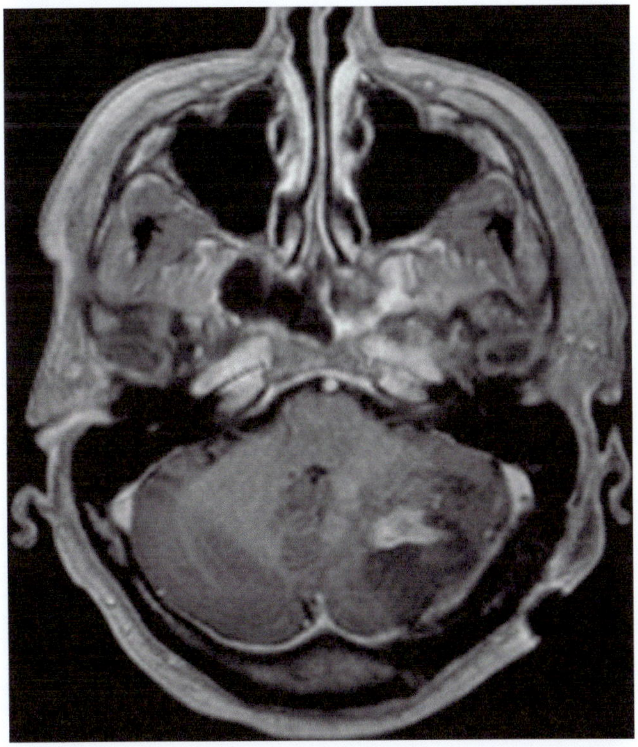

Fig. 10.24 Brain MRI post surgery showing the remaining extension of metastatic lesion of the left cerebellar region

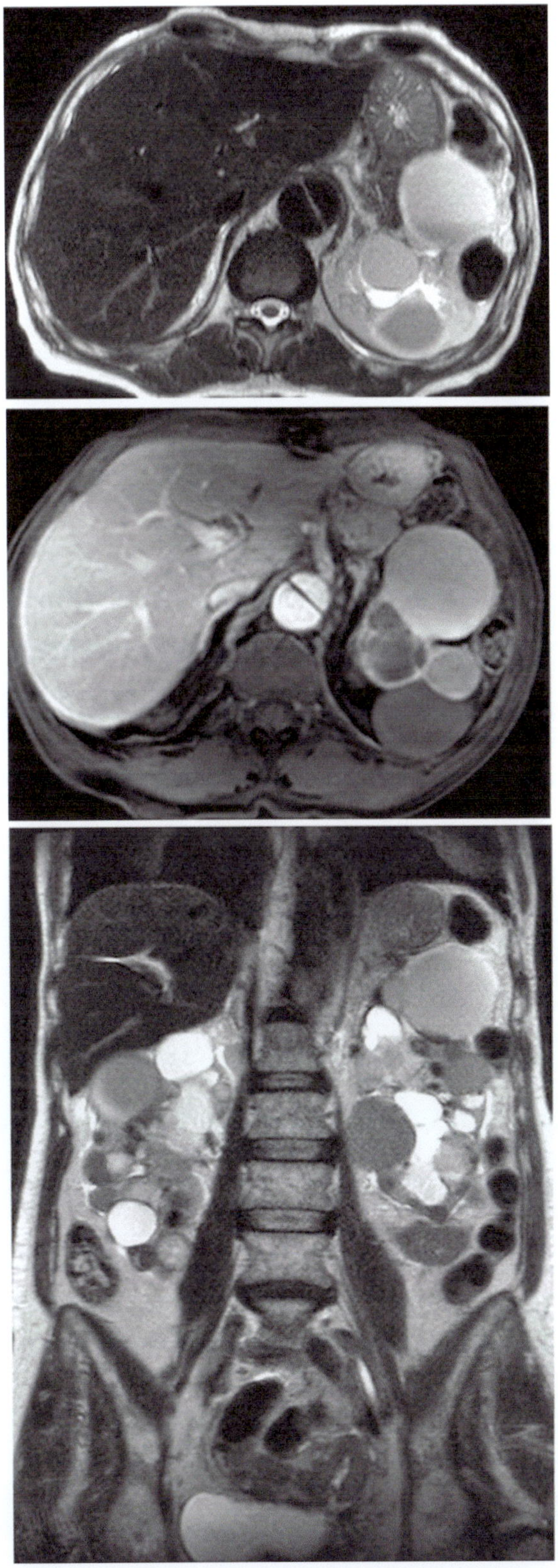

Fig. 10.25 Axial (*top*) and coronal (*bottom*) high resolution MR sequence of the abdomen show polycystic renal disease and incidental finding of an aortic dissection

Pulmonary Adenocarcinoma

Clinical History

Sixty-eight-year-old patient following incidental finding of a right lung mass on chest X-ray for chronic cough. CT guided biopsy confirmed a pulmonary adenocarcinoma. Study requested for staging and treatment planning.

Imaging Technique

PET: Whole-body PET acquired 60 min after injection of 370 MBq of ^{18}F-FDG.

MRI: Whole body atMR (T1 weighted), supine position. 3D FFE T1 weighted (eThrive) MRI followed by a whole body STIR acquisition.

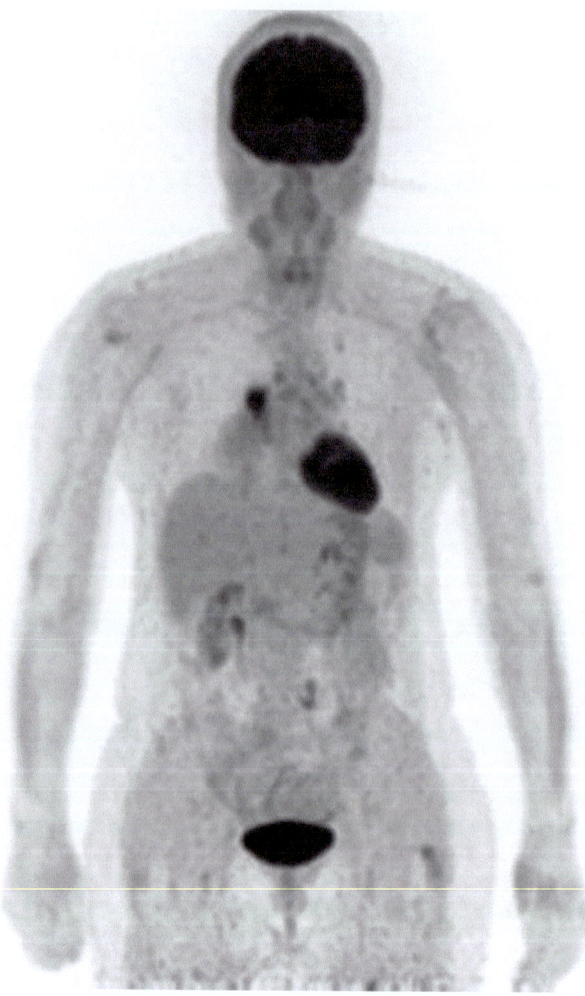

Fig. 10.26 Coronal projection of volume rendered MIP images of PET showing the hypermetabolic tumor lesion of the right lung with moderate FDG uptake of the surrounding pneumonia

Findings

PET/MR confirmed the presence of a hilar tumoral mass of the right lower lobe, associated with pneumonitis of the lower lobe secondary to partial obstruction of the bronchi by the tumor. Identification of multiple hypermetabolic lymph nodes of the mediastinum and subclavicular region

> **Teaching Points**
>
> PET images of PET/MR studies allow differentiating the extension of hypermetabolic tumor tissue from associated pneumonia with low or moderate FDG uptake.

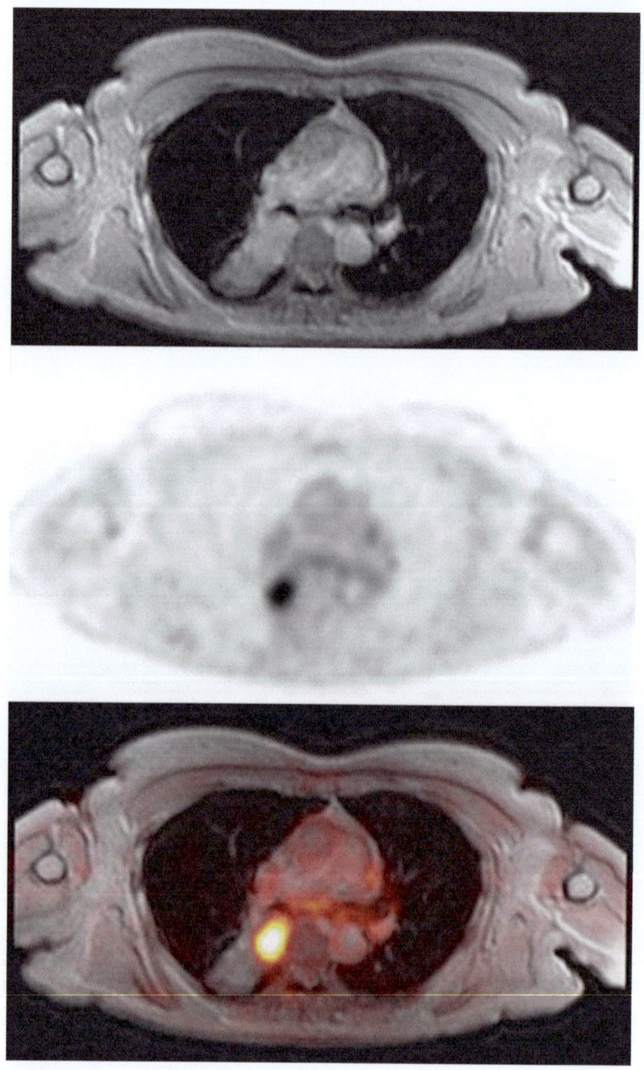

Fig. 10.27 Axial views from low resolution whole-body MR scan (*top*) and PET scan (*middle*) and fusion of the two images (*bottom*) showing the different FDG uptake between tumor and pneumonitis-induced condensation of pulmonary parenchyma

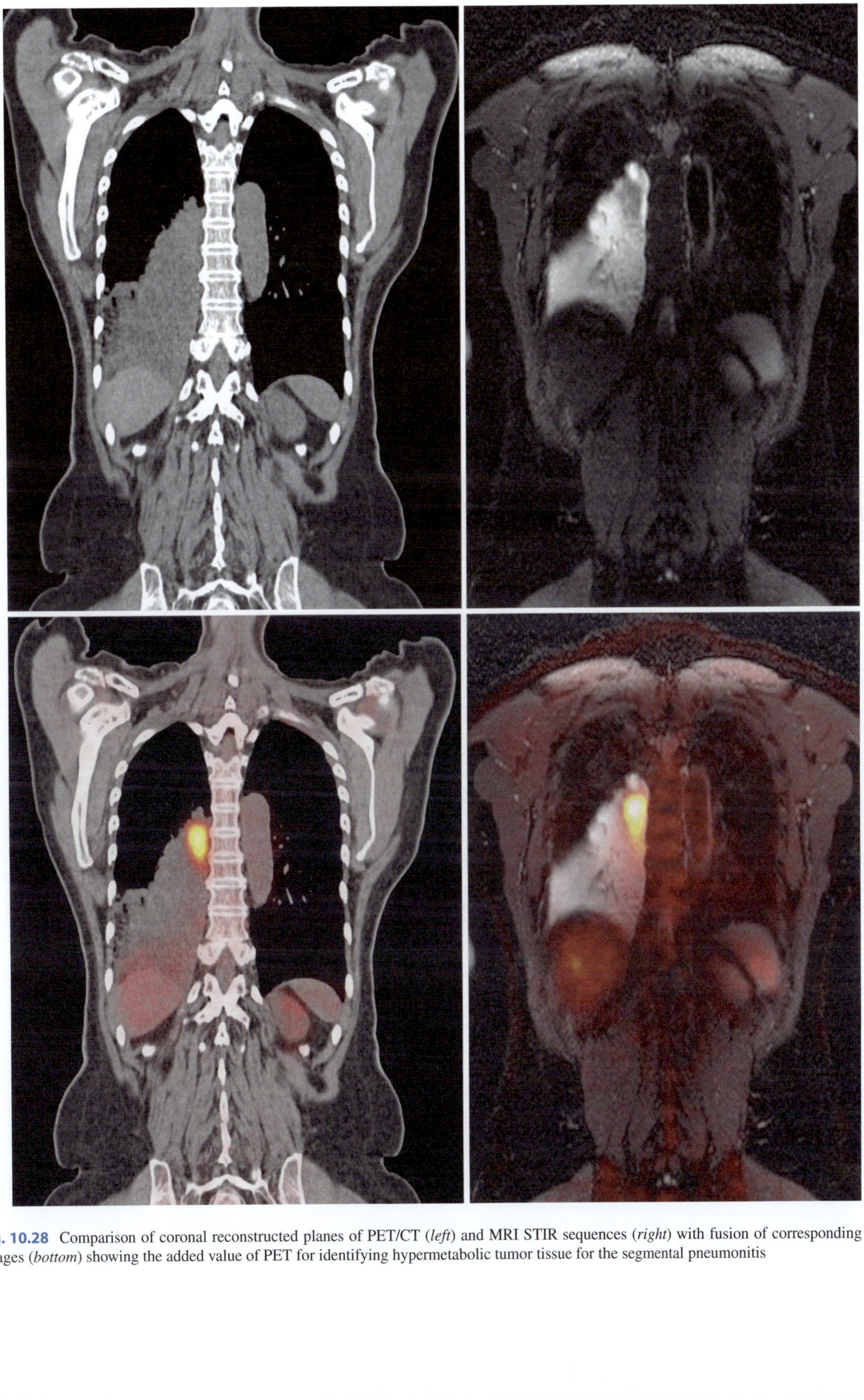

Fig. 10.28 Comparison of coronal reconstructed planes of PET/CT (*left*) and MRI STIR sequences (*right*) with fusion of corresponding PET images (*bottom*) showing the added value of PET for identifying hypermetabolic tumor tissue for the segmental pneumonitis

PET/MR in Acute Lymphocytic Leukemia (ALL)

Clinical History

A 44 year old patient with a pathological fracture of the lumbar spine previously stabilized with dorsal instrumentation. Histopathology revealed ALL-infiltration in the lumbar spine.

Imaging Technique

Whole body PET/MR images acquired 112 min after iv injection 408 MBq 18F-FDG, 77 kg.

8 beds × 5 min together with whole body cor T1w TSE and cor T2w STIR. Axial T1w VIBE fat saturated after Gadolinium over the region of the thorax, abdomen and pelvis.

Findings

A diffuse affection with bone marrow infiltration primarily of the lumbar and sacral spine is found in PET. MR demonstrates the extent of extra-osseous growth around the sacral bone.

Teaching Points

Combined PET/MR provides detailed information about the extent of the bone marrow infiltration. Smaller lesions might be missed by MR only but the high lesion-to-background ratio of PET facilitates their detection.

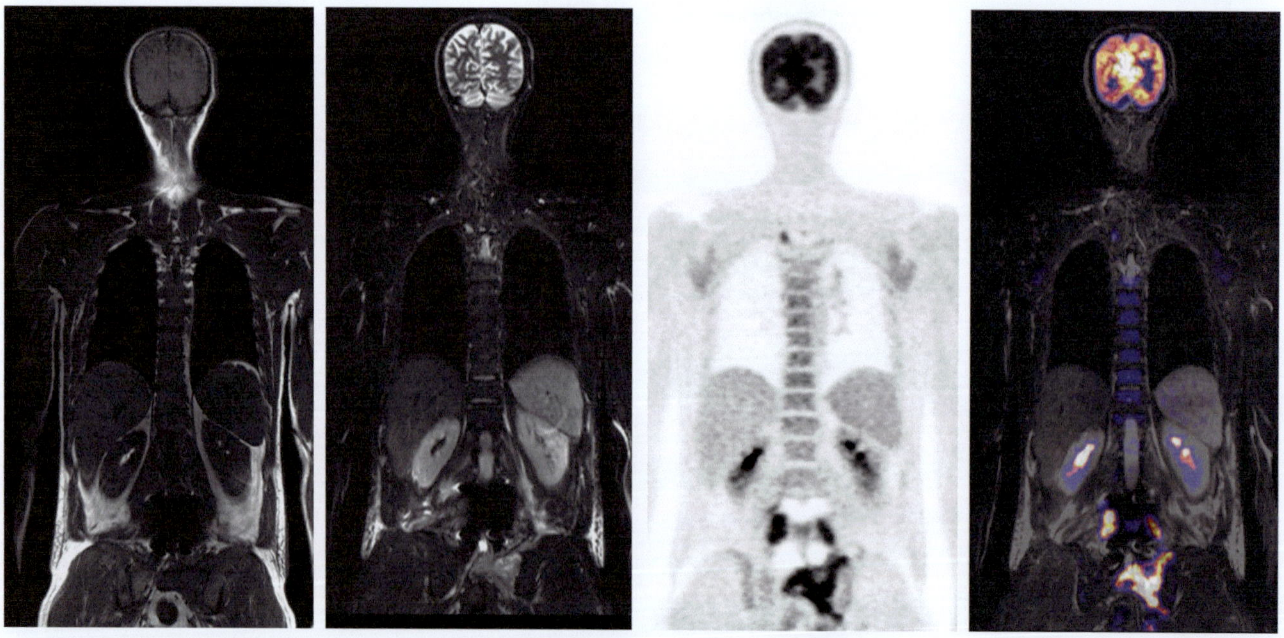

Fig. 10.29 Coronal T1w TSE (*far left*) and T2w STIR (*middle left*) show bone marrow infiltration in the left sacral bone, the left proximal femur, right ischium and the upper thoracic spine. Metal artifacts from the dorsal instrumentation obscure this region on MR images. PET (*middle right*) and fused PET/MR (*far right*) images demonstrate high uptake of 18F-FDG in the corresponding regions. The lesion in the upper thoracic spine might be missed on MR only, however the high lesion-to-background ratio on the PET images helps identifying it

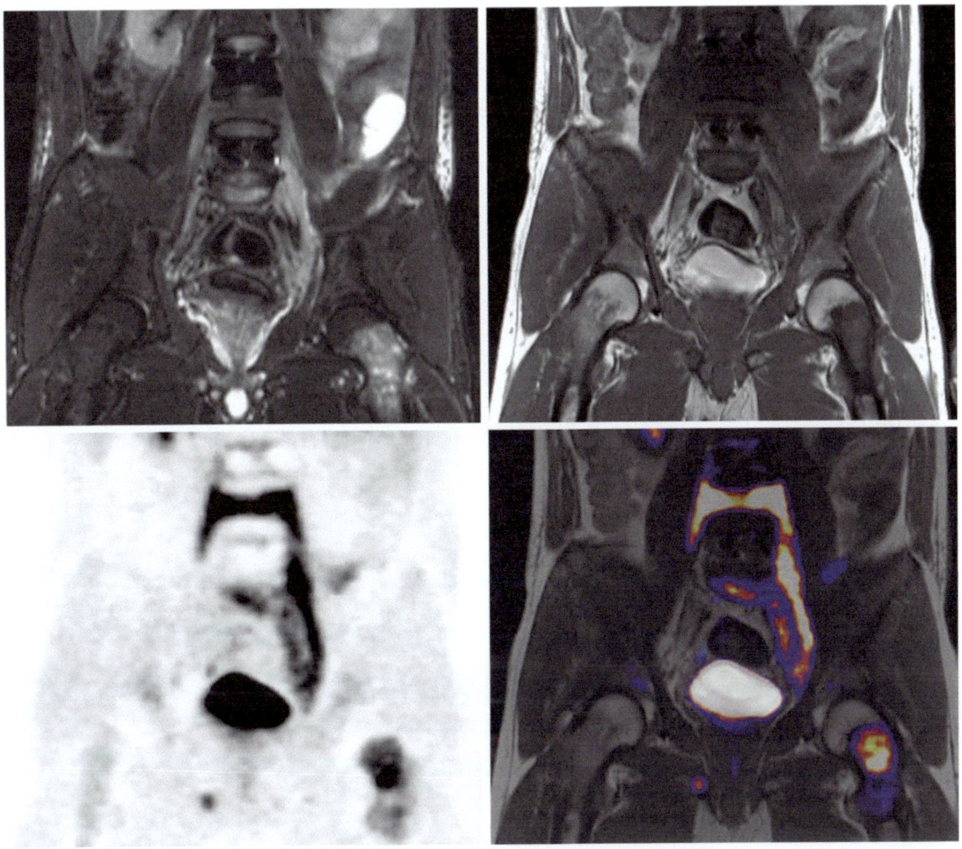

Fig. 10.30 Coronal T12w STIR and T1w TSE show a pathological fracture of L4 with artifacts from dorsal instrumentation in L3 and L5 (*upper row*). The T1w hypointense signal in L4 and the proximal left femur indicates complete infiltration of the vertebra by lymphoblastic cells. A small lesion is also found in the right pubic bone. In addition T2w STIR demonstrates a hyperintense extraosseous strand on the left side reaching from L4 to the sacral bone. Another small extraosseous formation is present on the left side. Both PET and fused image confirm high uptake of 18F-FDG in the corresponding regions (*lower row*)

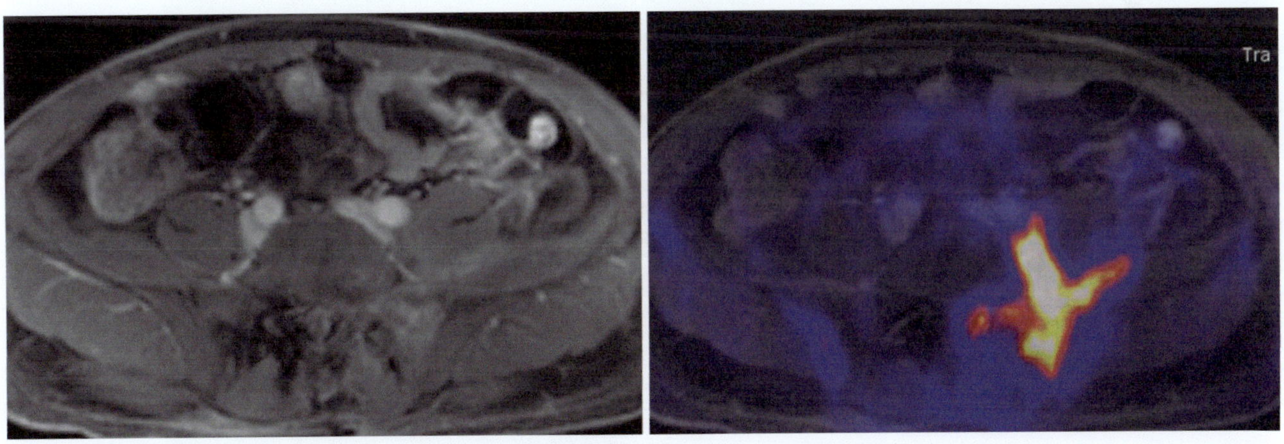

Fig. 10.31 The extraosseous tumor growth is better depicted in PET (*right*) compared to an axial T1w VIBE sequence (*left*) after Gadolinium with fat saturation. In this sequence only a diffuse low to moderate contrast enhancement could be found, whereas the high lesion-to-background ratio in PET outlines the spread more clearly

PET/MR for Biopsy Planning in NHL with Bone Infiltration

Clinical History

A 54 year old patient presents chronically elevated leucocytes and the suspicion of lymphoma. No suspicious lymph nodes were found on CT.

Imaging Technique

Whole body PET/MR images acquired 174 min after iv injection 444 MBq 18F-FDG, 95 kg.

4 beds × 4 min together with whole body cor T1w TSE and axial T2w HASTE fs. 1 bed (pelvis) a 4 min together with cor T2w STIR and axial T1w fs after Gadolinium.

Findings

T1w TSE and T2w STIR show a patchy bone marrow infiltration with islands of normal bone interposed between. Note the extensive artifacts from a hip prosthesis on the left side especially impairing the fat suppression.

Teaching Points

The combination of whole-body PET and MR can aid in guiding biopsy in patients with lymphoma especially in atypical cases like primary bone infiltration. The information of T1w TSE and T2w STIR delineate areas of bone infiltration against the normal bone marrow. In contrast, CT often shows no pathological finding.

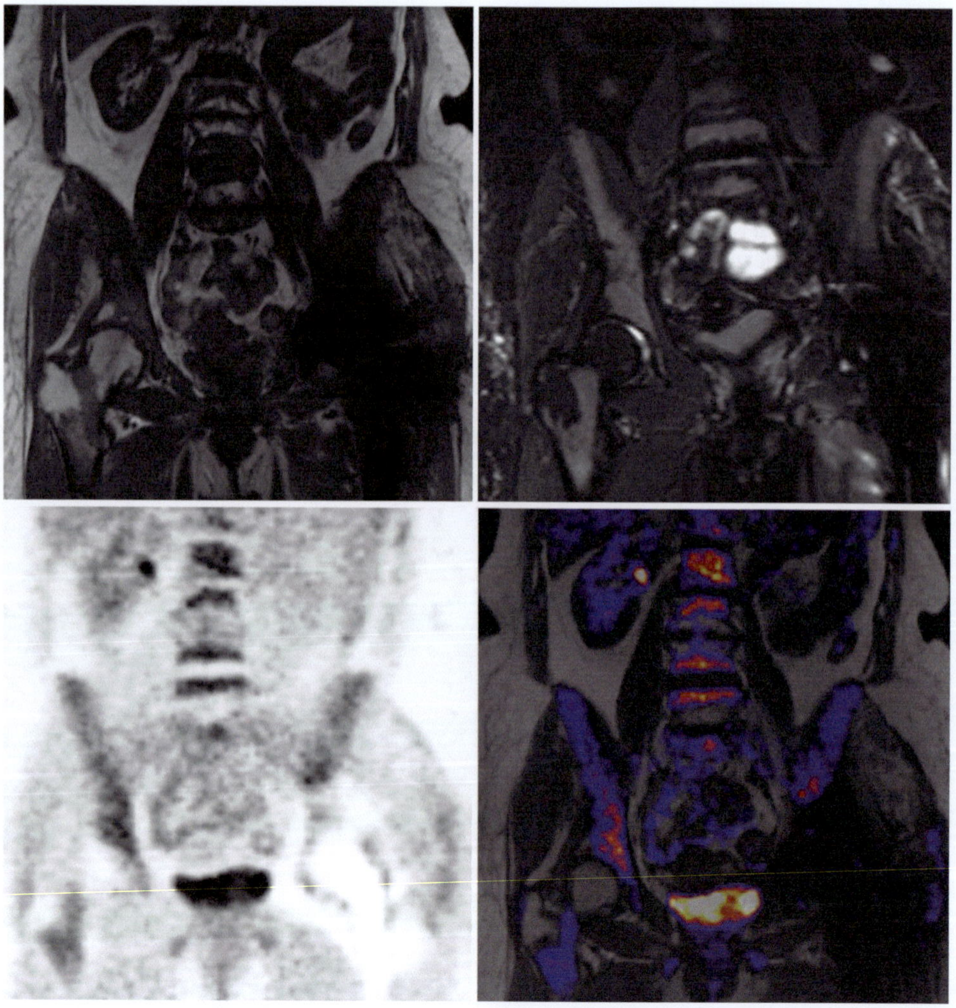

Fig. 10.32 Coronal T1w TSE and T2w STIR show patchy bone marrow infiltration of the lumbar spine and pelvis (*upper row*). Note the normal interposed bone marrow between the affected areas. Coronal PET shows moderate increase tracer uptake in the lumbar spine and pelvis. Fused PET and T1w TSE demonstrate good correlation between the uptake in PET and the hypointense regions in T1w (*lower row*)

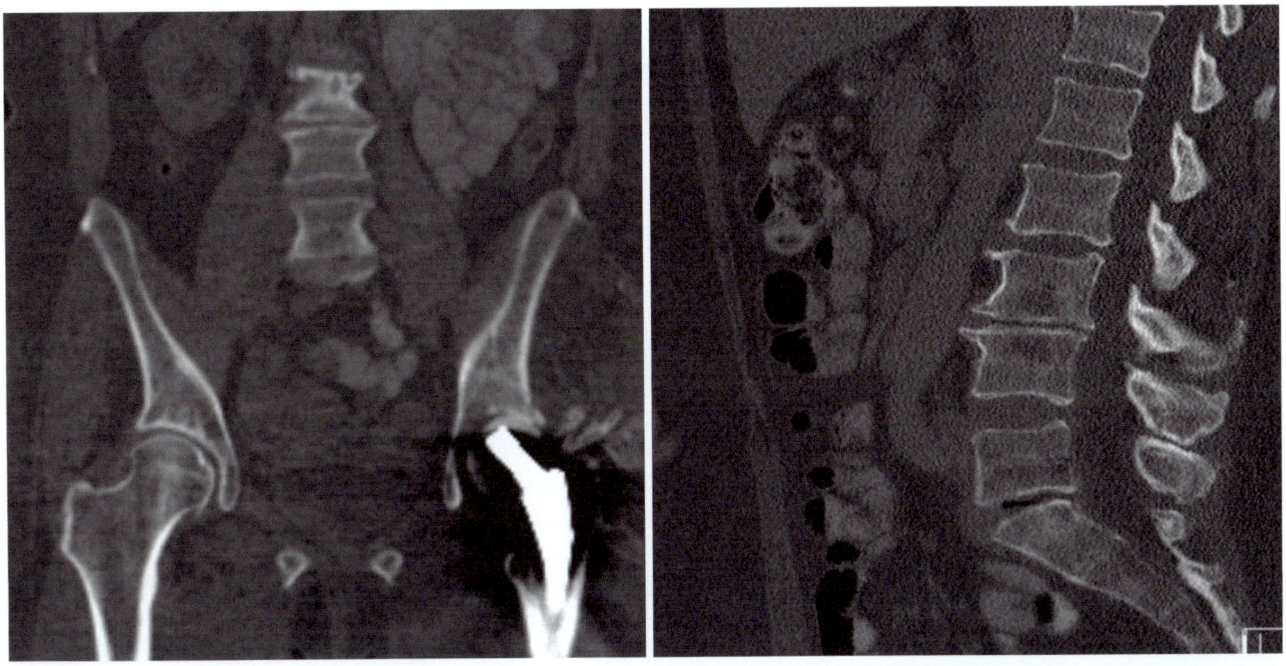

Fig. 10.33 In the coronal (*left*) and sagittal (*right*) reformatted bone window from CT no abnormalities could be detected underlining the value of bone marrow imaging in MRI

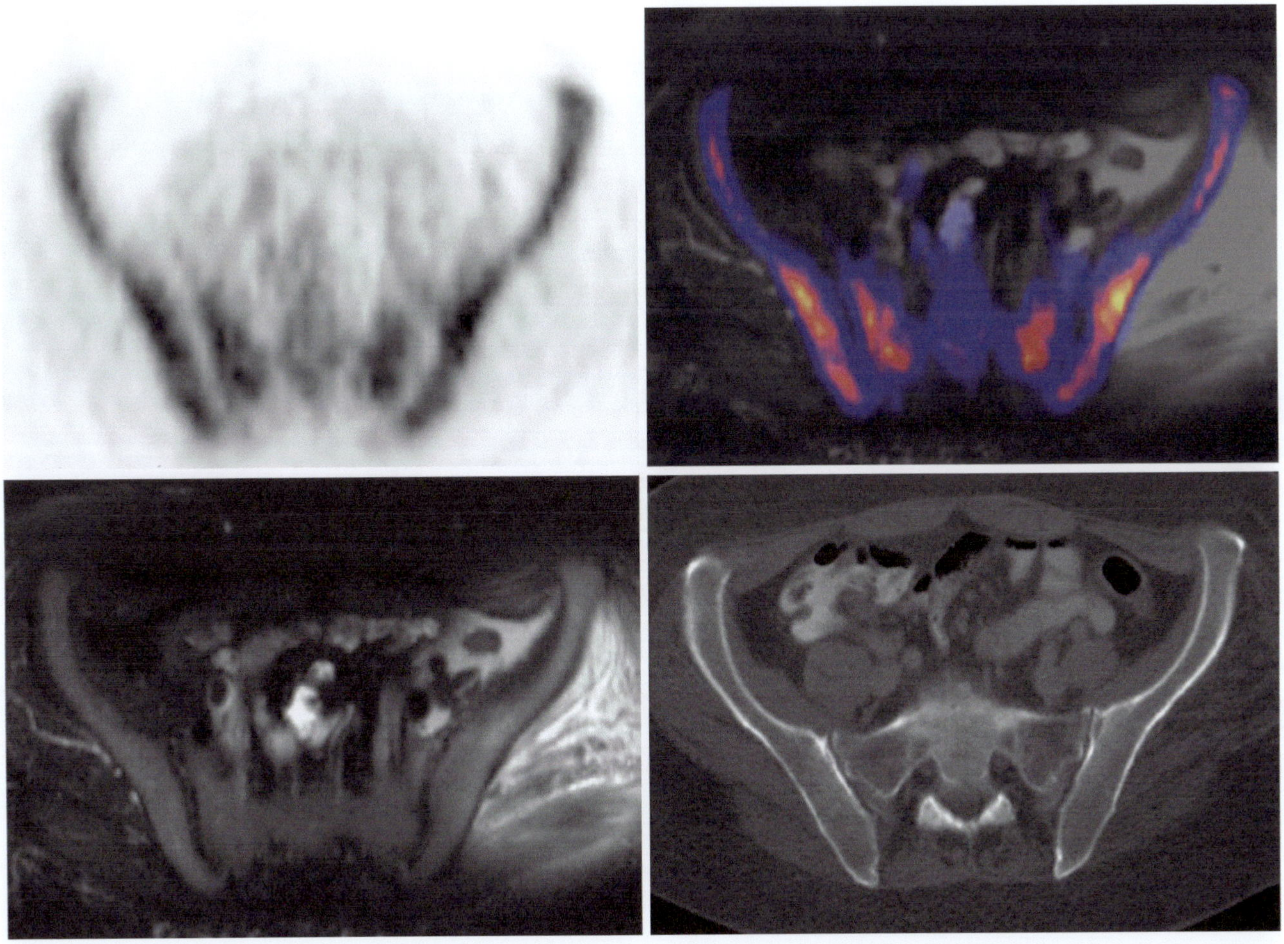

Fig. 10.34 Axial PET and fused images show a patchy infiltration of the pelvis and sacral bone (*upper row*). Diffuse hyperintensity in T2w HASTE fs in MRI demonstrate the replacement of fatty marrow in the corresponding region (*left, lower row*). In CT no abnormalities could be detected (*right, lower row*). Incomplete fat suppression is related to hip prosthesis on the left side

Recurrent T-NHL with Bone Infiltration

Clinical History

A 60 year old patient with prior T-NHL presents with pain in the right hip. CT demonstrates diffuse osteolyses in the right acetabulum rising the suspicious of a recurrence with bone infiltration.

Imaging Technique

Whole body PET/MR images acquired 117 min after iv injection 367 MBq 18F-FDG, 78 kg.

4 beds × 5 min together with whole body coronal T1w TSE and cor T2w STIR. Whole body axial T1w flash fat saturated after Gadolinium.

Findings

In contrast to CT T1w TSE clearly outlines the area of bone infiltration by recurrent NHL. It corresponds to an intense high uptake of 18F-FDG.

Teaching Points

The combination of PET and MRI can demonstrate the extent of bone marrow infiltration more clearly than PET/CT. Especially T1w TSE sequences outline the replacement of fatty bone marrow by malignant tissue better than CT.

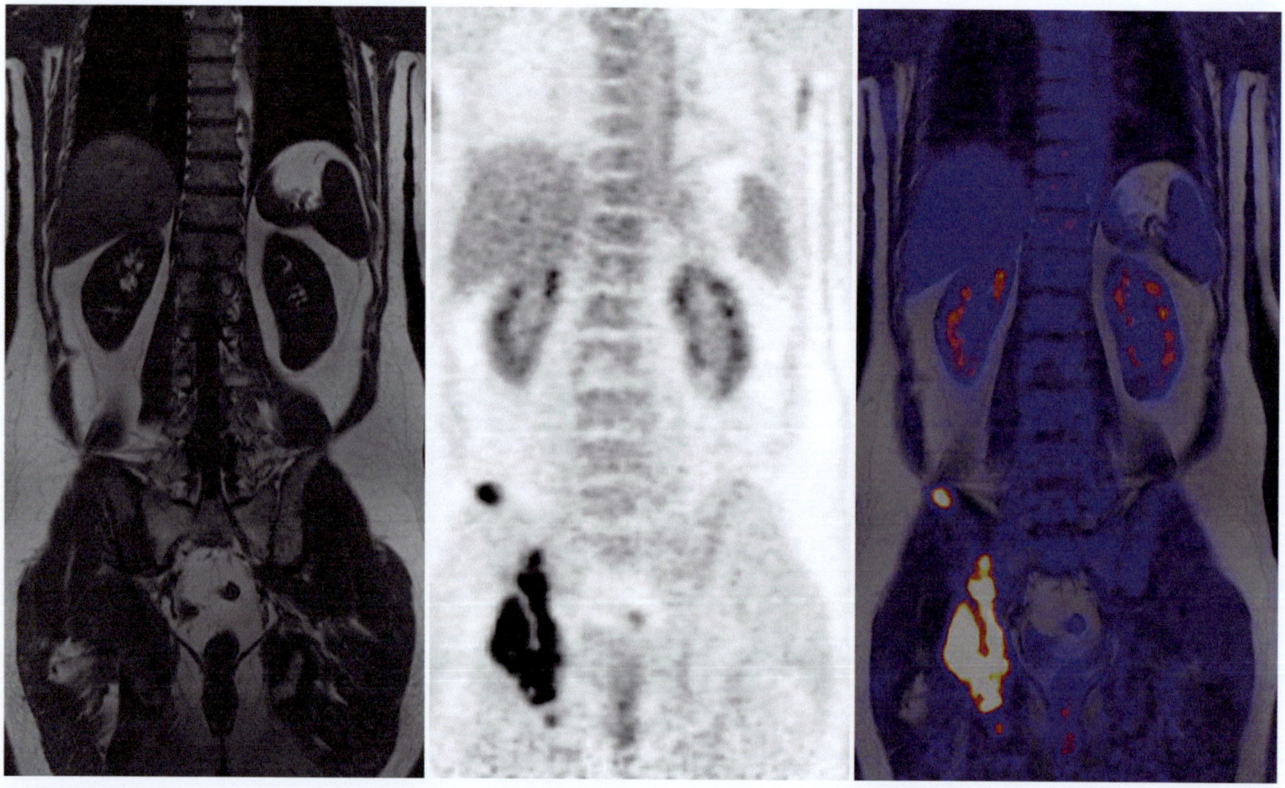

Fig. 10.35 Coronal T1w TSE (*left*) show a nodular hypointensity in the iliac crest on the right side and a diffuse bone marrow infiltration of the right acetabulum. Coronal PET demonstrate high focal uptake in the corresponding regions (*middle*). A good correlation between the findings in MR and PET is outlined in the fused dataset (*right*)

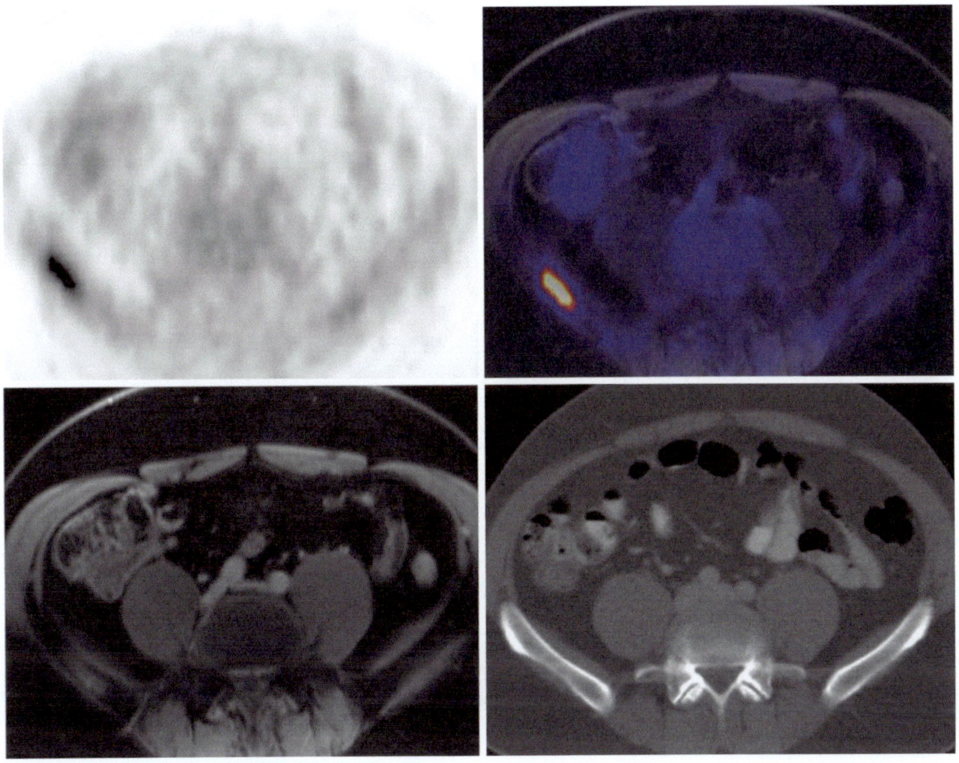

Fig. 10.36 Axial PET and fused PET images show a high uptake in the right pelvis (*upper row*). Intense contrast enhancement is found in the fat saturated T1w sequence after Gadolinium (*lower row*, *left*). The corresponding CT exhibits a faint sclerosis in the corresponding region (*lower row*, *right*)

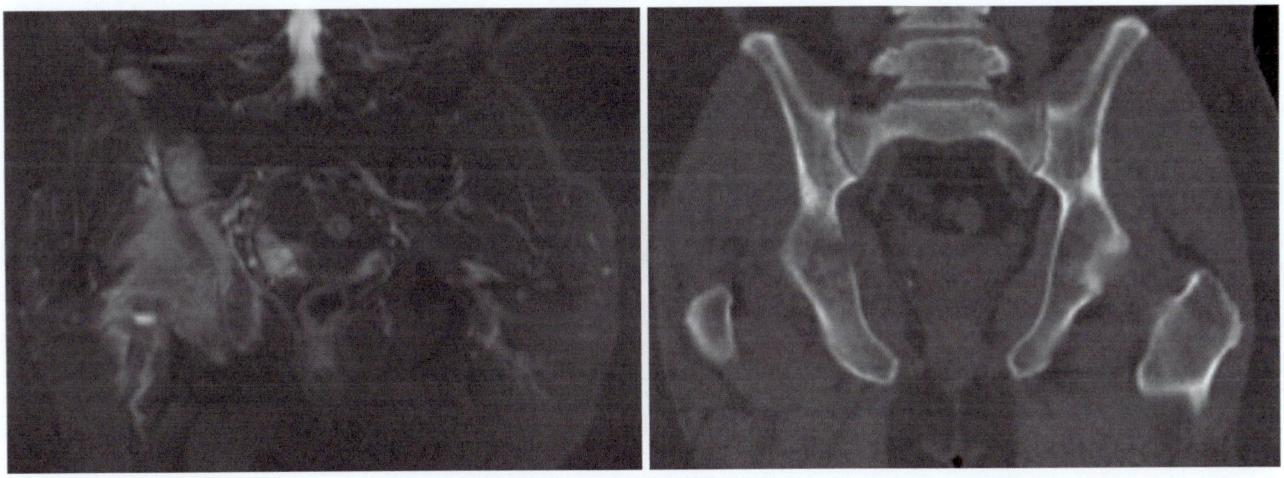

Fig. 10.37 A direct comparison of T2w STIR (*left*) and CT (*right*) demonstrates the superiority of MR in outlining the infiltration of bone marrow. In the CT lesions in the iliac crest and near the ileo-sacral joint cannot be visualized

Liver Metastasis of Adenocarcinoma of the Adrenal Gland

Clinical History

Thirty-five-year-old patient with adenocarcinoma of the left adrenal gland undergoing a staging examination.

Imaging Technique

Whole body PET/MR images acquired 46 min after iv injection of 359 MBq 18F-FDG, 67 kg.

4 beds × 4 min together with coronal T1w TSE and axial T2w haste fs. 1 bed (upper abdomen) a 15 min together with ax/cor T2 HASTE, ax EPI (DWI), ax T1-VIBE dynamic post i.v. Gd.

Findings

In the right liver lobe a large focal lesion that is hyperintense on T2-weighted sequence can be depicted. The lesion shows a hyperintense signal in diffusion-weighted imaging both at a low and a high *b*-value suggesting a restricted diffusion within a likely hypercellular lesion. There is intense focal uptake of 18F-FDG in PET. Both MRI and PET strongly indicate a liver metastasis.

Teaching Points

Diffusion-weighted MR imaging (DWI) is an important MR sequence for both detection and characterization of focal liver lesions. In malignant lesions often a restricted diffusion due to hypercellularity can be seen.

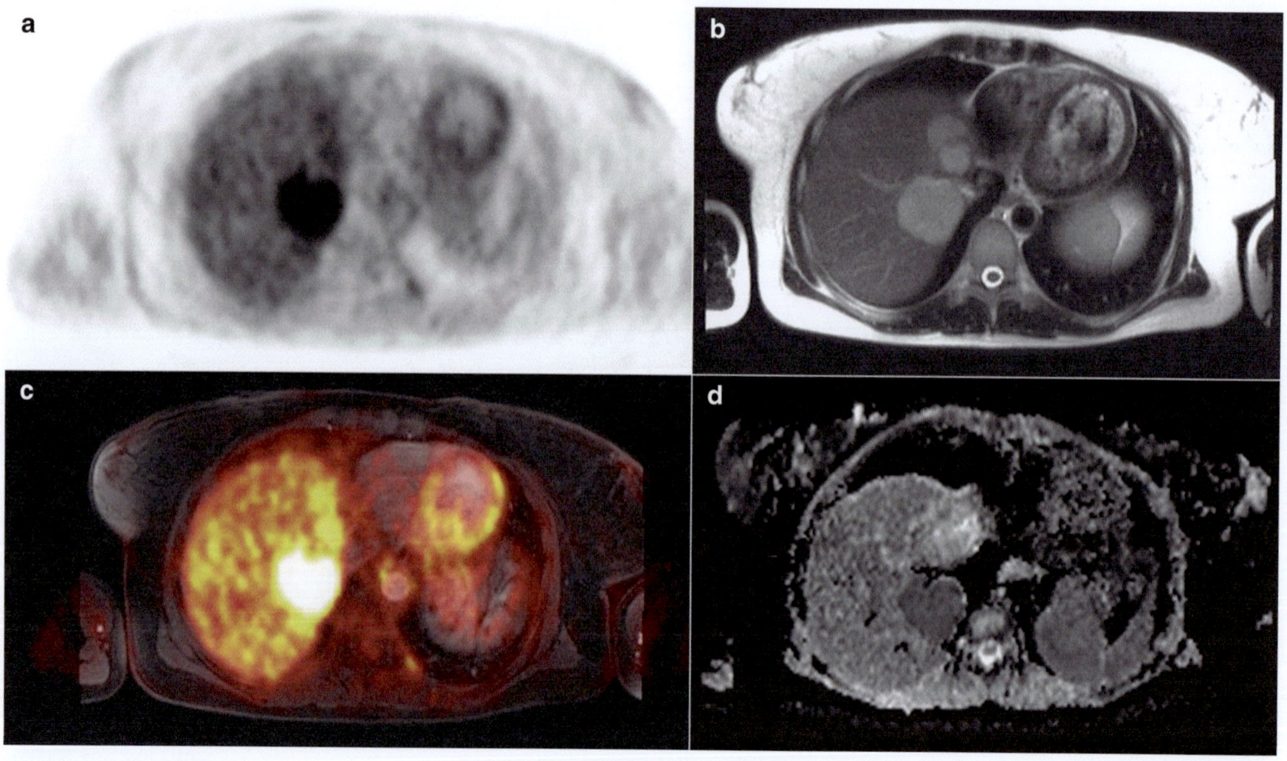

Fig. 10.38 In the right liver lobe a large focal lesion with intense focal uptake of 18F-FDG is seen (**a**). The lesion is hyperintense in a T2-weighted sequence (**b**). A low ADC-value (**d**) suggests a hypercelluar lesions. Both MRI and PET indicate one vital and one avital liver metastasis (**c** and **d**)

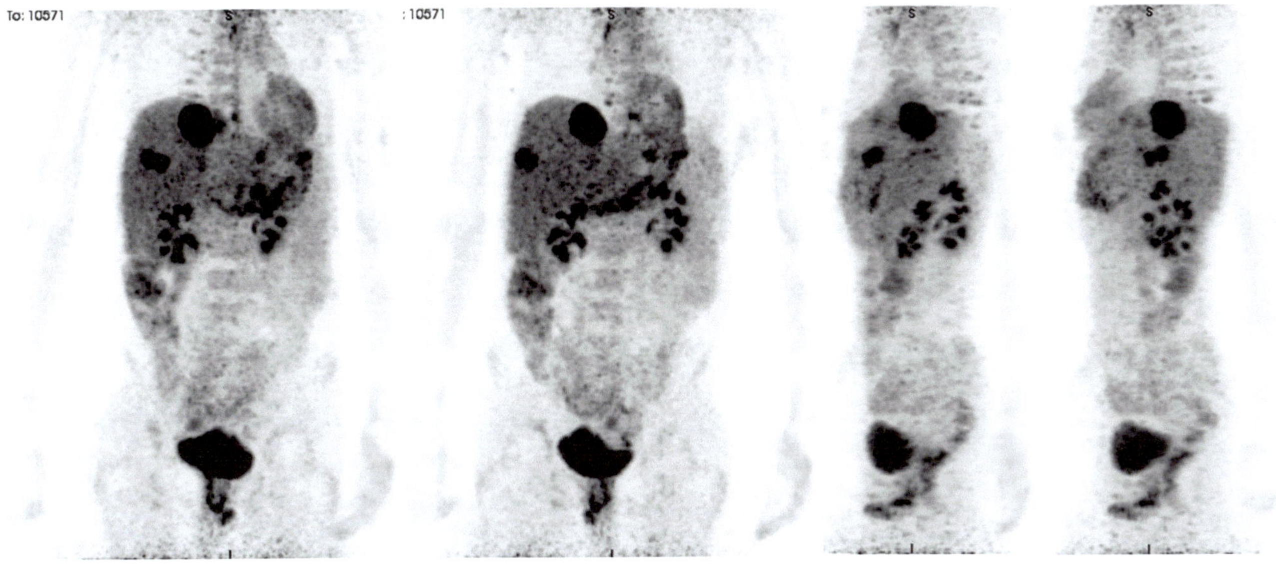

Fig. 10.39 Whole-body 18F-FDG-PET in the coronal plane. Except for the liver there is no evidence for metastases to other organs

Liver Metastases of Colorectal Cancer

Clinical History

Sixty-one-year-old patient with known liver metastases of colorectal cancer and a history of partial liver resection and radiofrequency ablation.

Imaging Technique

Whole body PET/MR images acquired 46 min after iv injection of 357 MBq 18F-FDG, 73 kg.

4 beds × 4 min together with coronal T1w TSE and axial T2w HASTE fs. 1 bed (upper abdomen) a 15 min together with ax/cor T2 HASTE, ax EPI (DWI), ax T1-VIBE dynamic post i.v. Gd.

Findings

Adjacent to the ablation defect in the left liver lobe a circular enhancement can be seen in the arterial phase after i.v. administration of contrast material. Another area of focal enhancement is seen in the right liver lobe. Both regions show an intense uptake of 18F-FDG in PET and are highly suspicious of newly developed liver metastases.

Teaching Points

Dynamic contrast-enhanced MR imaging together with PET is a valuable tool in the detection of liver metastases, especially in patients with previous treatment either by surgery or focal ablative techniques like radiofrequency ablation.

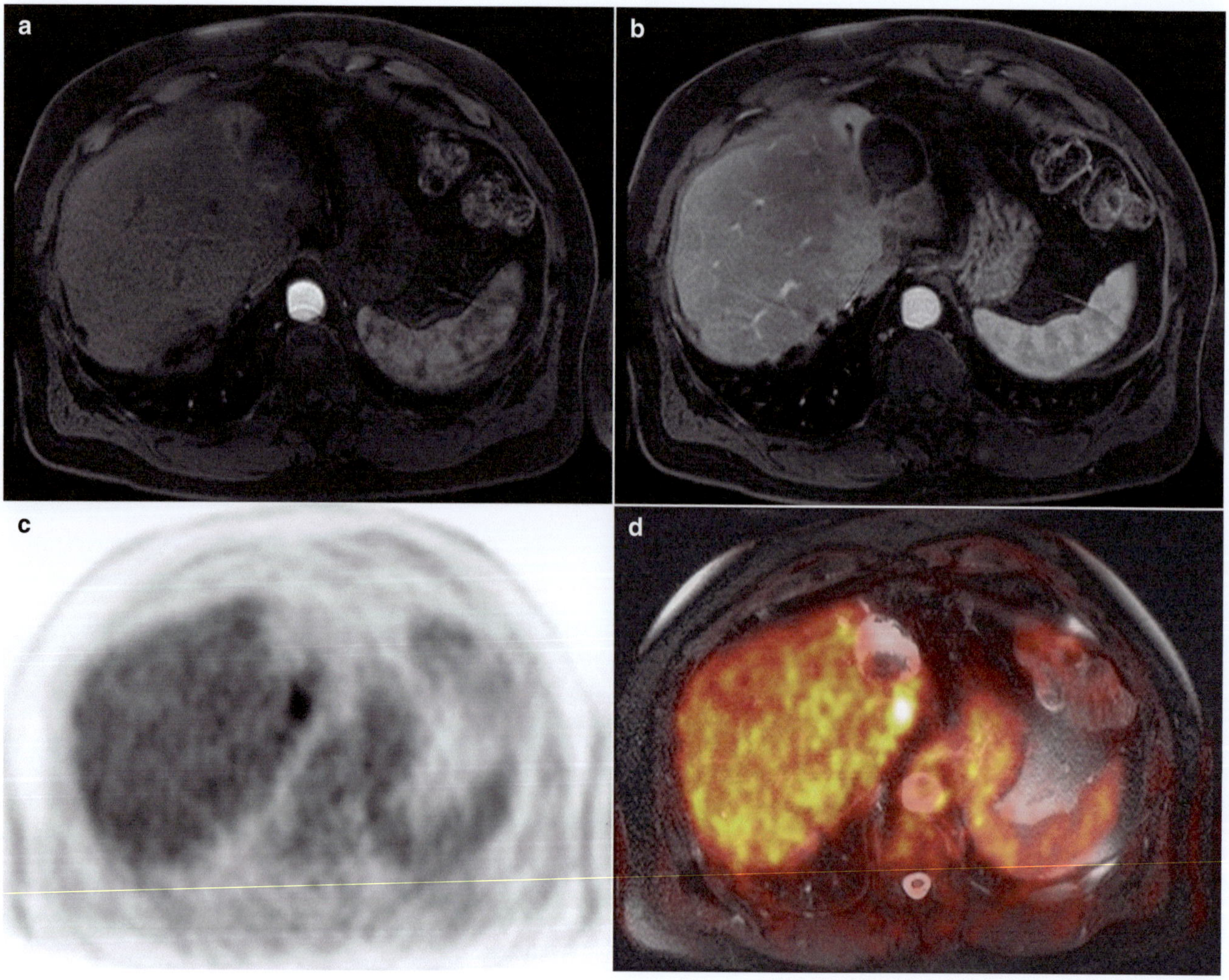

Fig. 10.40 Adjacent to the ablation defect in the left liver lobe a circular enhancement can faintly be seen in the early and late arterial phase after i.v. administration of contrast material (**a** and **b**). PET (**c**) and fusion (**d**) nicely delineate the area of recurrence

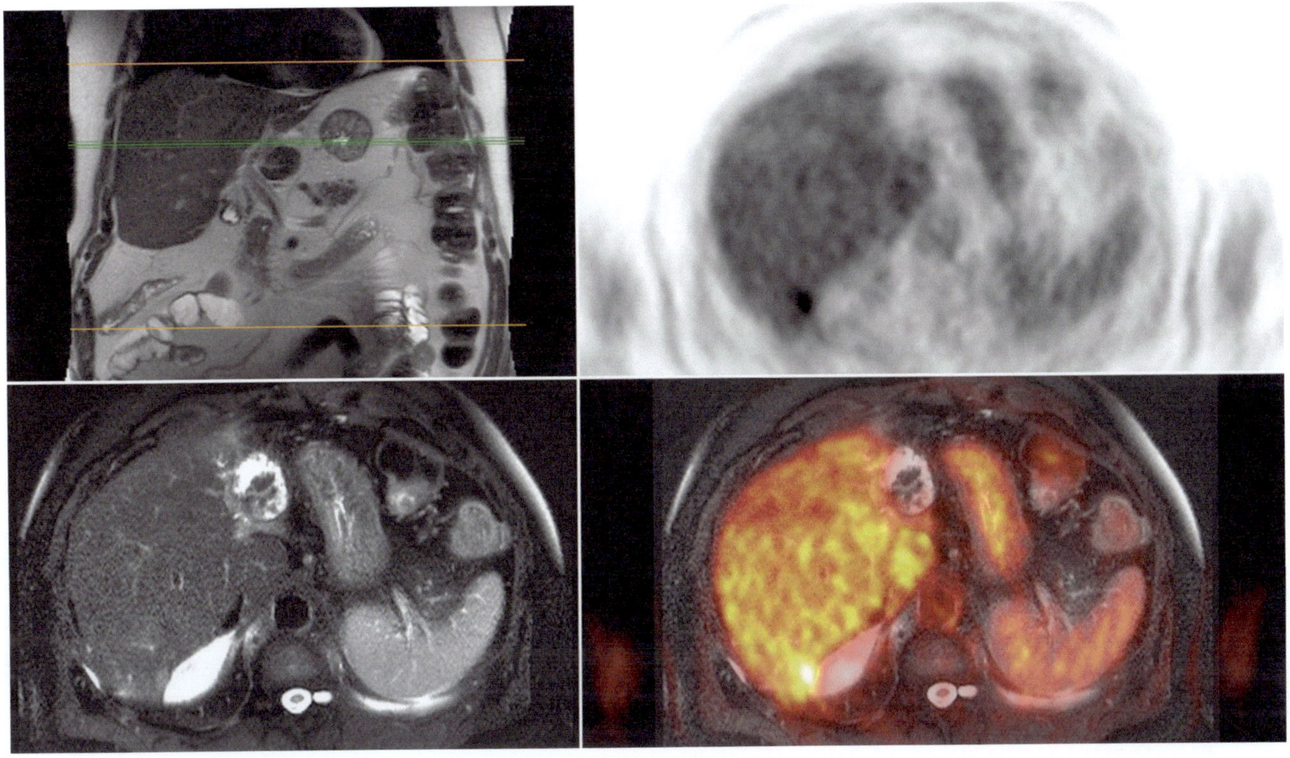

Fig. 10.41 Another PET positive lesion in the right lobe shows an faint T2w hyperintensity

Liver Metastasis of Rectal Cancer

Clinical History

Forty-six-year-old patient with rectal cancer undergoing a staging examination.

Imaging Technique

Whole body PET/MR images acquired 46 min after iv injection of 487 MBq 18F-FDG, 100 kg.

4 beds × 4 min together with coronal T1w TSE and axial T2w haste fs. 1 bed (upper abdomen) a 15 min together with ax/cor T2 HASTE, ax EPI (DWI), ax T1-VIBE dynamic post i.v. Gd.

Findings

In the left liver lobe a focal lesion with restricted diffusion and peripheral enhancement is seen. There is intense focal uptake of 18F-FDG in PET. Both MRI and PET strongly indicate a liver metastasis. No additional focal lesions are seen.

Teaching Points

In patients with colorectal cancer accurate staging of liver metastases is of paramount importance as patients eligible for resection of metastases can be treated curatively. Combination of a dedicated MR protocol of the liver and 18F-FDG PET imaging is helpful regarding the detection of liver metastases.

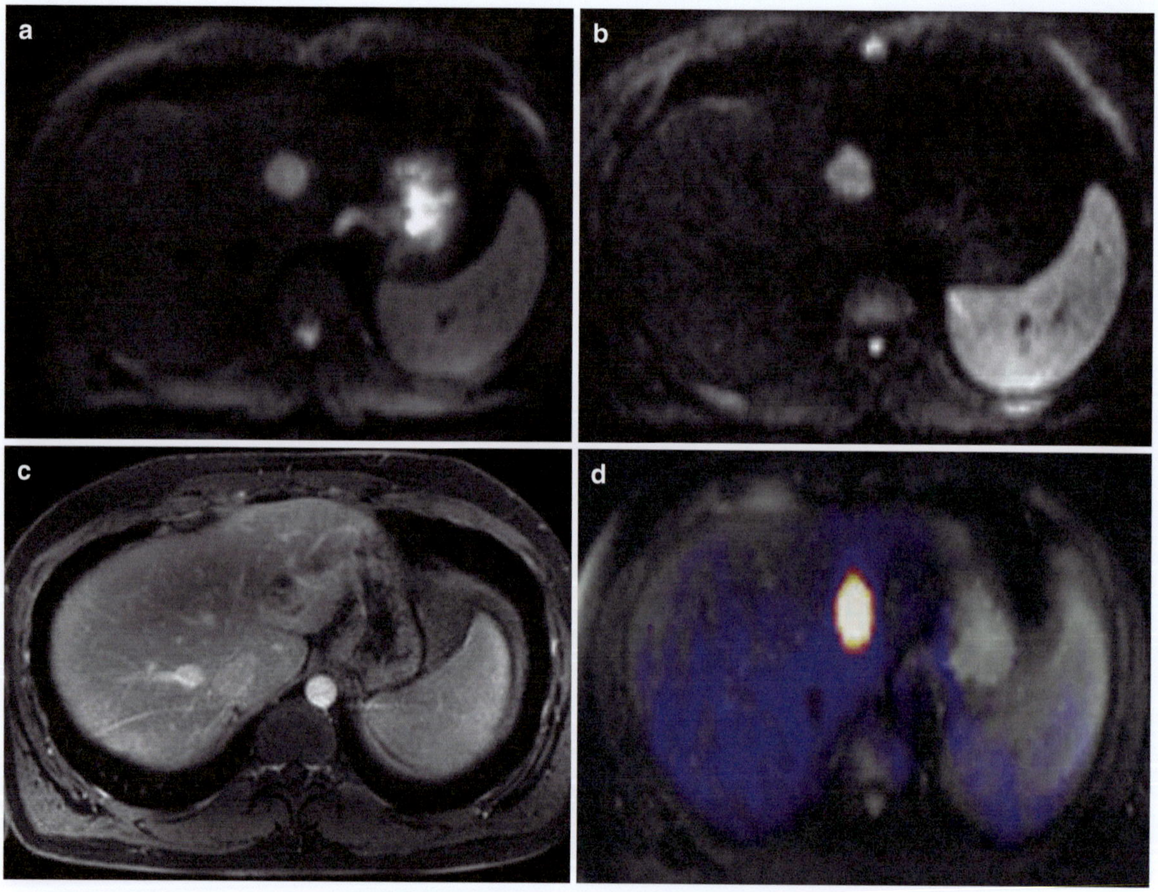

Fig. 10.42 In the left liver lobe a focal liver lesion is seen. It is hyperintense in DWI on both low (**a**) and high (**b**) *b*-value images reflecting restricted diffusion. In the portal venous phase the lesion shows peripheral enhancement (**c**). In addition intense focal uptake of 18F-FDG is seen (**d**). Both MRI and PET strongly indicate a liver metastasis

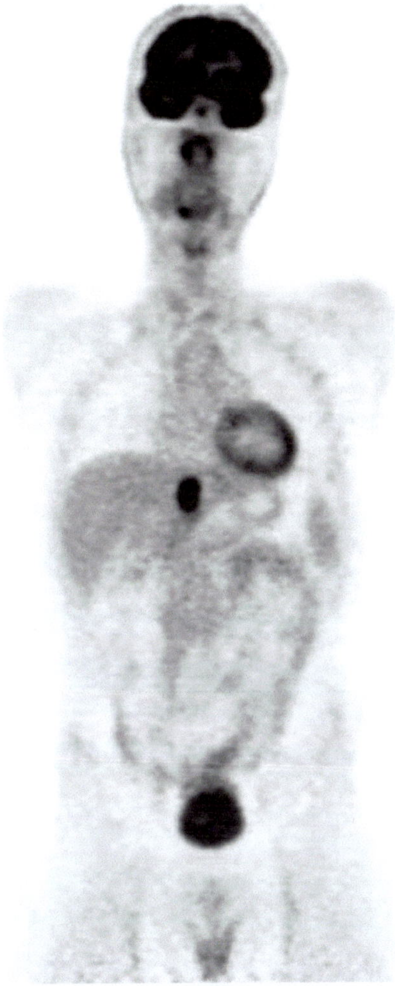

Fig. 10.43 Whole-body 18F-FDG-PET in the coronal plane. Except for the liver there is no evidence for metastases to other organs

References

1. Hutchings M, Barrington SF (2009) PET/CT for therapy response assessment in lymphoma. J Nucl Med 50(Suppl_1):21S–30S
2. Kwee TC, Van Ufford HMEQ, Beek FJ, Takahara T, Uiterwaal CS, Bierings MB et al (2009) Whole-body MRI, including diffusion-weighted imaging, for the initial staging of malignant lymphoma: comparison to computed tomography. Invest Radiol 44(10):683–690
3. Punwani S, Taylor SA, Bainbridge A, Prakash V, Bandula S, Vita ED et al (2010) Pediatric and adolescent lymphoma: comparison of whole-body STIR half-Fourier RARE MR imaging with an enhanced PET/CT reference for initial staging1. Radiology 255(1):182–190
4. Lin C, Luciani A, Itti E, El-Gnaoui T, Vignaud A, Beaussart P et al (2010) Whole-body diffusion-weighted magnetic resonance imaging with apparent diffusion coefficient mapping for staging patients with diffuse large B-cell lymphoma. Eur Radiol 20(8):2027–2038
5. Wu L-M, Chen F-Y, Jiang X-X, Gu H-Y, Yin Y, Xu J-R (2012) 18F-FDG PET, combined FDG-PET/CT and MRI for evaluation of bone marrow infiltration in staging of lymphoma: a systematic review and meta-analysis. Eur J Radiol 81(2):303–311
6. Abdulqadhr G, Molin D, Aström G, Suurküla M, Johansson L, Hagberg H et al (2011) Whole-body diffusion-weighted imaging compared with FDG-PET/CT in staging of lymphoma patients. Acta Radiol 52(2):173–180
7. Antoch G, Vogt FM, Freudenberg LS, Nazaradeh F, Goehde SC, Barkhausen J et al (2003) Whole-body dual-modality PET/CT and whole-body MRI for tumor staging in oncology. JAMA 290(24):3199–3206
8. Schmidt GP, Baur-Melnyk A, Herzog P, Schmid R, Tiling R, Schmidt M et al (2005) High-resolution whole-body magnetic resonance image tumor staging with the use of parallel imaging versus dual-modality positron emission tomography-computed tomography: experience on a 32-channel system. Invest Radiol 40(12):743–753
9. Liu J, Yang X, Li F, Wang X, Jiang X (2011) Preliminary study of whole-body diffusion-weighted imaging in detecting pulmonary metastatic lesions from clear cell renal cell carcinoma: comparison with CT. Acta Radiol 52(9):954–963
10. Lauenstein TC, Goehde SC, Herborn CU, Goyen M, Oberhoff C, Debatin JF et al (2004) Whole-body MR imaging: evaluation of patients for metastases1. Radiology 233(1):139–148
11. Schwenzer NF, Schraml C, Müller M, Brendle C, Sauter A, Spengler W et al (2012) Pulmonary lesion assessment: comparison of whole-body hybrid MR/PET and PET/CT imaging—pilot study. Radiology 264(2):551–558

Thyroid and Endocrine Tumors

11

M. Eiber, F. Gärtner, K. Scheidhauer,
and M. Souvatzoglou

Contents

M. Eiber (✉)
Department of Radiology, Klinikum Rechts der Isar,
Technische Universität München, Munich, Germany
e-mail: matthias.eiber@tum.de

F. Gärtner • K. Scheidhauer • M. Souvatzoglou
Department of Nuclear Medicine,
Technische Universität München, Munich, Germany

Thyroid and Endocrine Tumors

In thyroid cancer ^{18}F-FDG is well established for detection of noniodine-avid disease in patients with elevated Tg levels [1, 2]. This has led to a substantial improvement of patient management especially for cases of recurrent tumor [3]. From a prognostic perspective it is known that patients with FDG-avid, high-volume disease (>125 mL) as assessed with CT and PET have markedly reduced survival [4]. Thus FDG PET is a tool for assisting in the clinical decision making for either localized or systemic therapy other than the use of ^{131}I in patients with negative iodine scans and elevated hTg and in patients with suspected local recurrence after thyroidectomy [5]. One important prerequisite of using ^{18}F-PET/CT for these patients is that no intravenous contrast media should be administered when combined with a ^{131}I-scan or when potentially a radio-iodine-therapy is planned no intravenous contrast should be administered for the diagnostic CT [6, 7]. Here PET/MR can offer the possibility to add a diagnostic morphological dataset to the PET/examination as Gd-based contrast media do not interfere with the use of a ^{131}I-scan or therapy. Additionally PET/MR is expected to be a useful tool in surgical planning and radioactive iodine therapy decisions.

For neuroendocrine tumors of the abdomen the use of PET/MR offers potential advances especially for detection of the primary tumor and potential liver metastases. Recently studies [8, 9] showed that ^{68}Ga- radiolabeled somatostatin analog and combination of PET and MR performed significantly more accurate (sensitivity, specificity, NPV, and PPV of 91, 96, 87, and 97 %) compared to PET/CT (74, 88, 69, and 93 %, respectively). It is assumed that MRI compensates for the drawbacks in PET in small hepatic lesions where diffusion-weighted imaging can provide high lesion-to-liver contrast. Additional gain in diagnostic performance is also expected for determining the extent primary pancreatic tumors and thus helping in therapeutic decisions [10, 11]. Especially for neuroendocrine pancreatic cancer MR is often superior to CT in the detection of small lesions implying an important role of PET/MR in this patient population [12, 13].

O. Ratib et al. (eds.), *Atlas of PET/MR Imaging in Oncology*,
DOI 10.1007/978-3-642-31292-2_11,

Metastatic Pulmonary Carcinoid

Clinical History

Twenty-nine-year-old male patient with a neuroendocrine tumor of the right upper lobe of the lung, bilobectomy was performed 6 years ago. Resection of a bone metastasis in the proximal right tibia was performed 3 years ago.

Imaging Technique

Whole body PET/MR images acquired 42 min after i.v. injection of 131 MBq [68Ga]-DOTATOC, weight 82 kg. 8 bed positions × 4 min (head to lower legs). MR-Sequences: Whole body: Dixon for attenuation correction, cor T1 TSE. Liver: ax/cor T2 BLADE.

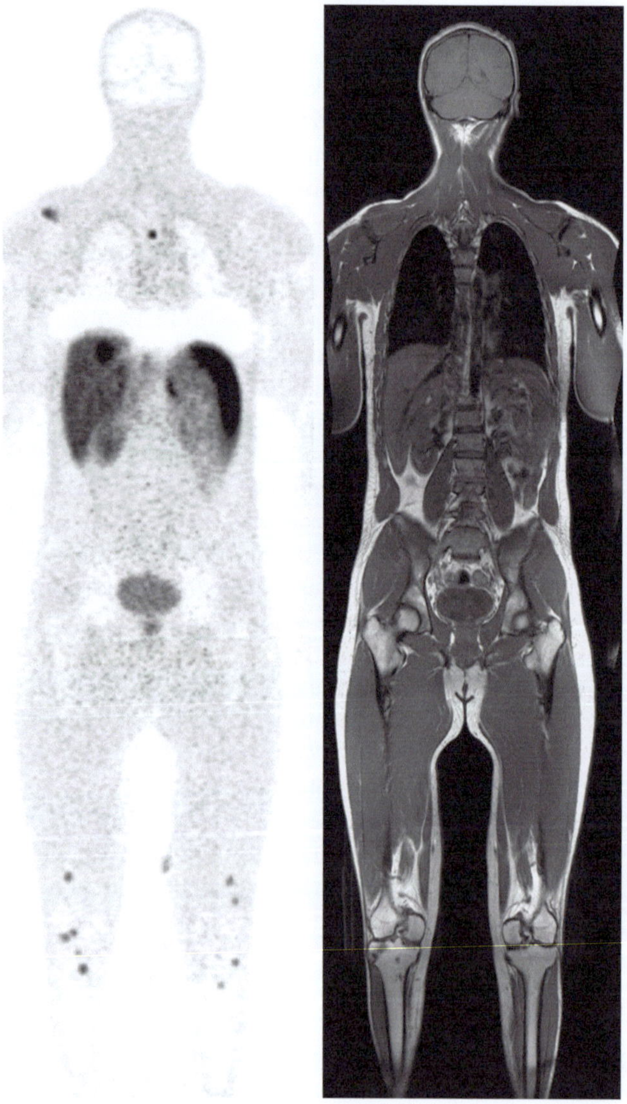

Fig. 11.1 *Left*: MIP of the [68Ga]-DOTATOC tracer distribution, showing multiple pathologic foci in the bones and in the liver. *Right*: whole-body T1-weighted coronal slice for anatomic overview. Notice attenuation correction artifact of the upper abdomen due to respiratory motion

Findings

PET shows disseminated bone metastases with avid tracer uptake, correlating with suspicious hypointense signal alterations on the T1-weighted MR images. Additionally, multiple somatostatin-receptor positive liver metastases are seen, showing hyperintense correlates in the T2-weighted MR images.

Teaching Points

Somatostatin receptor PET/MR is feasible for whole-body staging of patients with neuroendocrine tumors. This patient underwent peptide receptor radiotherapy (PRRT) with Lu-177-DOTATATE.

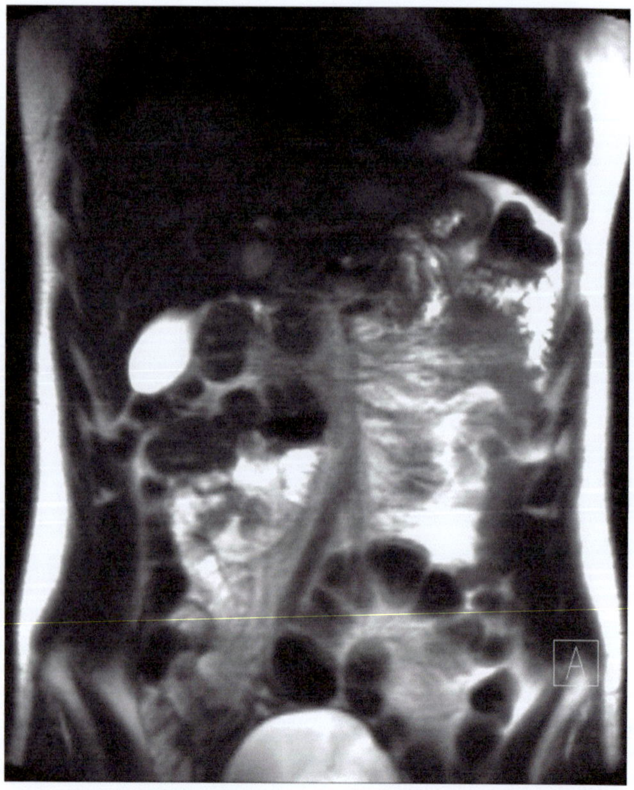

Fig. 11.2 Coronal T2-weighted MRI (BLADE) of the abdomen. Multiple pathologic signal enhancements are seen in the liver, consistent with multiple hepatic metastases

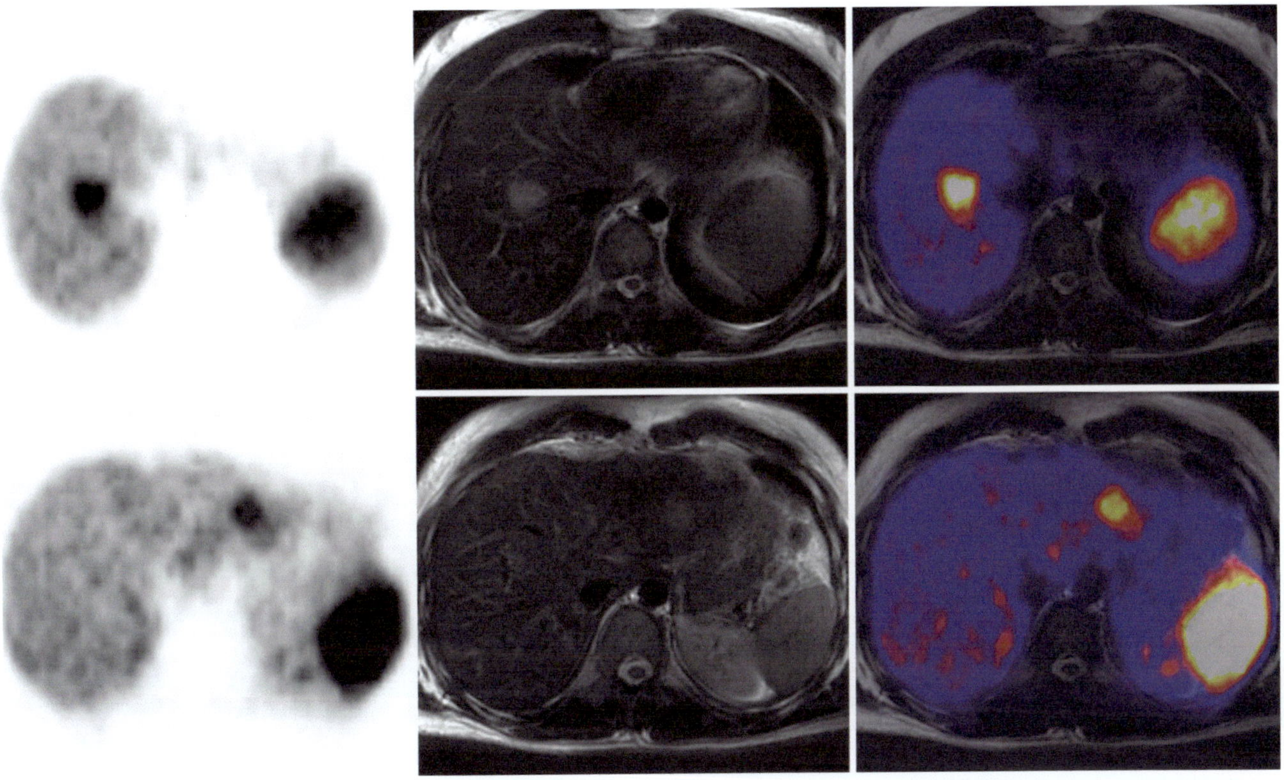

Fig. 11.3 *Left column*: Two axial slices (*top row* and *bottom row*) showing somatostatin-receptor positive liver metastases with intense tracer uptake (PET). *Middle column*: T2-weighted MR images show multiple hyperintense masses in the liver, corresponding to the areas of increased somatostatin receptor expression, consistent with liver metastases. Furthermore, additional multiple smaller hyperintense lesions are seen on the MR images, also suspicious for malignancy. *Right column*: PET/MR fusion

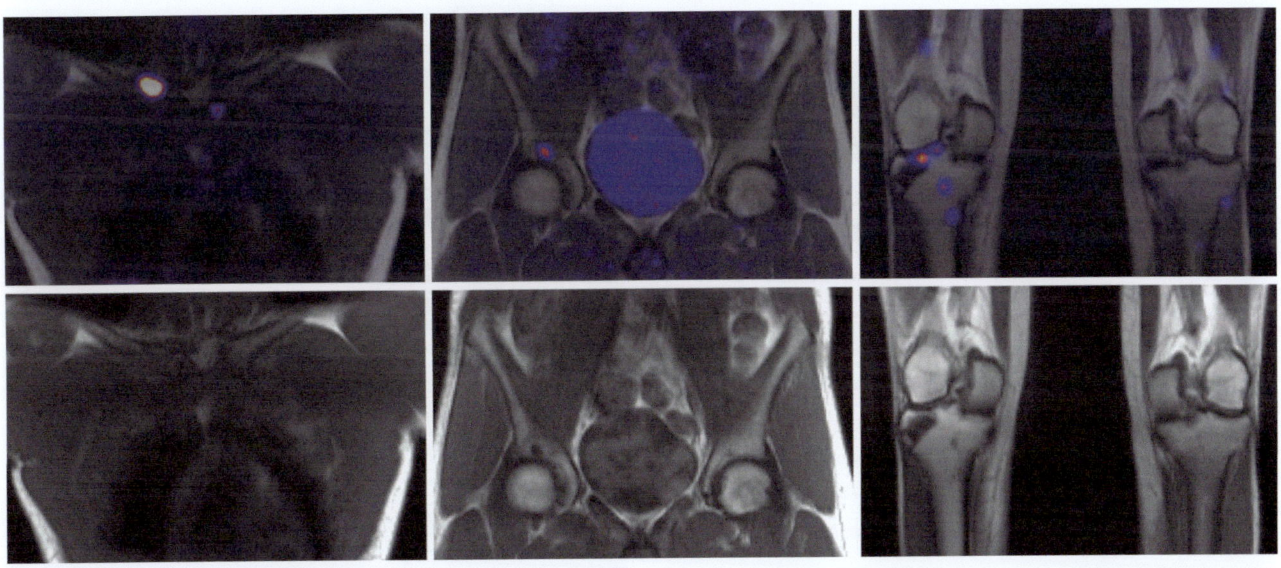

Fig. 11.4 Examples of the multiple bone metastases in this patient. *Top row*: coronal PET/MR fusion. *Bottom row*: coronal T1-weighted MR images. *Left column*: Metastasis in the right clavicle showing intense somatostatin receptor overexpression. *Middle column*: Metastasis in the right acetabulum, showing a a clear hypointense correlate in the T1w MR image. *Right column*: multiple somatostatin-receptor positive bone metastases in the right proximal tibia. Additionally, a large hypointense defect is observed in the T1w MR images in the lateral part of the proximal right tibia, showing no tracer uptake, consistent with postoperative changes

Metastatic Medullary Thyroid Cancer

Clinical History

Eighty-six-year-old male patient with history of total thyroidectomy (medullary thyroid cancer) 12 years ago and radiotherapy of a bone metastasis (4th lumbar vertebra) 2 years ago. Currently ongoing therapy with somatostatin analogs.

Imaging Technique

Whole body PET/MR images acquired 103 min after i.v. injection of 107 MBq [68Ga]-DOTATOC, weight 67 kg. 3 bed positions × 4 min (head to pelvis). MR-Sequences: Partial body: Dixon for attenuation correction, cor T1 TSE. Liver: ax/cor T2 BLADE, ax T1 VIBE, ax DWI.

Findings

Local recurrence and bone metastases showing intense overexpression of the somatostatin-receptor. Disseminated liver metastases are also observed, showing only low to moderate receptor expression.

> **Teaching Points**
> DOTATOC PET/MR can be used for assessment of somatostatin-receptor expression of neuroendocrine tumors. Especially in the liver, DWI can help to identify small or receptor-negative lesions.

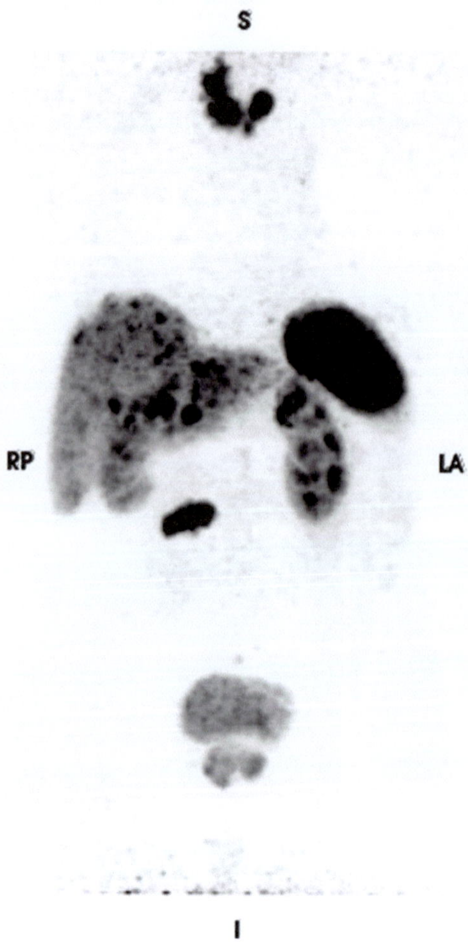

Fig. 11.5 The MIP overview shows pathologic tracer accumulation in the neck, bone (lumbar spine, pelvis) and inhomogeneous uptake in the liver

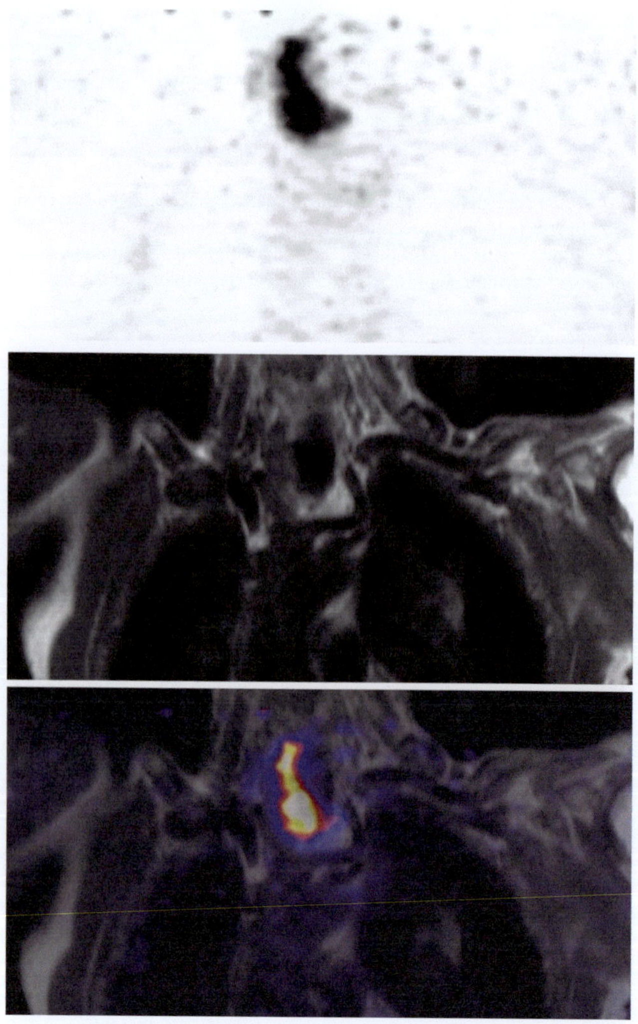

Fig. 11.6 Local recurrence in the area of the right thyroid bed with intense somatostatin receptor expression (PET, *top*). A hypointense mass is seen on coronal T1-weighted MR-images (*middle*). *Bottom*: PET/MR fusion

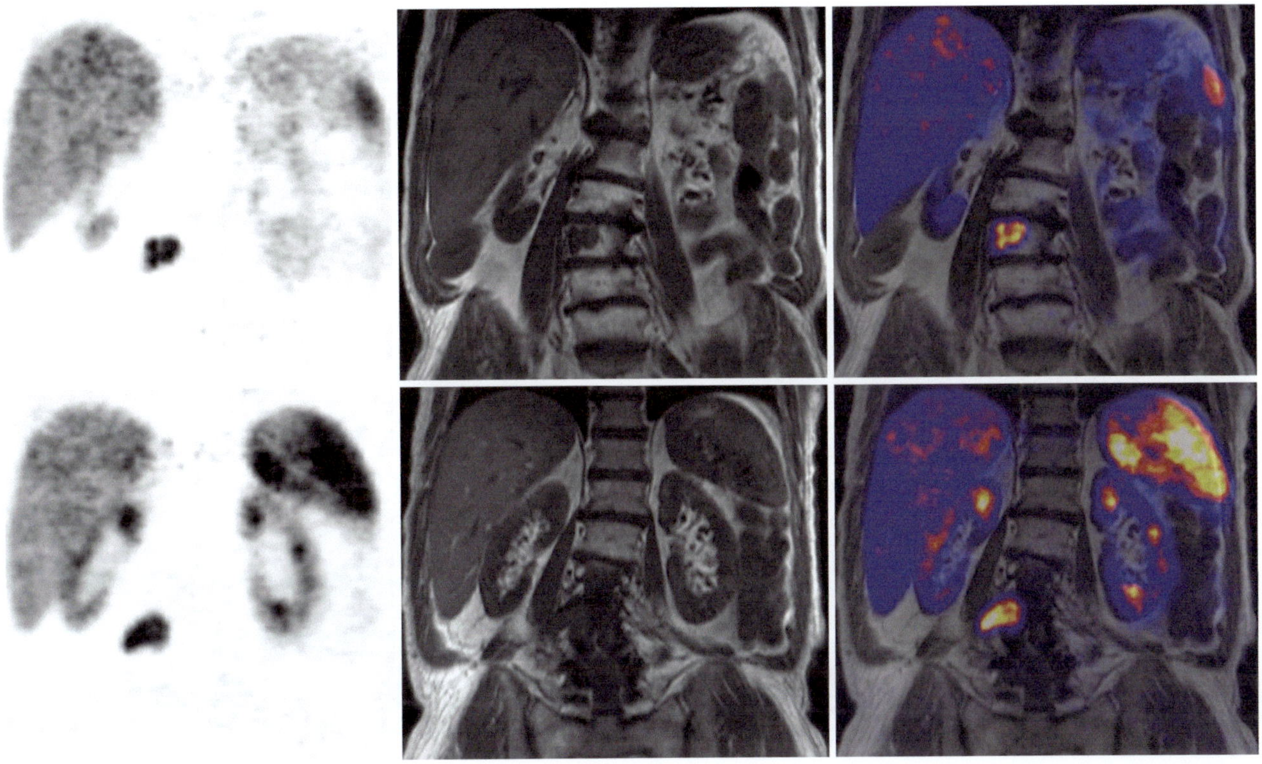

Fig. 11.7 Two coronal views (*top* and *bottom row*) showing a bone metastasis in the 4th lumbar vertebra (lumbalization of the 1st sacral vertebra). *Left*: PET shows intense overexpression of the somatostatin receptor. *Middle*: Hypointense mass in the 4th lumbar vertebra with extrasseous soft tissue extension to the right side. *Right*: PET/MR fusion

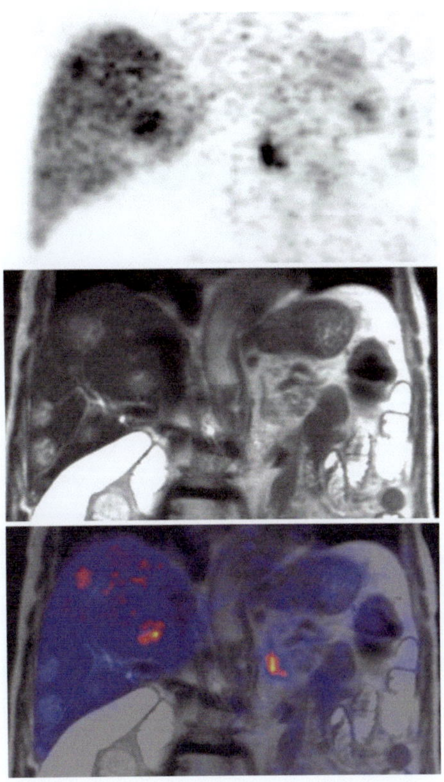

Fig. 11.8 Multiple liver metastases, partly somatostatin receptor positive. *Top*: coronal PET. *Middle*: coronal T2 BLADE MRI. *Bottom*: PET/MR fusion

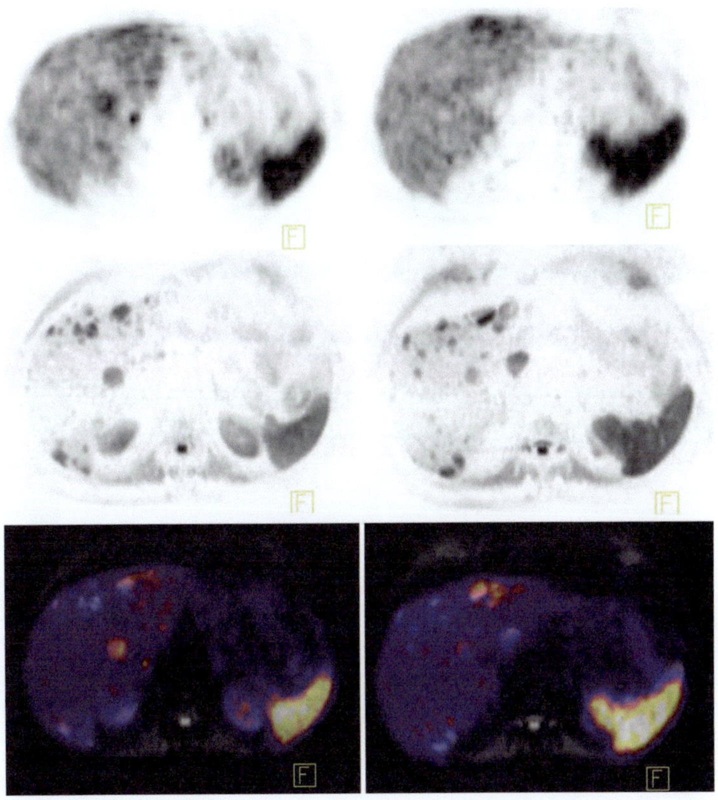

Fig. 11.9 Two axial slices (*left* and *right column*) showing multiple liver metastases. *Top*: some metastases show low to moderate expression of the somatostatin receptor (PET). *Middle*: diffusion-weighted MRI (DWI, $b=800$) additionally shows disseminated small, receptor negative metastases. *Bottom*: PET/MR fusion

Benign Finding on Somatostatin Receptor PET/MR

Clinical History

Fifty-one-year-old male patient after resection of a medullary thyroid carcinoma (left thyroid lobe, T2 N0 M0 R0) including neck dissection two years ago. The serum calcitonin was 72 ng/ml at the time of PET/MR imaging.

Imaging Technique

Partial body PET/MR images acquired 84 min after i.v. injection of 129 MBq [68Ga]-DOTATOC, weight 70 kg. 3 bed positions × 4 min (head to pelvis). MR-Sequences: Dixon for attenuation correction, cor T1w, sag T1w (spine) and sag T2w (spine) sequences.

Findings

Moderate tracer accumulation in the 8th thoracal vertebra. No further foci of pathological tracer accumulation. The finding correlates with a hyperintensity in the T1w images and in the fat-weighted Dixon images, corresponding to an hemangioma. The study was rated negative for metastases.

Teaching Points

MRI is useful to further characterize bone lesions, which may increase sensitivity for bone metastases, but on the other hand may also increase specificity by identifying false positive lesions.

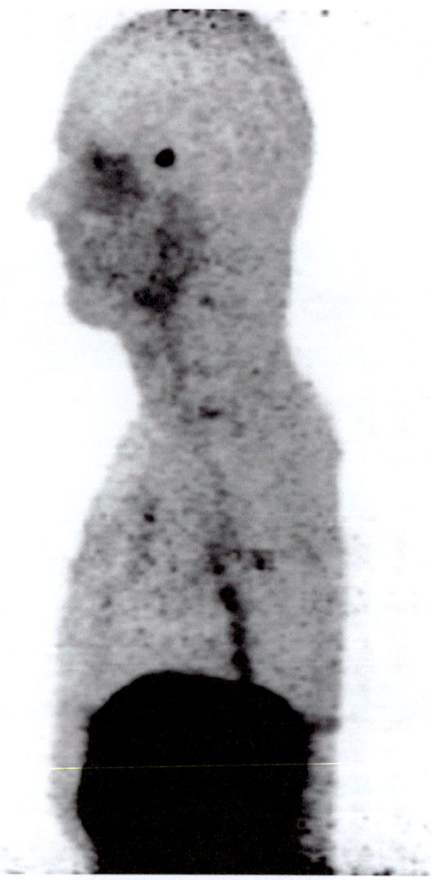

Fig. 11.10 Moderate focal uptake of [68Ga]-DOTATOC in the thoracic spine (MIP, lateral view). No other pathologic lesions were observed in the PET data

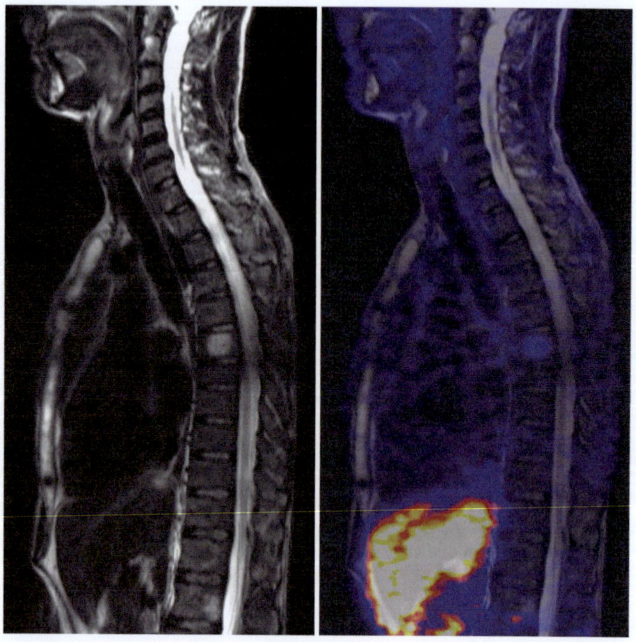

Fig. 11.11 The focal lesion projects on a hyperintense lesion in the 8th thoracal vertebra on the T2w images. *Left*: MRI T2w, sagittal view. *Right*: PET/MR fusion, sagittal view

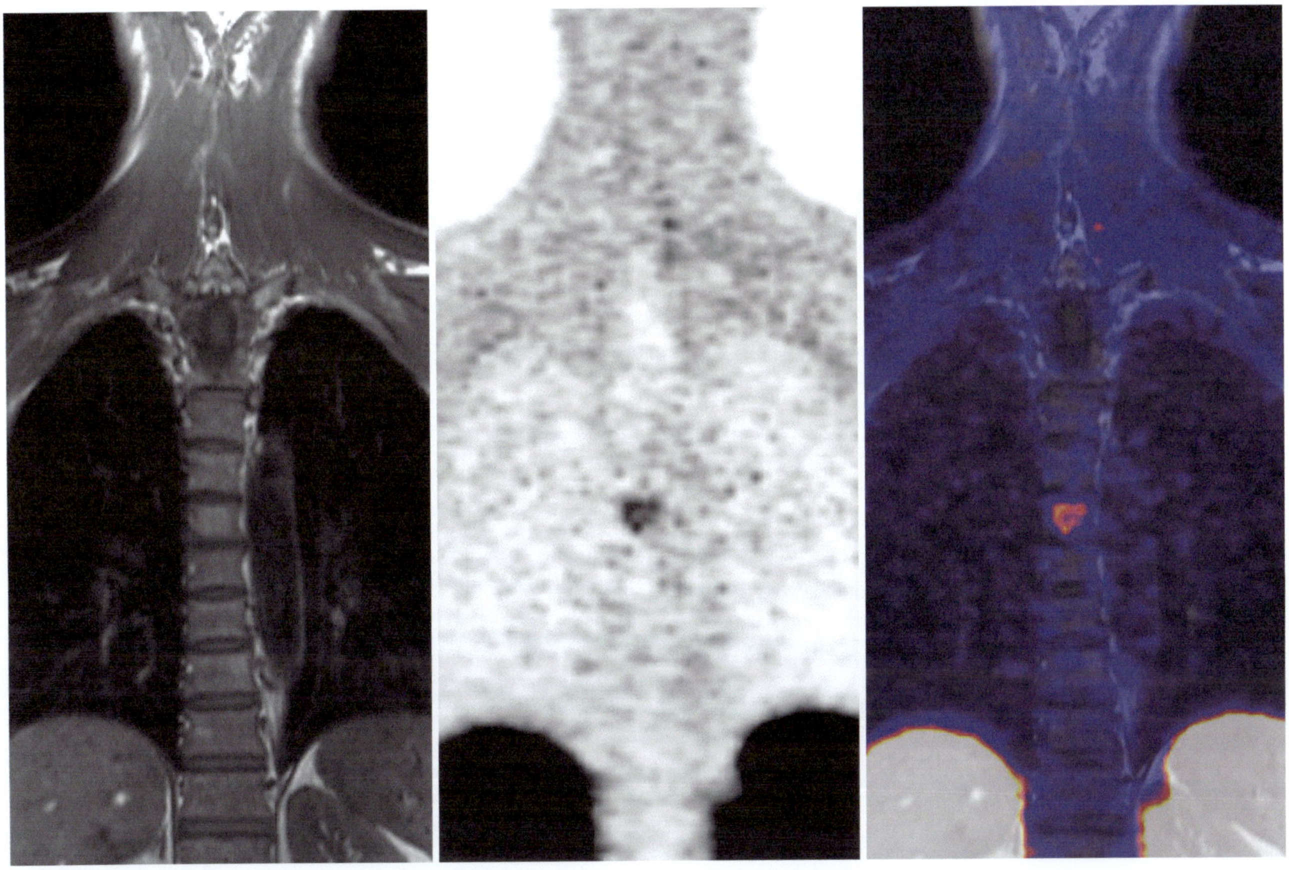

Fig. 11.12 The same lesion (8th thoracal vertebra) on T1w MRI images. *Left*: coronal T1w MRI. *Middle*: PET, coronal view. *Right*: PET/MR fusion

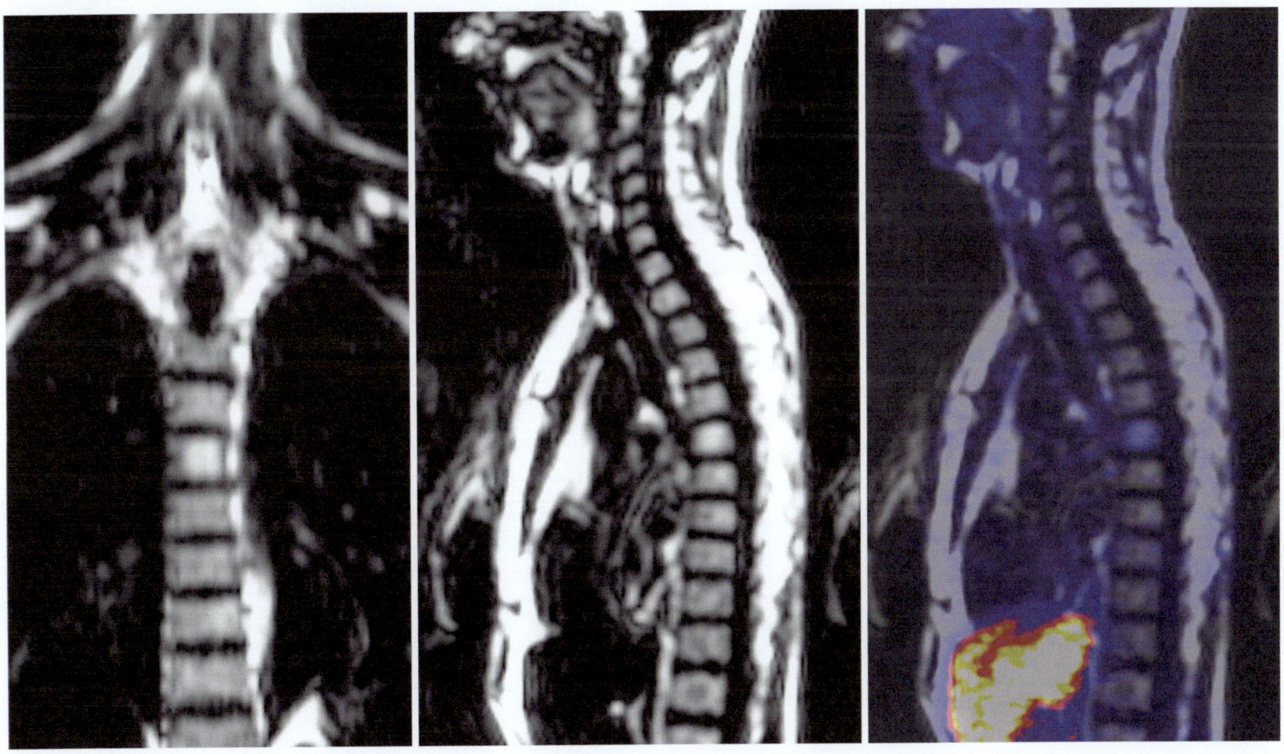

Fig. 11.13 The lesion in the 8th thoracal vertebra is also hyperintense on the fat-weighted Dixon images (acquired for attenuation correction), consistent with high fat content, consistent with a hemangioma. *Left*: coronal fat-weighted Dixon image. *Middle*: sagittal fat-weighted Dixon image. *Right*: sagittal PET/MR fusion

Papillary Thyroid Cancer

Clinical History

Twenty-three-year-old male patient with papillary thyroid cancer pT3pN1R0 (03/2012). He received ^{131}I therapy for ablation in April 2012. He presented with increased Tg levels (hTg: 3.6 ng/ml, TSH>100 μIU/ml) and therefore ^{131}I scintigraphy after administration of 40 MBq ^{131}I was performed (Fig. 11.14). To exclude FDG-avid, ^{131}I negative metastases, 18F-FDG PET/MR was performed while planning a second ^{131}I therapy.

Imaging Technique

PET/MR 97 min p.i. of 317 MBq 18F-FDG, 70 kg, 5 bed positions 4 min per bed position. T1 VIBE Dixon for attenuation correction.

MR component: neck: ax T2 STIR, ax T1 TSE –/+ Gd cor T1 SPIR post Gd trunk: ax T1 VIBE fs.

Findings

Diagnostic ^{131}I scan (Fig. 11.14) and 18F-FDG PET/MR (Fig. 11.15) do not exhibit any pathological increased focal uptake. However in the ^{131}I planar and SPECT/CT scan performed after treatment with 206 mCi of ^{131}I increased focal ^{131}I uptake is shown in right cervical lymph nodes (Fig. 11.16). The lymph nodes cannot be distinguished on CT images of SPECT/CT, however they can be identified on MR images of PET/MR (Fig. 11.17).

Teaching Points

When exact anatomical localization of thyroid cancer manifestations is an issue, the MR component of PET/MR can be a valuable tool as the diagnostic performance of CT is limited in this condition due to the inability to use contrast enhancement. Latter would lead to iodine contamination limiting treatment with ^{131}I. Further, iodine negative 18F-FDG avid lesions could be identified with PET/MR.

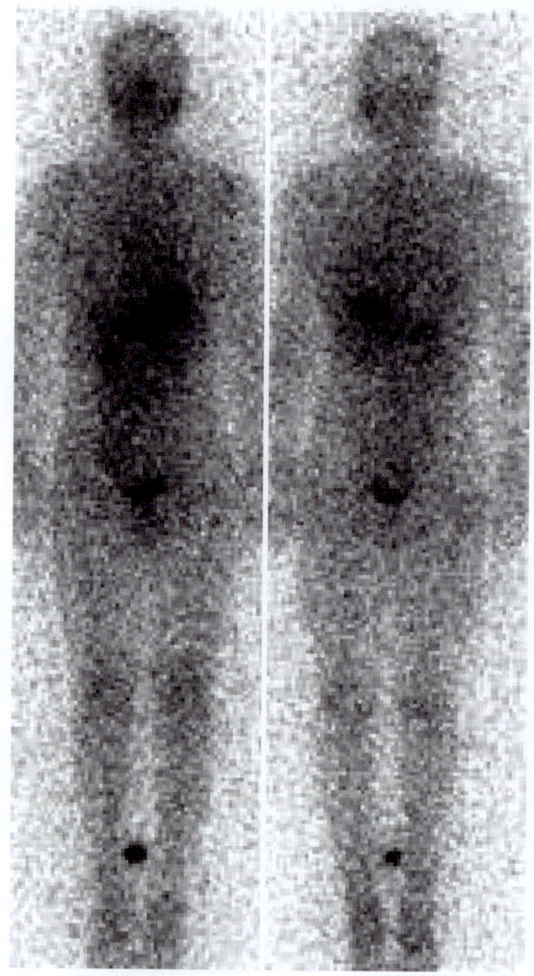

Fig. 11.14 Diagnostic ^{131}I scan (40 MBq ^{131}I) does not show any pathological focal ^{131}I uptake

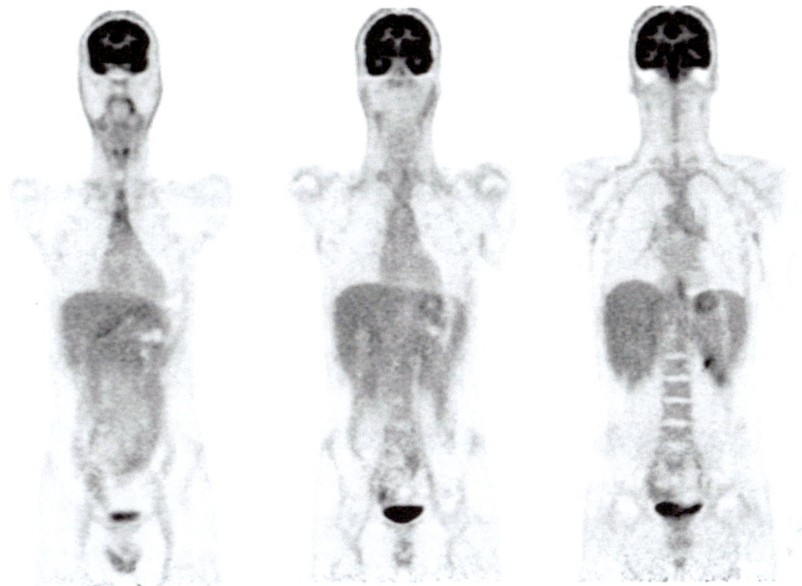

Fig. 11.15 Three coronal planes of the PET component of PET/MR without any evidence for a correlate for the increased hTg level

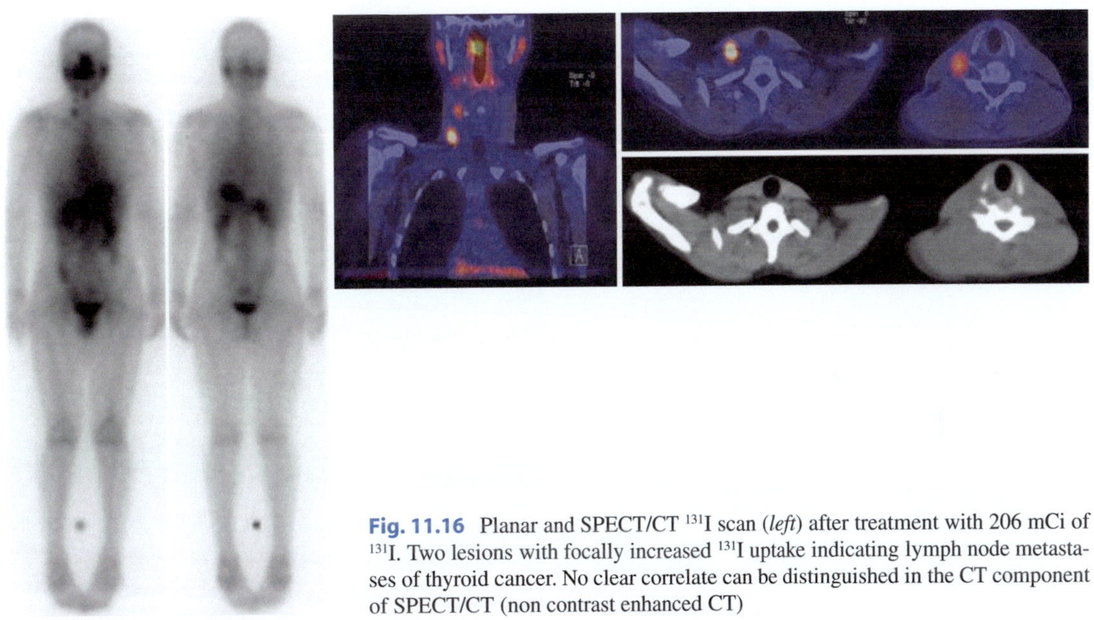

Fig. 11.16 Planar and SPECT/CT ^{131}I scan (*left*) after treatment with 206 mCi of ^{131}I. Two lesions with focally increased ^{131}I uptake indicating lymph node metastases of thyroid cancer. No clear correlate can be distinguished in the CT component of SPECT/CT (non contrast enhanced CT)

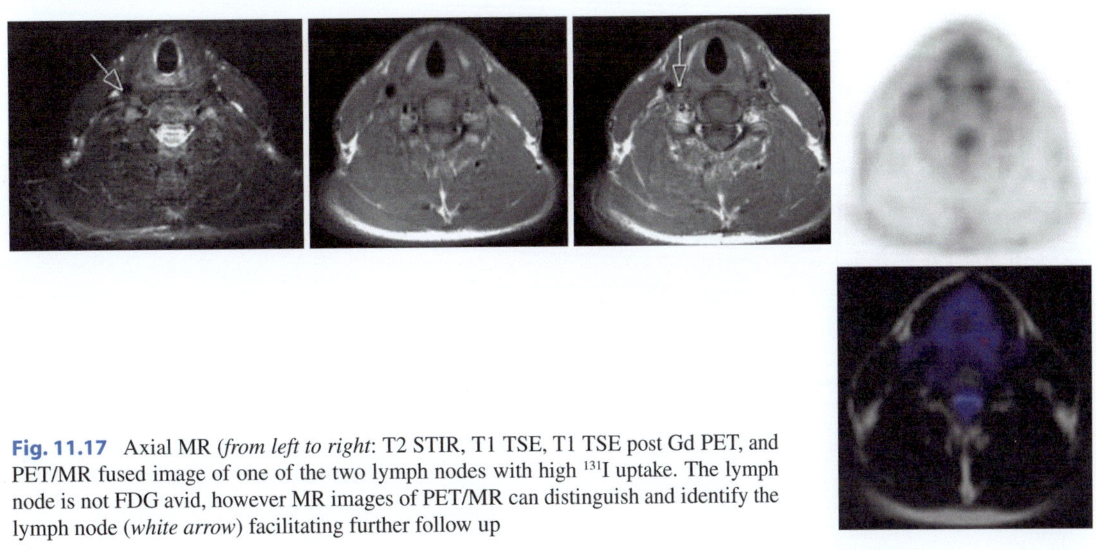

Fig. 11.17 Axial MR (*from left to right*: T2 STIR, T1 TSE, T1 TSE post Gd PET, and PET/MR fused image of one of the two lymph nodes with high ^{131}I uptake. The lymph node is not FDG avid, however MR images of PET/MR can distinguish and identify the lymph node (*white arrow*) facilitating further follow up

Lymph Node Metastasis of Thyroid Cancer

Clinical History

Seventy-six-year-old male patient after thyreoidectomy and ablative radioiodine treatment because of papillary thyroid cancer pT3pN1b(2/37)R0. Patient is referred for restaging due to a sonographically conspicuous lymph node in the left supraclavicular region. Thyreoglobulin in serum is not elevated, however there are thyreoglobulin antibodies. Diagnostic 131I scintigraphy (planar and SPECT/CT) with 379 MBq 131I and 18F-FDG PET/MR were performed.

Imaging Technique

PET/MR 78 min p.i. of 428 MBq 18F-FDG, 91 kg, 4 bed positions 4 min per bed position. T1 VIBE Dixon for attenuation correction.

MR component: Neck: ax T2 STIR, ax T1 TSE −/+ GD, cor T1 SPIR post GD, cor T1 TSE, trunk: ax T1 VIBE fs.

Findings

131I scintigraphy did not show any pathological focal uptake, however CT component of SPECT/CT demonstrates an enlarged lymph node in the left supraclavicular region (Fig. 11.18). PET/MR confirms the enlarged lymph node exhibiting an increased glucose utilization, suspicious for malignancy. No other lesions suspicious for malignant manifestations were shown (Figs. 11.19 and 11.20). Whole body PET/MR showed suspicion of a singular metastasis of thyroid cancer. Surgical lymph node excision followed, histopathology confirmed metastasis of papillary thyroid cancer.

Teaching Points

PET/MR is a valuable tool for evaluating iodine negative thyroid cancer. The whole body imaging capability of this technique allows better screening of distant lesions and adjustment of targeted therapy.

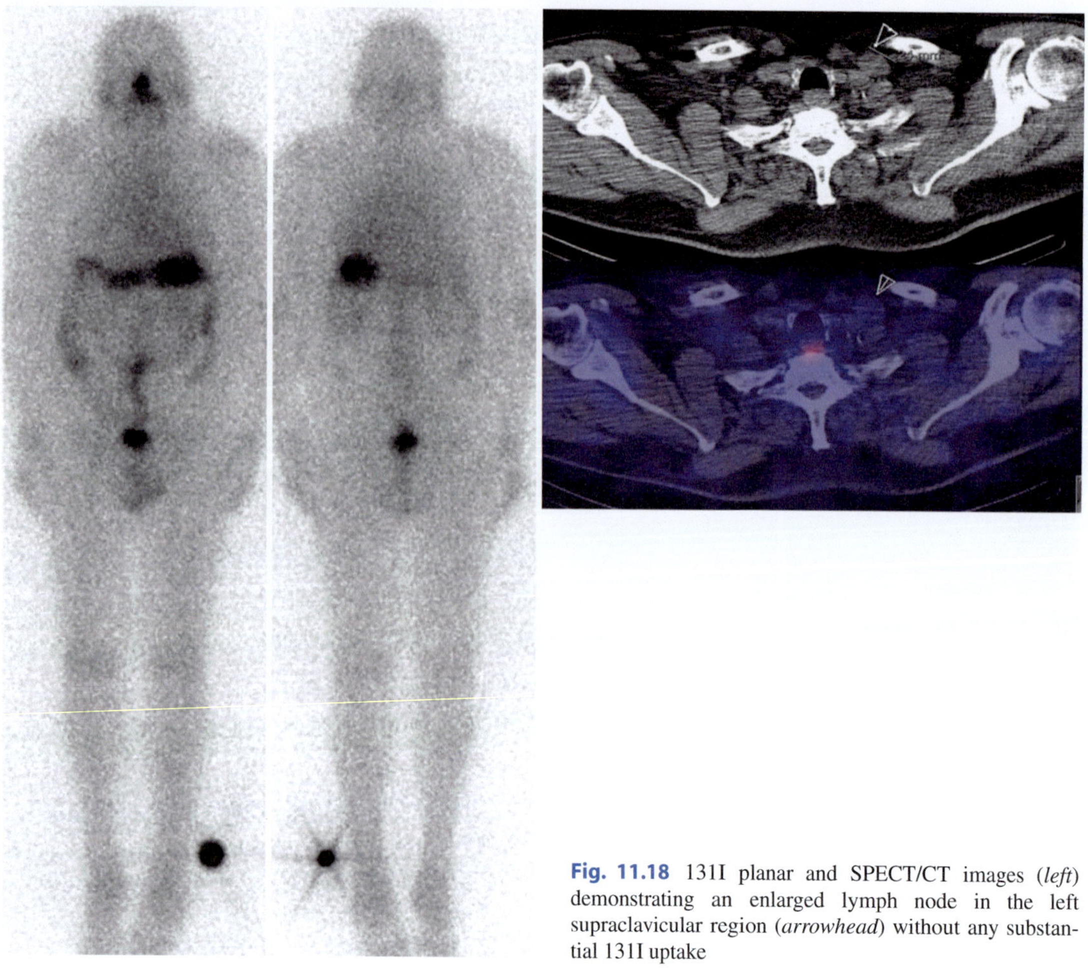

Fig. 11.18 131I planar and SPECT/CT images (*left*) demonstrating an enlarged lymph node in the left supraclavicular region (*arrowhead*) without any substantial 131I uptake

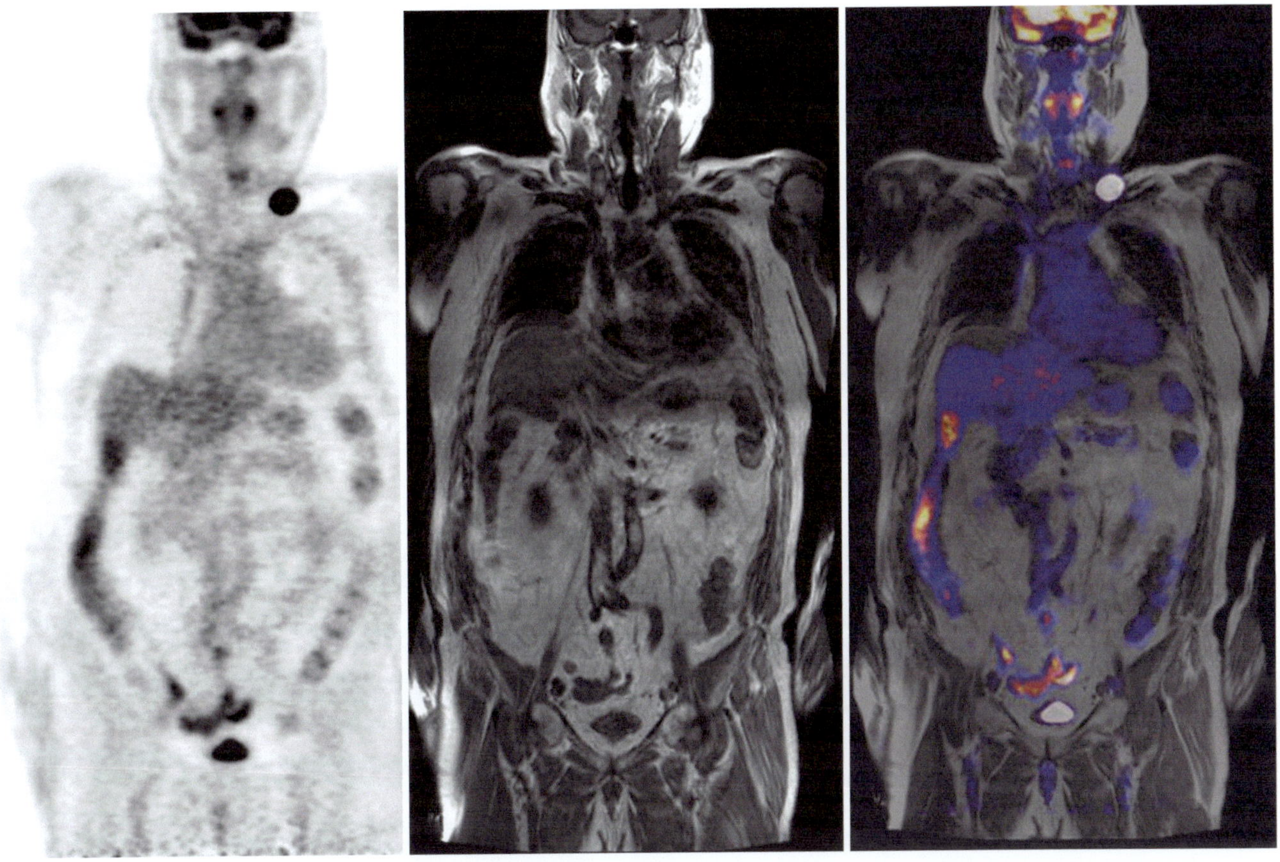

Fig. 11.19 PET, cor T1 TSE and fused image of the 18F-FDG PET/MR study. Increased focal uptake in the left supraclavicular lymph node, indicative of metastatic disease. No other suspicious lesions were observed

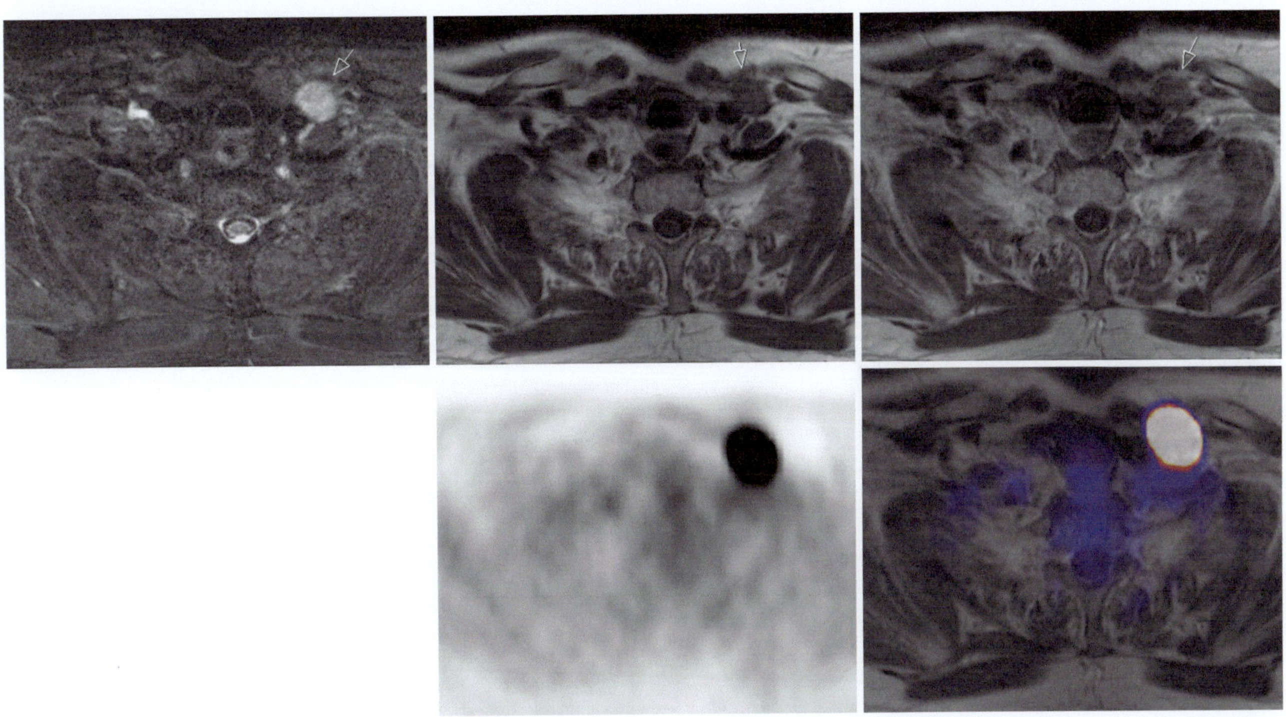

Fig. 11.20 ax T2 STIR, ax T1 TSE, ax T1 TSE post Gd, ax PET and ax fused PET/MR of the PET/MR study. The pathologically enlarged lymph node shows the typical T2 hyperintense/T1 isointense signal (*arrows*)

Hürthle Cell Thyroid Cancer

Clinical History

Restaging of a 67 year old male patient with Hürthle cell thyroid carcinoma after thyroidectomy, pT4pN0(0/16)R1, and radioiodine treatment for ablation, presenting with increasing thyreoglobulin levels (4 ng/ml) and negative post-therapeutic 131I scintigraphy.

Imaging Technique

PET/MR 90 min p.i. of 448 MBq 18F-FDG, 92 kg, 4 bed positions 4 min per bed position. T1 VIBE Dixon for attenuation correction.

MR component: neck: ax T2 STIR, ax T1 TSE –/+ Gd cor T1 STIR post Gd cor T1 TSE.

Findings

Increased focal 18F-FDG uptake in the region of the formal right thyroid bed indicating local recurrence of the thyroid carcinoma (Figs. 11.21 and 11.22). No other suspicious lesions were observed.

Teaching Points

This case emphasizes the value of PET/MR in iodine negative manifestations of thyroid cancer such as in Hürthle cell carcinoma. The excellent tumor/background ratio of the lesion demonstrated in the PET component of PET/MR facilitates detection of the lesion.

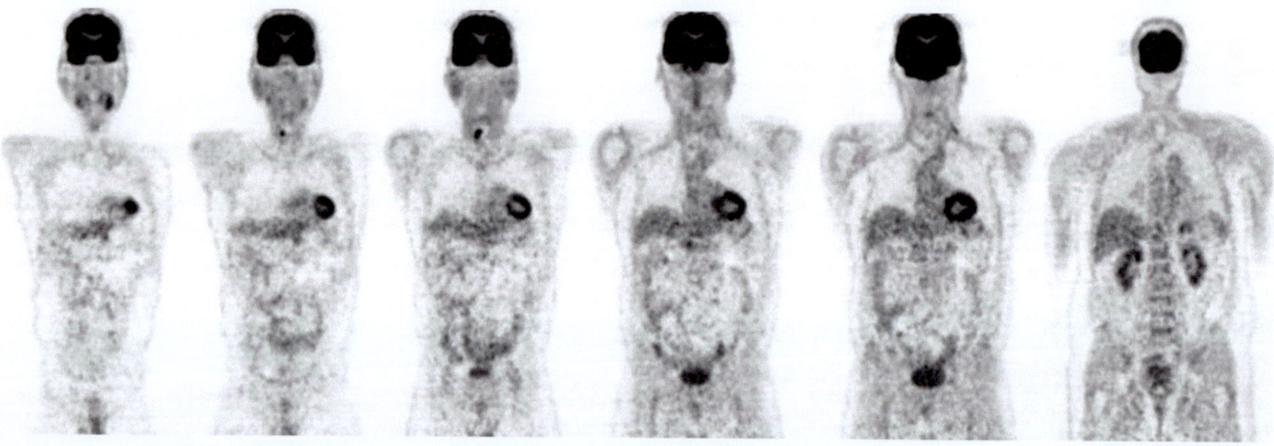

Fig. 11.21 Different coronal levels (from ventral to dorsal) of the PET component of the PET/MR. Increased focal uptake on the right formal thyroid bed indicating local recurrence.

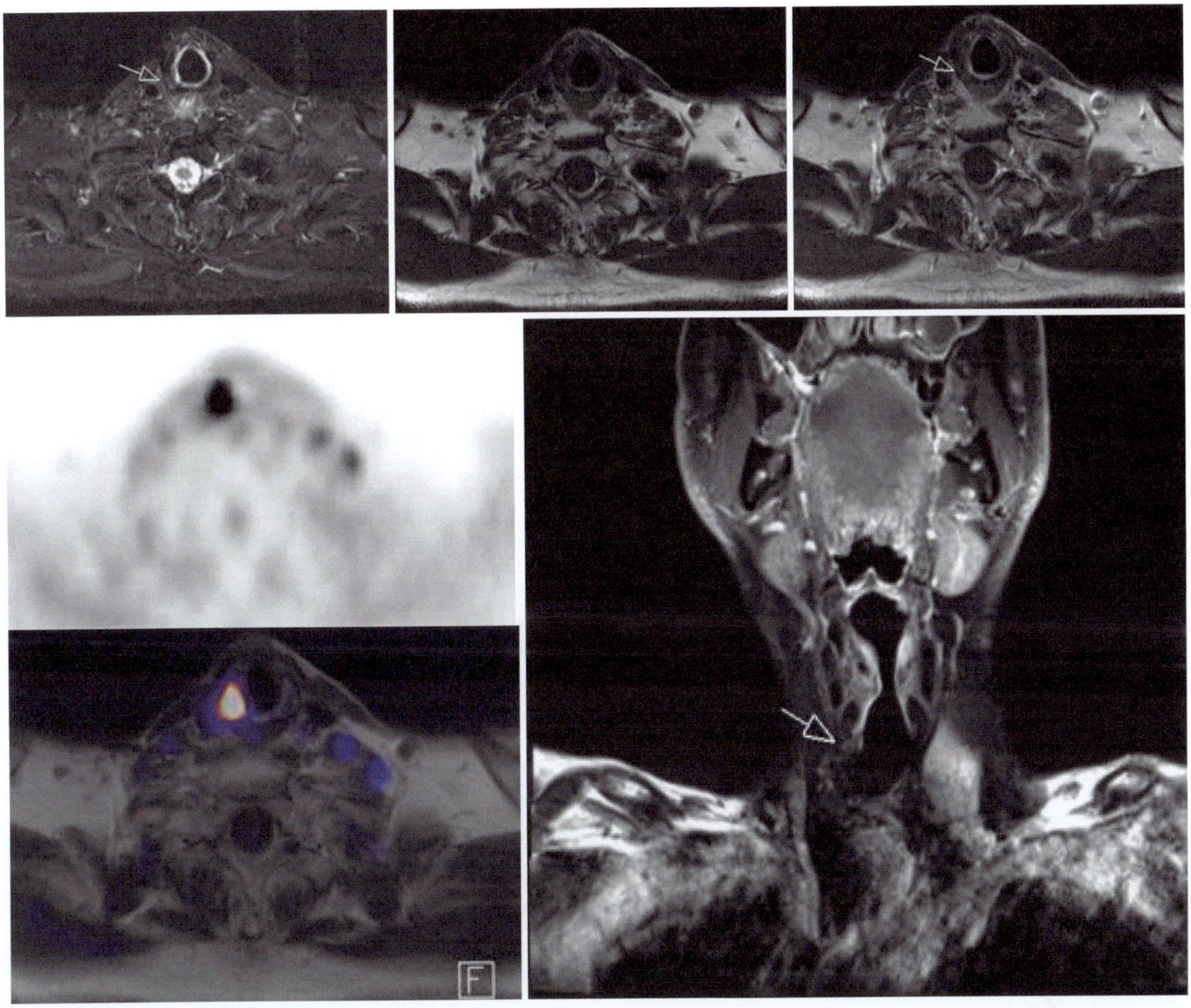

Fig. 11.22 *Upper row*: image of ax T2 STIR, ax T1 TSE and ax T1 TSE post Gd showing a T2 hyperintense signal alteration in the formal right thyroid bed enhancing after contrast media application (*arrows*). *Lower row*: image of ax PET and ax PET/MR fusion as well as cor T1 SPIR post Gd showing a contrast enhancing signal alteration in the formal thyroid bed (*arrow*) corresponding to the hypermetabolic lesion demonstrated in PET. Please note the very high tumor/background ratio in the PET image facilitating detection of local recurrence

References

1. Macapinlac HA (2001) Clinical usefulness of FDG PET in differentiated thyroid cancer. J Nucl Med 42(1):77–78
2. Schlüter B, Bohuslavizki KH, Beyer W, Plotkin M, Buchert R, Clausen M (2001) Impact of FDG PET on patients with differentiated thyroid cancer who present with elevated thyroglobulin and negative 131I scan. J Nucl Med 42(1):71–76
3. Wang W, Macapinlac H, Larson SM, Yeh SDJ, Akhurst T, Finn RD et al (1999) [18F]-2-Fluoro-2-deoxy-d-glucose positron emission tomography localizes residual thyroid cancer in patients with negative diagnostic 131I whole body scans and elevated serum thyroglobulin levels. JCEM 84(7):2291–2302
4. Grünwald F, Kälicke T, Feine U, Lietzenmayer R, Scheidhauer K, Dietlein M et al (1999) Fluorine-18 fluorodeoxyglucose positron emission tomography in thyroid cancer: results of a multicentre study. Eur J Nucl Med 26(12):1547–1552
5. Seiboth L, Van Nostrand D, Wartofsky L, Ousman Y, Jonklaas J, Butler C et al (2008) Utility of PET/neck MRI digital fusion images in the management of recurrent or persistent thyroid cancer. Thyroid 18(2):103–111
6. Mosci C, Iagaru A (2011) PET/CT imaging of thyroid cancer. Clin Nucl Med 36(12):e180–e185
7. Abraham T, Schöder H (2011) Thyroid cancer—indications and opportunities for positron emission tomography/computed tomography imaging. Semin Nucl Med 41(2):121–138
8. Buchmann I, Henze M, Engelbrecht S, Eisenhut M, Runz A, Schäfer M et al (2007) Comparison of 68Ga-DOTATOC PET and 111In-DTPAOC (Octreoscan) SPECT in patients with neuroendocrine tumours. Eur J Nucl Med Mo Imaging 34(10): 1617–1626
9. Schreiter NF, Nogami M, Steffen I, Pape U-F, Hamm B, Brenner W et al (2012) Evaluation of the potential of PET/MRI fusion for detection of liver metastases in patients with neuroendocrine tumours. Eur Radiol 22(2):458–467
10. Ruf J, Lopez Hänninen E, Böhmig M, Koch I, Denecke T, Plotkin M et al (2006) Impact of FDG-PET/MRI image fusion on the detection of pancreatic cancer. Pancreatology 6(6):512–519
11. Tatsumi M, Isohashi K, Onishi H, Hori M, Kim T, Higuchi I et al (2011) 18F-FDG PET/MRI fusion in characterizing pancreatic tumors: comparison to PET/CT. Int J Clin Oncol 16(4):408–415
12. Kalra MK, Maher MM, Mueller PR, Saini S (2003) State-of-the-art imaging of pancreatic neoplasms. Br J Radiol 76(912): 857–865
13. Fidler JL, Johnson CD (2001) Imaging of neuroendocrine tumors of the pancreas. Int J Gastrointest Cancer 30(1–2):73–85

Benign, Degenerative and Inflammatory Diseases

12

A.J. Beer, O. Ratib, I. Dregely, M. Eiber, M. Essler, S. Foerster, S. Nekolla, C. Rischpler, J.-P. Willi, and I. Yakushev

Contents

Benign, Degenerative and Inflammatory Diseases

^{18}F-FDG PET studies were shown to be quite sensitive to inflammation as well to a variety of benign diseases that induce focal increase in metabolism [1–3]. While in most countries PET imaging of these diseases are not reimbursed, it remains a potential alternative imaging modality for selected cases. FDG-PET remains a sensitive diagnostic modality for detection of infectious diseases and exploring sources of fever of unknown origin. In this chapter several diseases are presented, but also examples of identification and characterization of vascular plaques [4]. While ^{18}F-FDG is being reported as a potential marker of plaque inflammatory process and therefore may help identify unstable plaques and be a predictor of cardiovascular events, alternative PET tracers are also being evaluated for better characterization of vascular plaques [4–6].

Another application domain of PET and therefore could potentially benefit from hybrid PET/MR is the assessment of neurodegenerative diseases and differentiation of diagnostic classification based on anatomical distribution of brain metabolic activity. Many studies reported the added value of ^{18}F-FDG in dementia in complementarity to MRI findings [7–9]. Future development of new specific tracers will bring additional potential applications of for PET imaging in combination with MRI [10, 11].

A.J. Beer (✉) • M. Eiber
Department of Radiology, Klinikum Rechts der Isar, Technische Universität München, Munich, Germany

O. Ratib • J.-P. Willi
Division of Nuclear Medicine and Molecular Imaging, Department of Medical Imaging, Geneva University Hospitals, Geneva, Switzerland
e-mail: osman.ratib@hcuge.ch

I. Dregely • M. Essler • S. Foerster • S. Nekolla
C. Rischpler • I. Yakushev
Department of Nuclear Medicine, Technische Universität München, Munich, Germany

O. Ratib et al. (eds.), *Atlas of PET/MR Imaging in Oncology*,
DOI 10.1007/978-3-642-31292-2_12, © Springer-Verlag Berlin Heidelberg 2013

Atherosclerotic Plaque at Carotid Bifurcation

Clinical History

Fifty-nine-year-old man with history of an intermittent weakness of the left hand. An ultrasound examination of the right internal carotid artery shows a slight stenosis.

Imaging Technique

PET/MR image acquired 140 min after iv injection of 421 MBq 18F-FDG.

1 bed position × 15 min together with axial TOF, T2w TSE, T1w TSE native and post injection of 17 ml of Gd-DTPA MR contrast agent (CA). Head/neck and dedicated phased-array carotid coil.

Findings

A mild stenosis of right carotid artery slightly above bifurcation is observed. Axial high resolution TSE images show morphology of outward plaque remodeling. Different MR contrast weightings allow distinguishing plaque constituents. Faint uptake of 18F-FDG tracer at plaque location indicates possible inflammatory status of the plaque.

Teaching Points

In atherosclerosis characterization of the so-called "vulnerable" plaque at risk for disruption is critical to predict adverse events. PET/MR allows for identification of atherosclerotic plaque morphology and functional status.

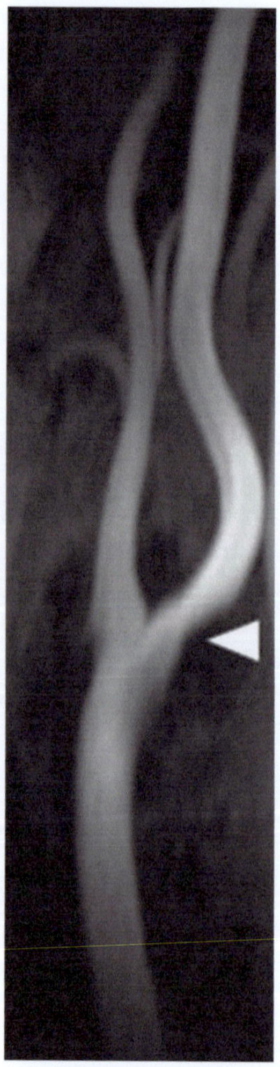

Fig. 12.1 Slight stenosis observed at carotid artery slightly above bifurcation (*arrowhead*) shown on a MIP projection of axial time-of-flight MR images, acquired without the use of contrast agent

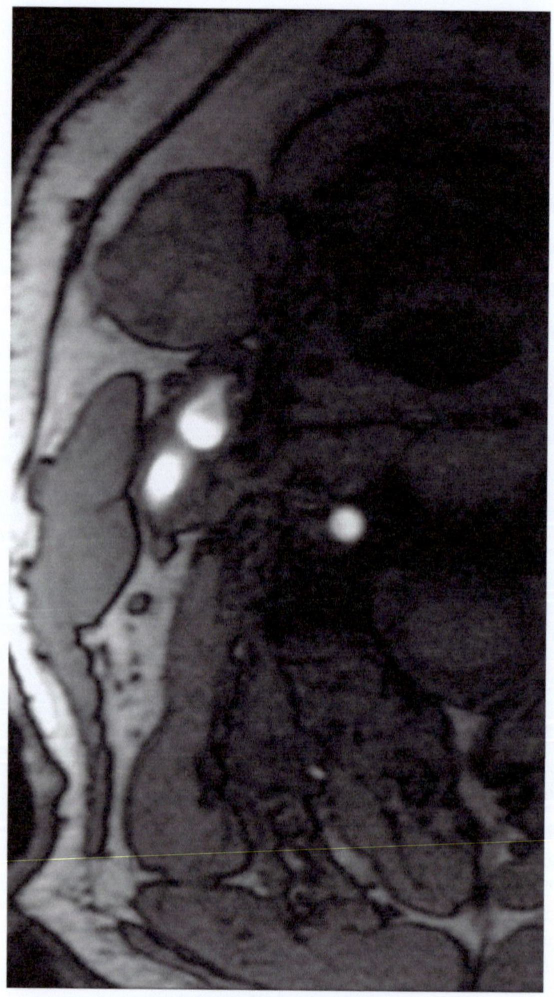

Fig. 12.2 Axial TOF MR images show slightly restricted lumen due to a plaque, which extends also outward to the vessel lumen

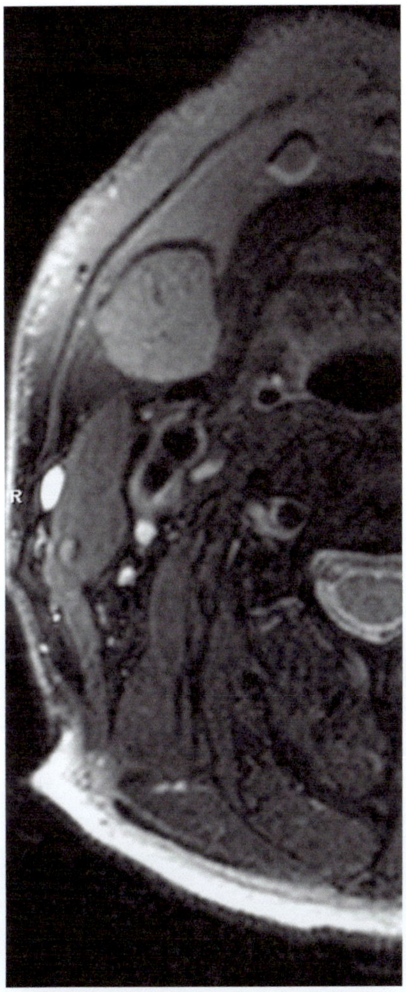

Fig. 12.3 Bright signal on T2 weighted images show intact fibrous cap as well as additional fibrous constituents in plaque

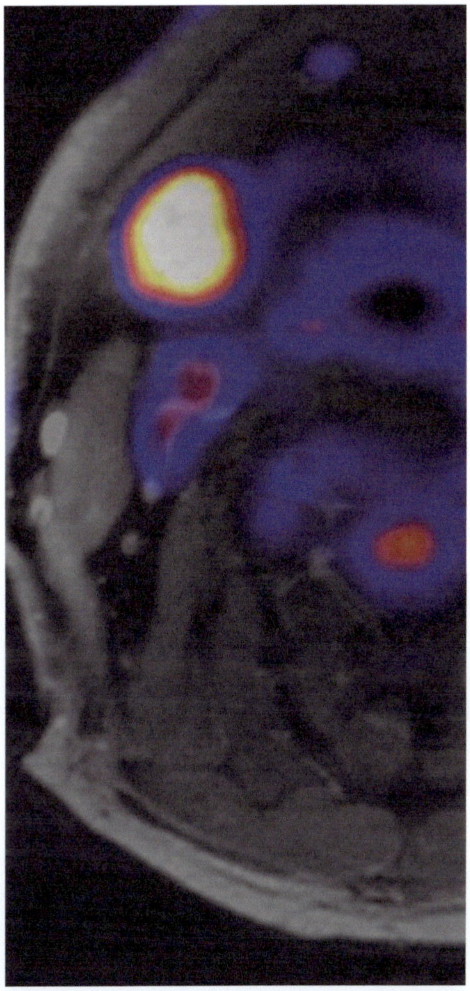

Fig. 12.5 Fusion of PET and post CA T1w TSE shows a perfect anatomical co-registration of the faint 18F-FDG tracer uptake at the location of the plaque (PET images is calibrated in SUV values, intensity scale 1–3 SUV)

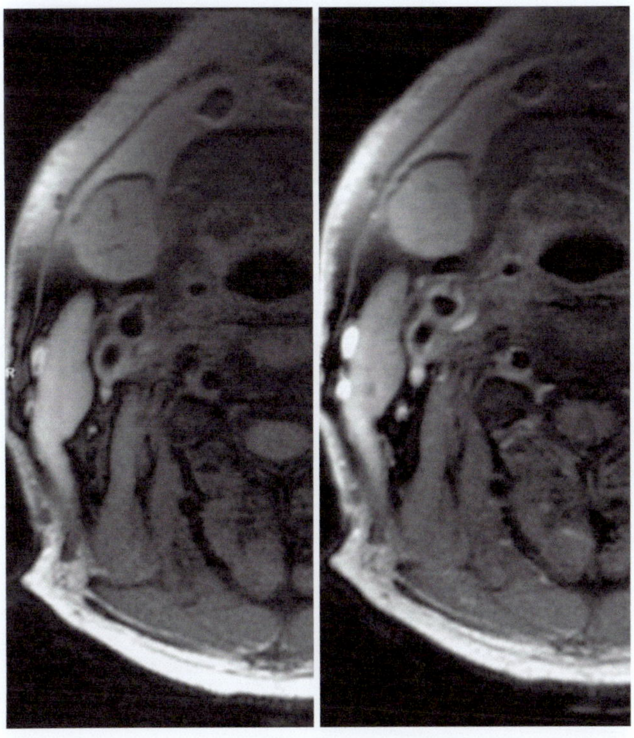

Fig. 12.4 Lipid is bright on native T1 weighted images (*left image*), if calcium was present it would be dark. Signal enhancement on T1 weighted post CA image (*right image*) indicates fibrous tissue, lipid or calcified areas do not enhance

Stress Fracture

Clinical History

Fifty-nine-year-old female patient with osteosynthetic supply of the right ankle after a complex fracture 1.5 years ago. The patients suffers from increasing pain of the right foot developing over the last few months. A prior X-ray was negative.

Imaging Technique

PET/MR of the right foot acquired 126 min after iv injection 326 MBq 18F-Flouride, 78 kg.

1 bed × 10 min together with sagittal T1w TSE/ PDw fs, axial T1w TSE/ PDw fs and coronal T2w TSE. Flex coil.

Findings

Bone marrow edema and high osteoblastic activity in PET indicate an active process in the cuboid bone. Only mild edema and minor uptake combined with a clear stress fracture line are signs of a more chronic process in the calcaneus.

> **Teaching Points**
>
> 18F-Flouride PET and MRI can provide complementary information in patients with chronic foot pain. The combination of T1w TSE outlining a potential fracture line and the extent of osteoblastic activity is helpful in the differentiation between an active and chronic process.

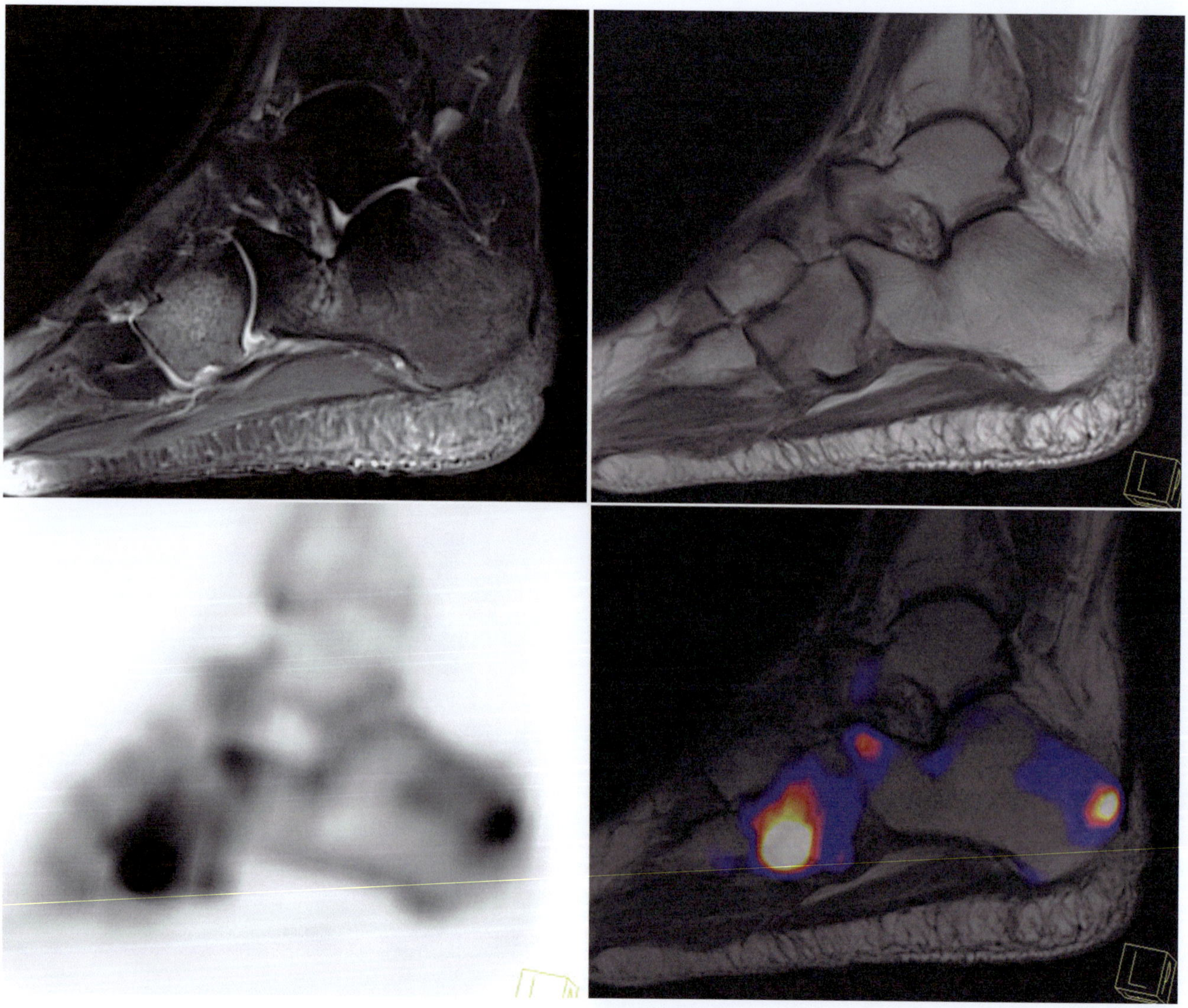

Fig. 12.6 Sagittal PDw image (*top left*) reveals an extensive hyperintensity in the cuboid bone. Minor bone marrow edema is also found in the dorsal part of the calcaneus. Sagittal T1w TSE shows a hypointense *curved line* in the calcaneus adjacent to the achilles tendon consistent with a stress fracture. In addition a beginning hypointense line can be found in the anterior part of the cuboid bone (*top right*). An intense uptake of 18F-Flouride is found in the cuboid bone indicating high osteoblastic activity. The low and circumscribed uptake in the dorsal part of the calcaneus indicates a more chronic process (*bottom*)

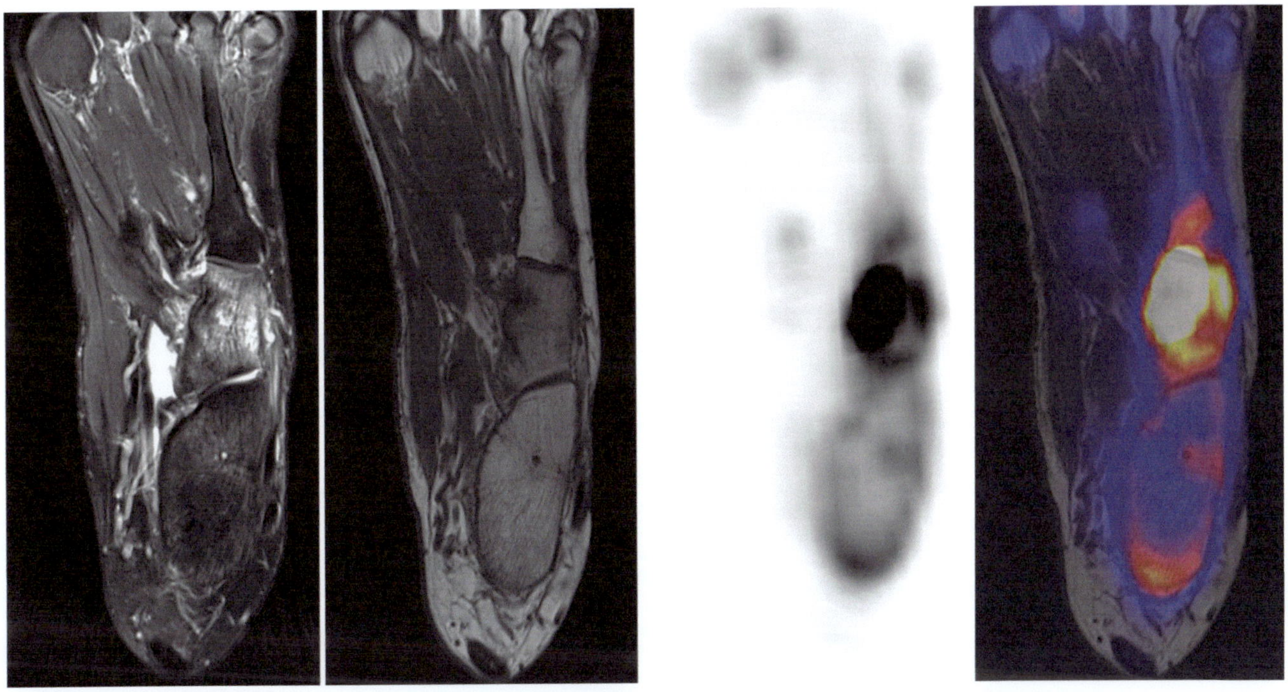

Fig. 12.7 Axial PDw fs and T1w TSE show an extensive bone marrow edema in the cuboid bone. The beginning fracture line present in the sagittal image is only partially visualized (*left images*). 18F-Flouride PET and fused image demonstrate high osteoblastic activity in the cuboid bone (*right images*)

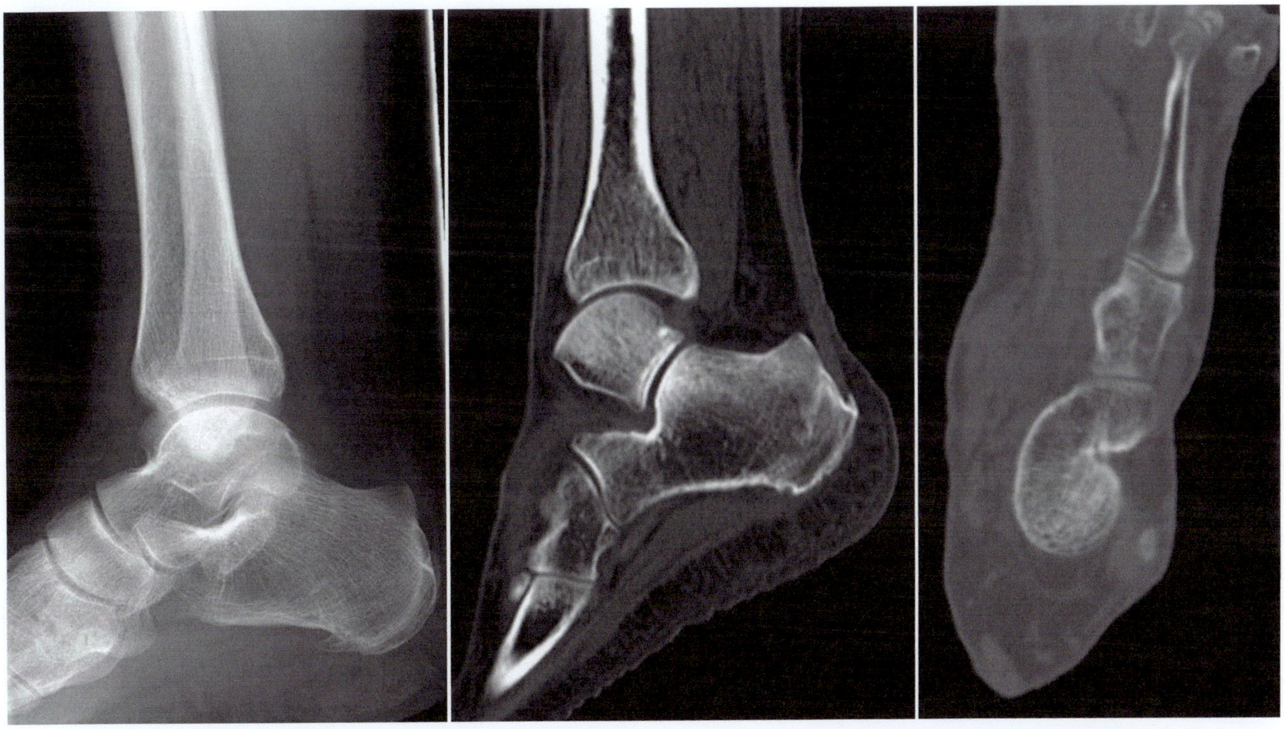

Fig. 12.8 A prior x-ray of the right ankle is completely normal (*left*). Sagittal reformatted multi-slice computed tomography (MS-CT) shows a curved hyperdense line in the posterior part of the calcaneus analogous to the findings in T1w TSE (*middle*). The axial reformatted MS-CT cannot outline the beginning fracture line in the cuboid bone (*right*)

Multicystic Disease

Clinical History

65 y.o. patient with polycystic disease and status post renal transplant due to renal insufficiency. Diagnostic staging for possible lymphoma.

Imaging Technique

PET: Whole-body PET acquired 60 min after injection of 369 MBq of ^{18}F-FDG, 57 kg/157 cm patient, with 5.2 mmol/L of fasting glycemia.

MRI: Whole body atMR (T1 weighted), supine position. 3D TSE T2 weighted whole-body MRI.

Findings

PET/MR images confirmed the diffuse polycystic disease with only mild focal uptake of some retro-peritoneal and para-aortic lymph nodes with strong evidence of any malignant disease.

> **Teaching Points**
>
> In patients with renal insufficiency and complex clinical history, high resolution MR of hybrid PET/MR can replace PET/CT studies for whole-body staging.

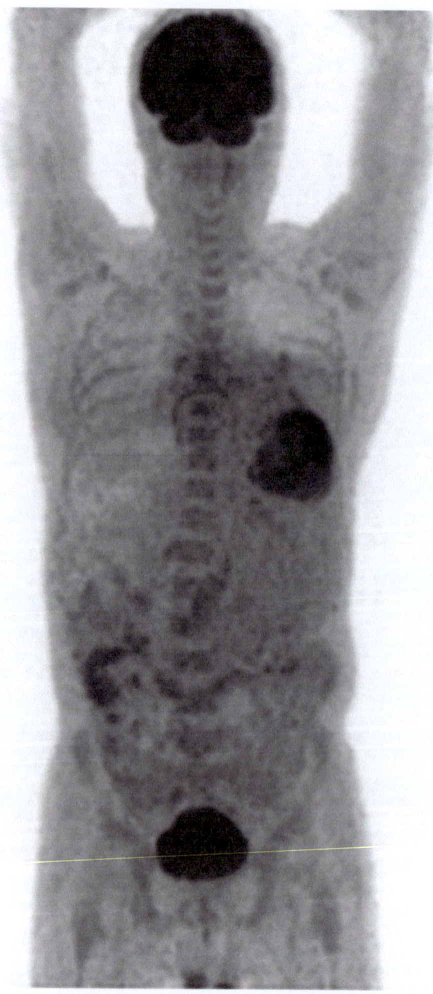

Fig. 12.9 Coronal MIP reconstruction of PET images shows diffuse focal spots of mild FDG uptake in the abdomen

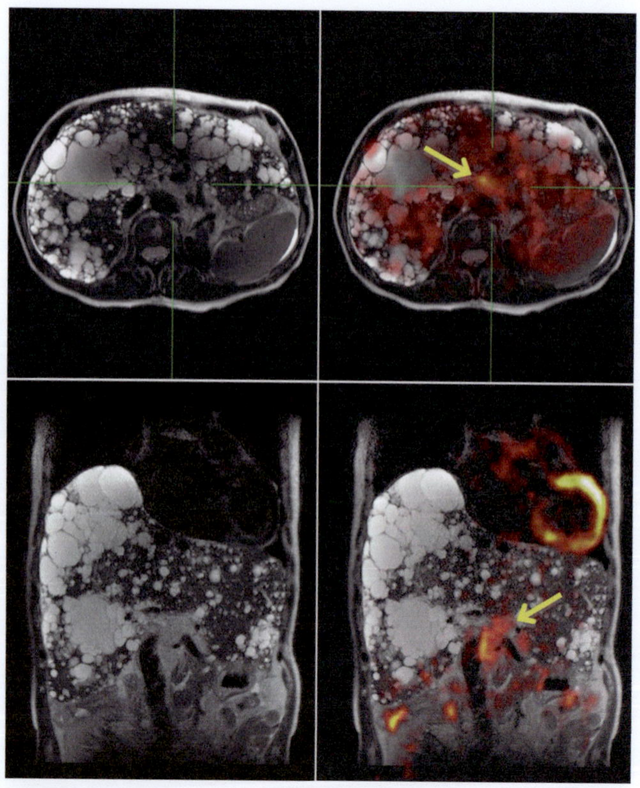

Fig. 12.10 Axial and coronal respiratory-gated HASTE images (*left*) fused with PET images (*right*), showing mild uptake (*arrow*) of enlarged retro-peritoneal lymph nodes (SUV max 3.2)

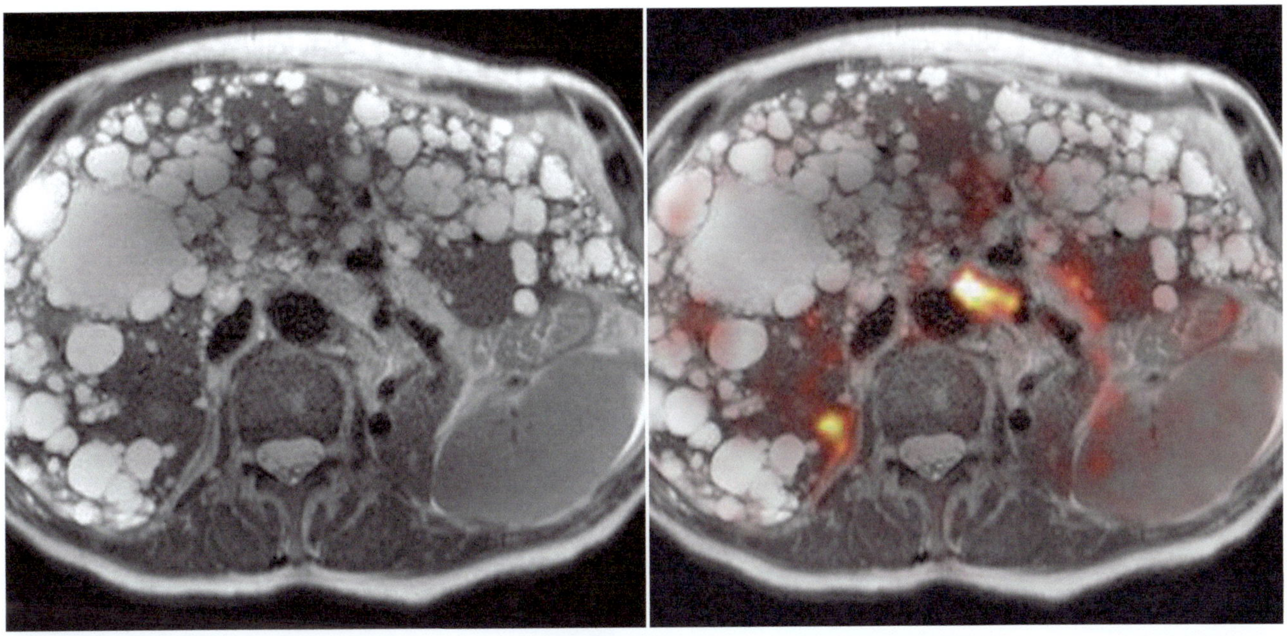

Fig. 12.11 Axial T2 HASTE MR images showing diffuse polycystic disease fused with PET image showing focal FDG uptake in a para-aortic enlarged lymph-node

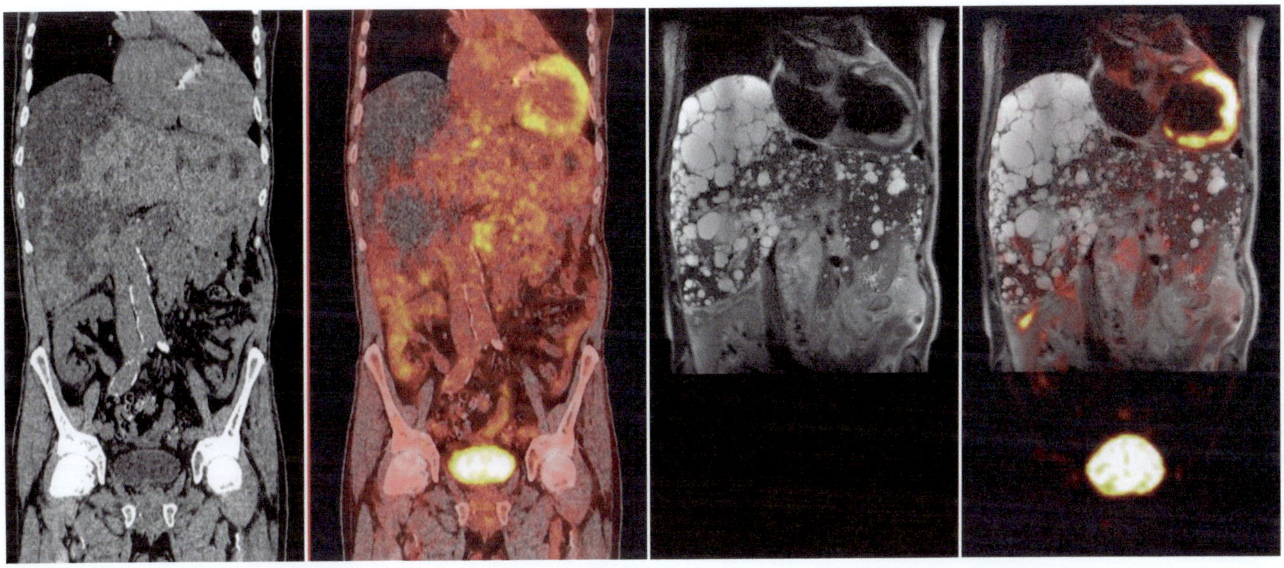

Fig. 12.12 Comparison of coronal PET/CT (*left*) and high resolution coronal abdominal HASTE images of PET MR study (*right*)

Kaposi Sarcoma

Clinical History

61 y.o. patient with known Kaposi sarcoma in an endemic African form associated with HHV8 virus often associated with HIV positive subjects.

Imaging Technique

PET: Whole-body PET acquired 60 min after injection of 377 MBq 18F-FDG, 83 kg/169 cm patient.

MRI: Whole body atMR (T1 weighted), supine position. 3D TSE T2 weighted whole-body MRI.

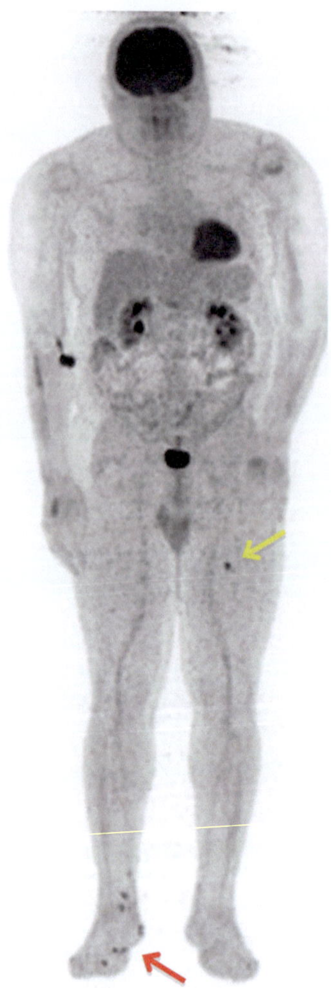

Fig. 12.13 Coronal MIP reconstruction of PET images shows focal FDG uptake on the right foot (*red arrow*) and single focal lesion of the left thigh (*yellow arrow*)

Findings

PET/MR images multiple subcutaneous lesions with high FDG uptake corresponding to the Kaposi sarcoma lesions, with only one distant hypermetabolic lesion of the left thigh.

> **Teaching Points**
>
> In soft-tissue lesions, MRI can provide a wealth of different imaging sequences for better characterization and localization of focal hypermetabolic lesions seen on PET.

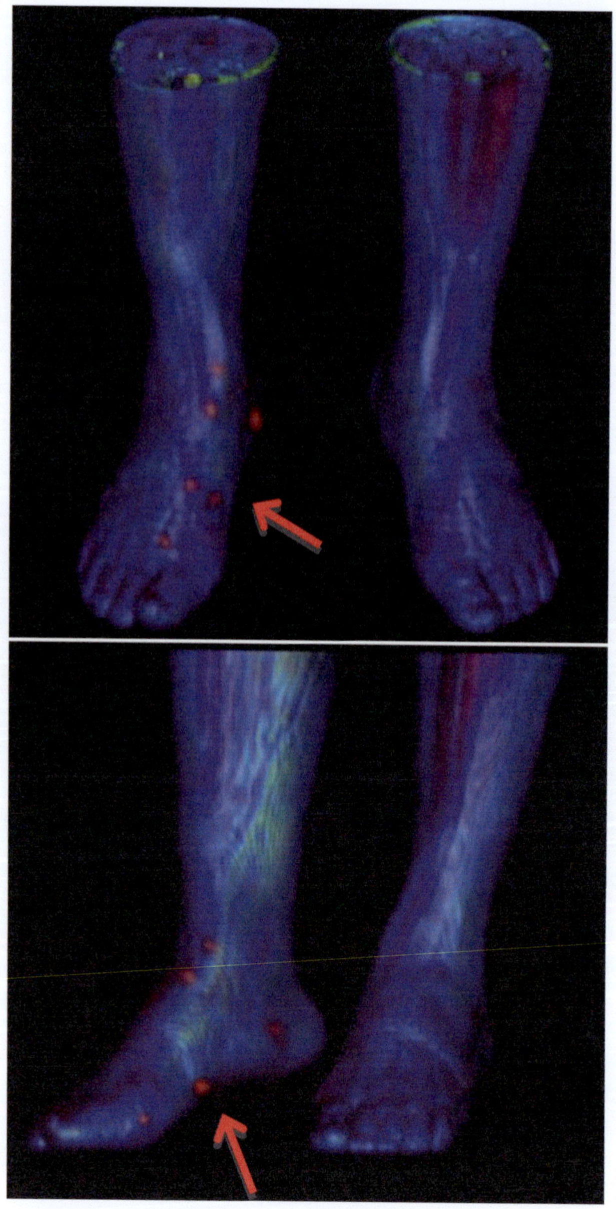

Fig. 12.14 3D volume rendering of PET/MR images showing the location of Kaposi lesions on the right foot (*red arrow*)

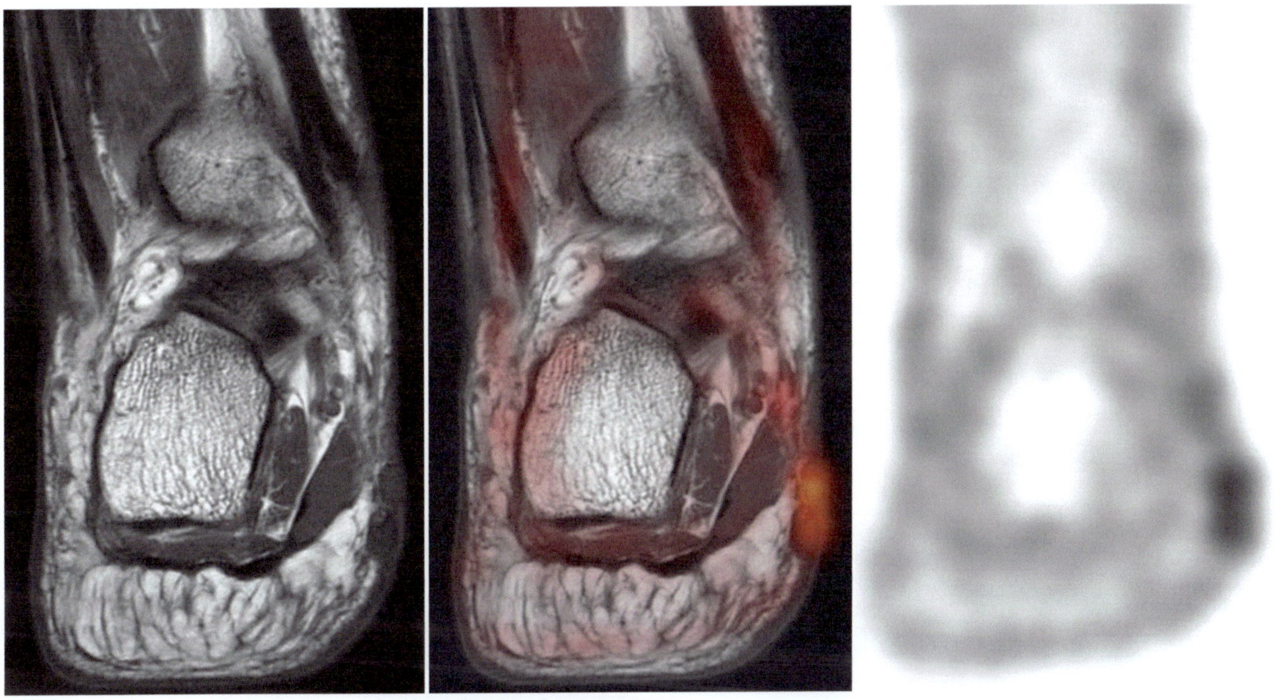

Fig. 12.15 Coronal high resolution T1 weighted TSE image of the right talus, fused with the corresponding PET image showing two subcutaneous hypermetabolic nodules corresponding to Kaposi sarcoma lesions

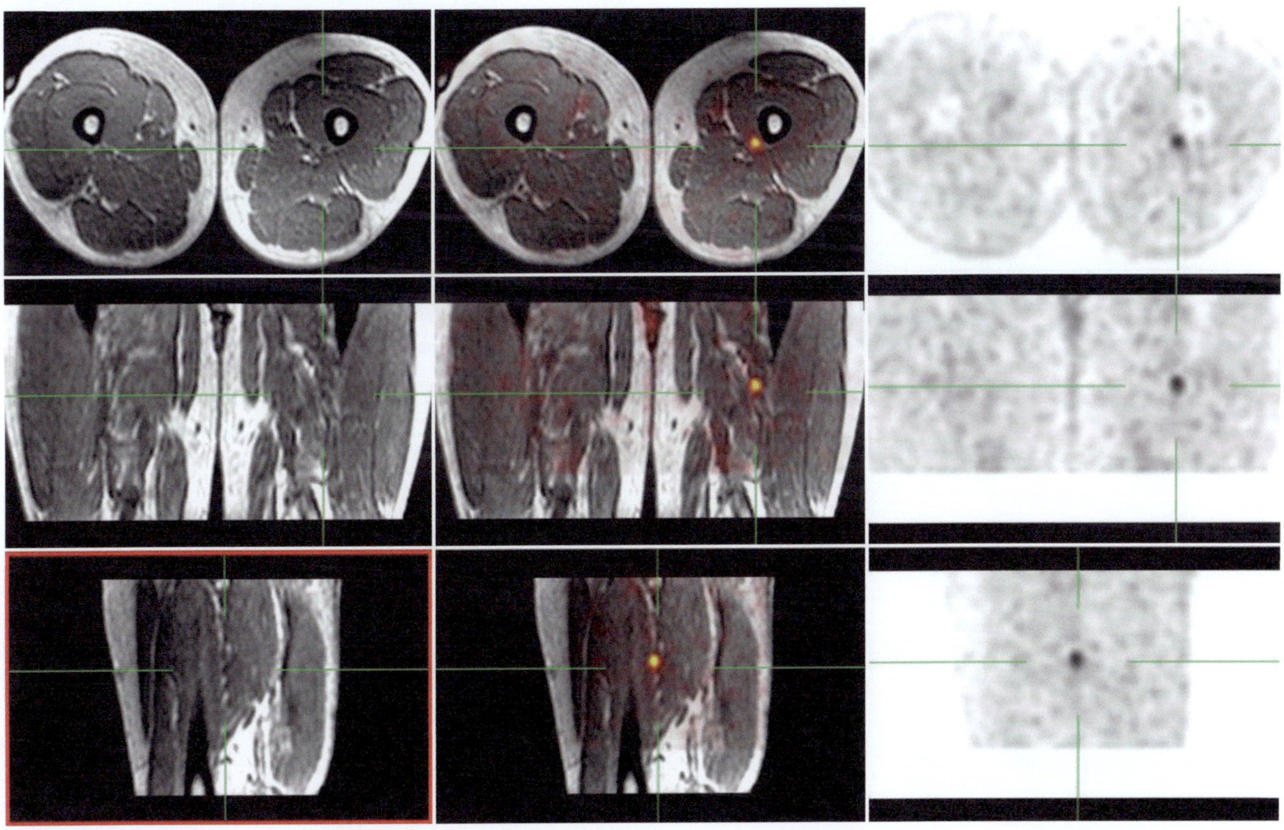

Fig. 12.16 Multiplaner reformatting (MPR) of T1 weighted TFE PET/MR images showing the focal FDG uptake in the left thigh corresponding to a <10 mm nodule

Maffucci Syndrome

Clinical History

29 y.o. patient with a Maffucci syndrome (a rare non-hereditary syndrome characterized by the presence of multiple enchondromas associated with multiple hemangiomas) who underwent several surgical interventions for bone lesions of the lower limbs. Study requested for assessment of a rapidly growing lesion of the left shoulder.

Imaging Technique

PET: Whole-body PET acquired 60 min after injection of 370 MBq of ^{18}F-FDG.

MRI: Whole body atMR (T1 weighted), supine position. 3D TSE T2 weighted whole-body MRI.

Findings

PET/MR images confirmed the wide spread of endochondroma lesions across the whole body with mild to moderate FDG uptake. A growing lesion of the left shoulder showed moderate homogeneous FDG uptake with no evidence of malignant transformation.

Teaching Points

Multi-parametric criteria from MRI tissue characteristics and patterns of FDG uptake can help differentiate benign from malignant lesions in soft tissue tumors.

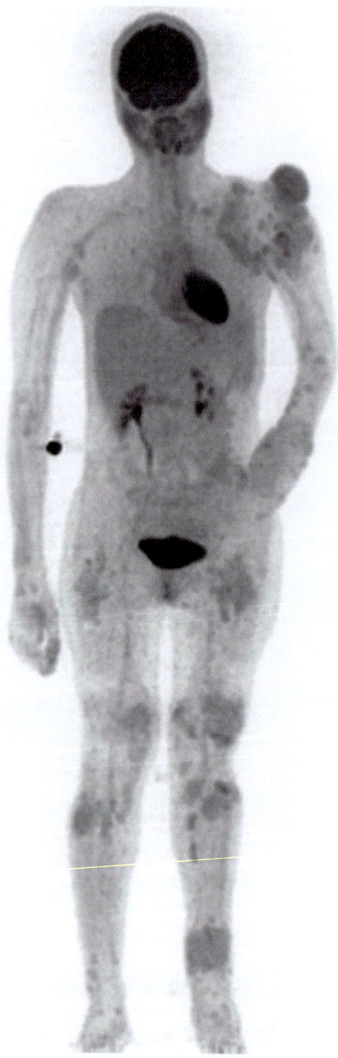

Fig. 12.17 Coronal MIP reconstruction of PET images shows multiple diffuse lesions with mild to moderate tracer uptake in enchondroma lesions of the limbs

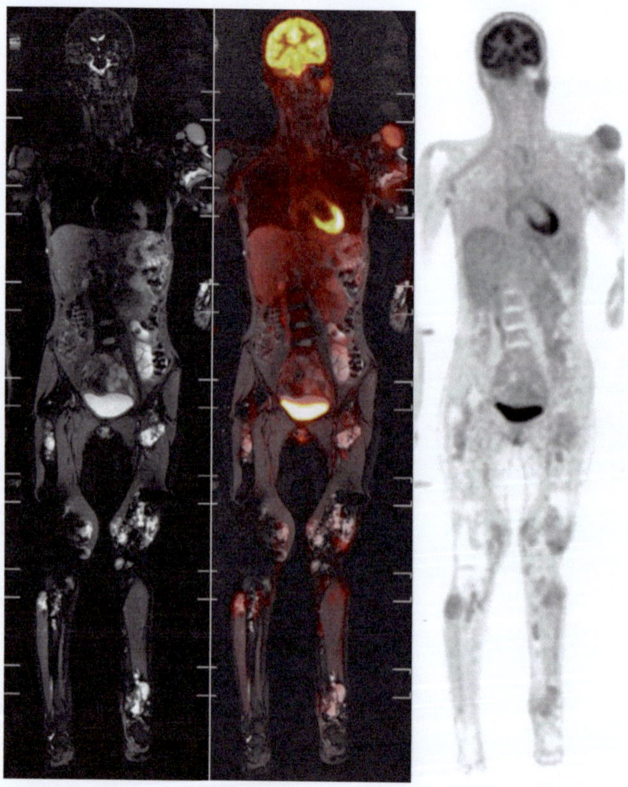

Fig. 12.18 Coronal STIR MR (*left*) and corresponding whole-body PET image (*right*) with fused images in the middle. Not the important metal artifacts of metal implants in the right knee and left limb

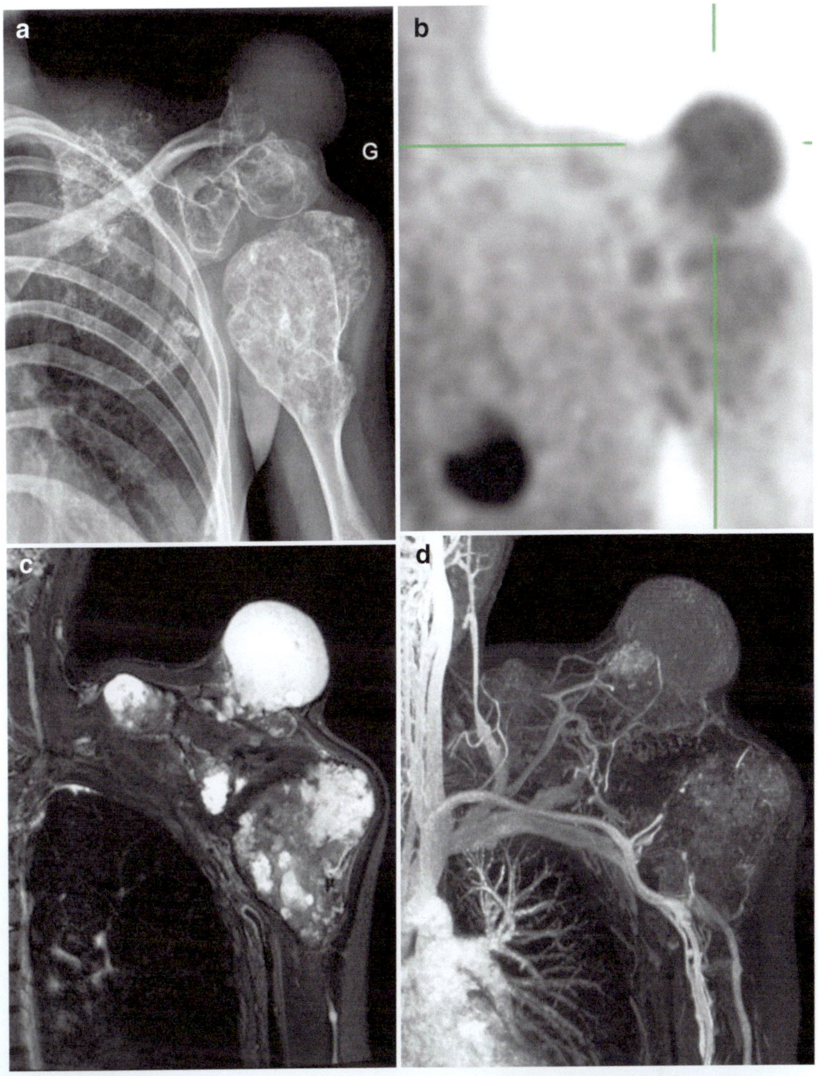

Fig. 12.19 Comparison of different imaging modalities: (**a**) conventional X-ray, (**b**) PET, (**c**) T1 weighted gadolinium enhanced TSE MRI (**d**) MR angiogram

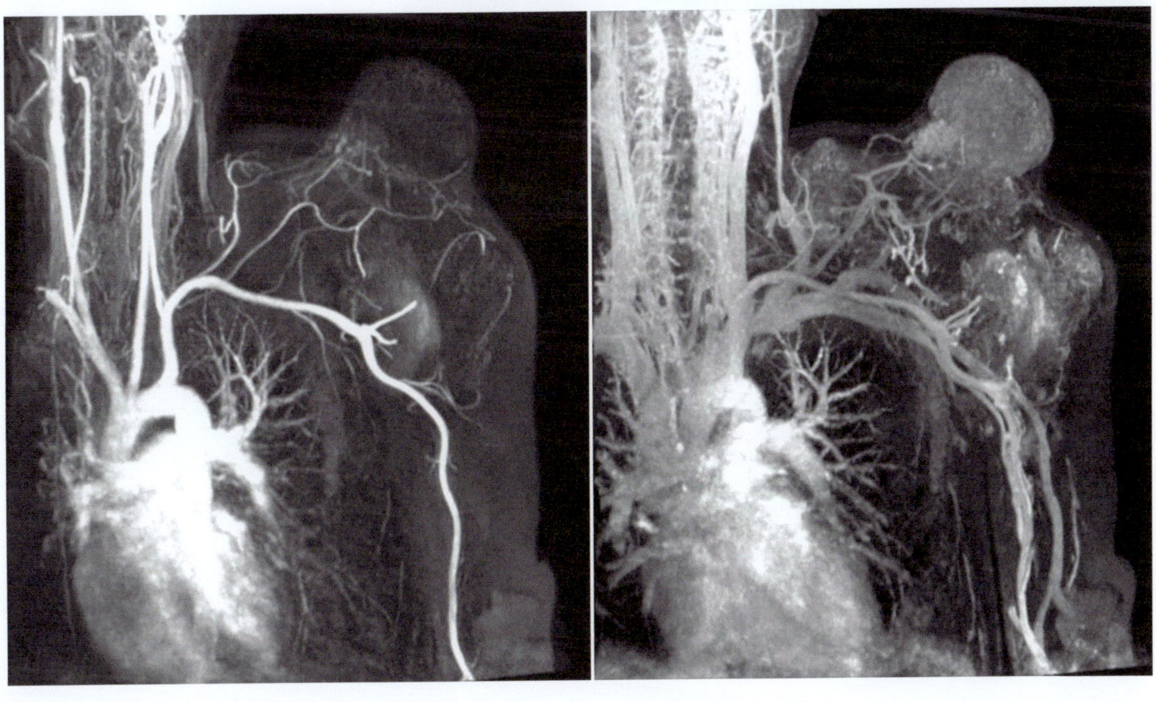

Fig. 12.20 Arterial (*left*) and venous (*right*) phase of MR angiogram of the left shoulder

Giant Cell Vasculitis

Clinical History

Seventy-two-year-old patient presenting with elevated CRP and chest pain.

Imaging Technique

PET/MR images of the whole body were acquired 108 min after iv injection 420 MBq18F-FDG.

Coronal T2w STIR MRI, GRE MRI before and after application of CM.

Findings

Increased glucose metabolism in the vessel wall of the descending thoracic aorta was found to correlate with hyperintense changes seen in T2w MRI.

> **Teaching Points**
>
> FDG-PET detects pathological tracer uptake in vascular wall which confirms active vasculitis. MRI helps to localize vascular uptake and allows correlation with morphological changes of the vessel wall.

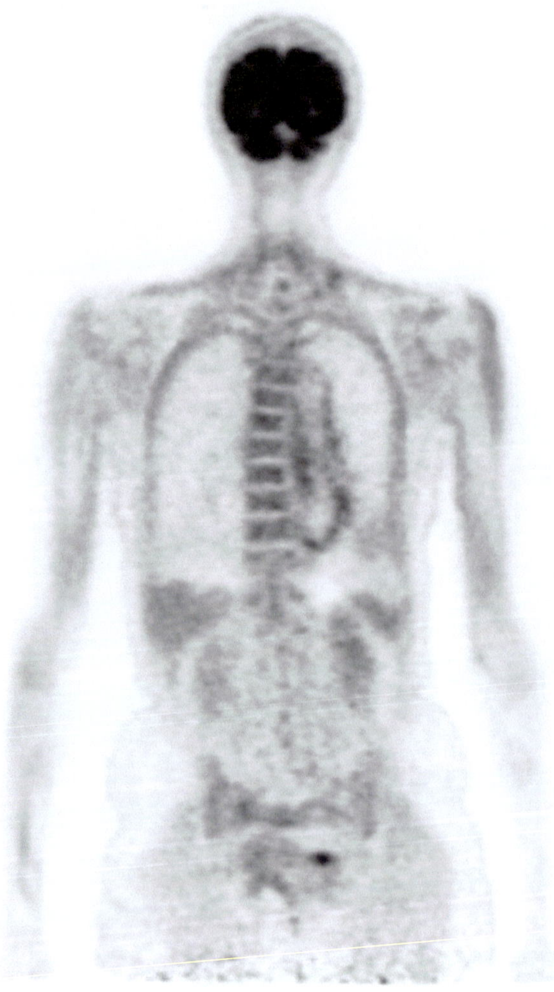

Fig. 12.21 FDG-PET shows increased glucose metabolism in the wall of the descending thoracic aorta

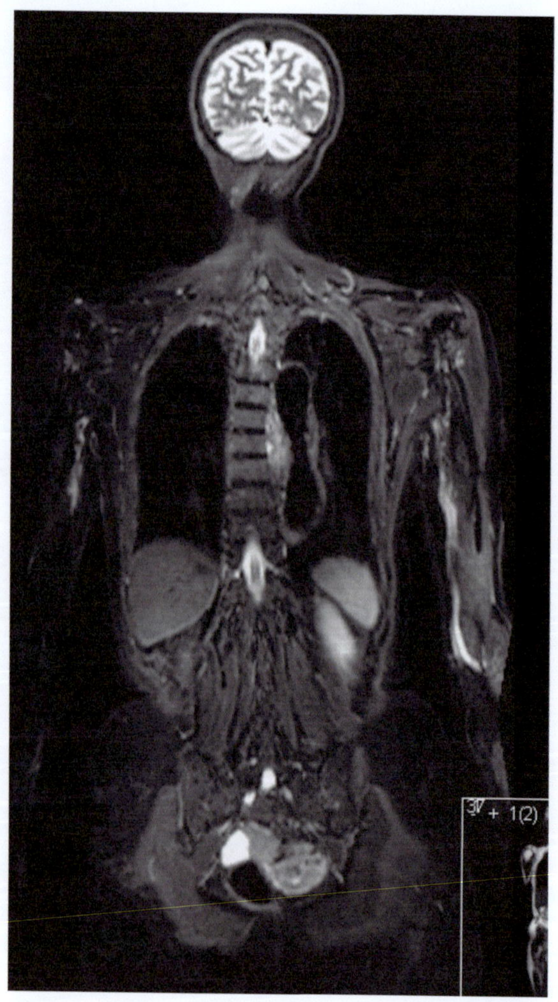

Fig. 12.22 Coronal T2w STIR MRI shows thickening of the wall of the descending thoracic aorta

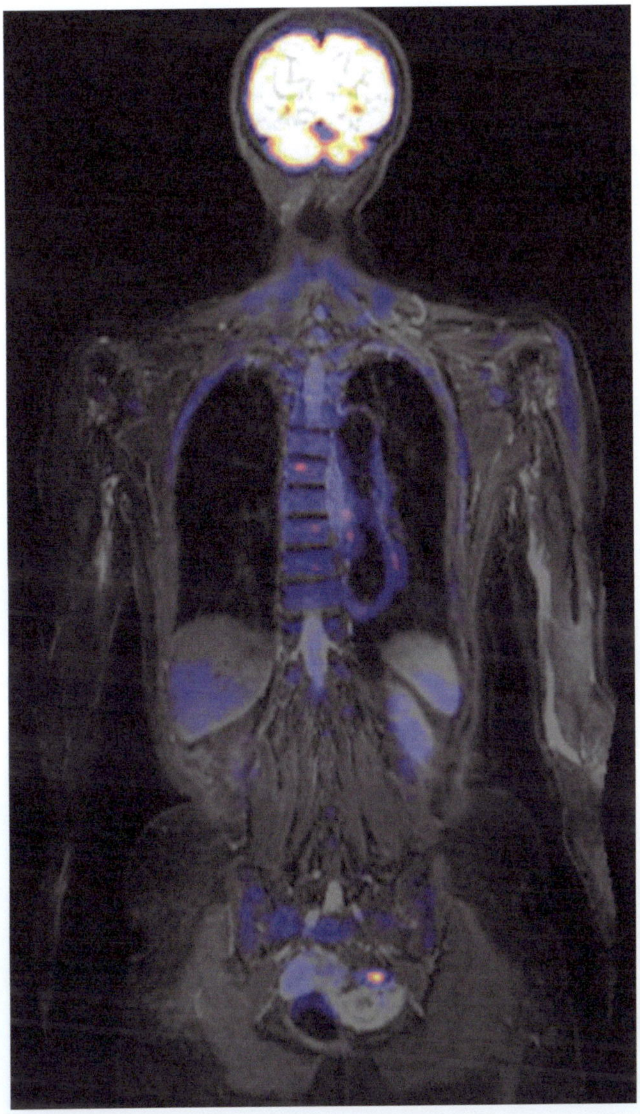

Fig. 12.23 Colocalization of FDG-uptake and morphological changes are demonstrated by coregistration of MR and PET

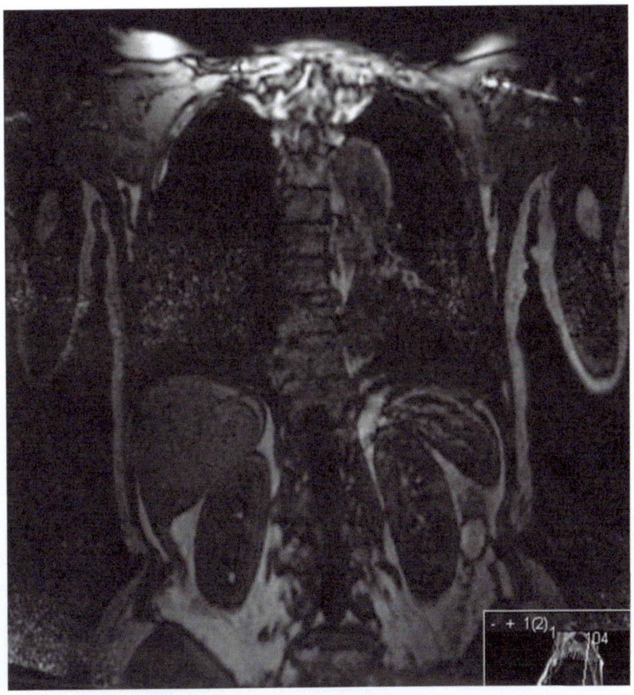

Fig. 12.24 GRE MRI before injection of contrast media

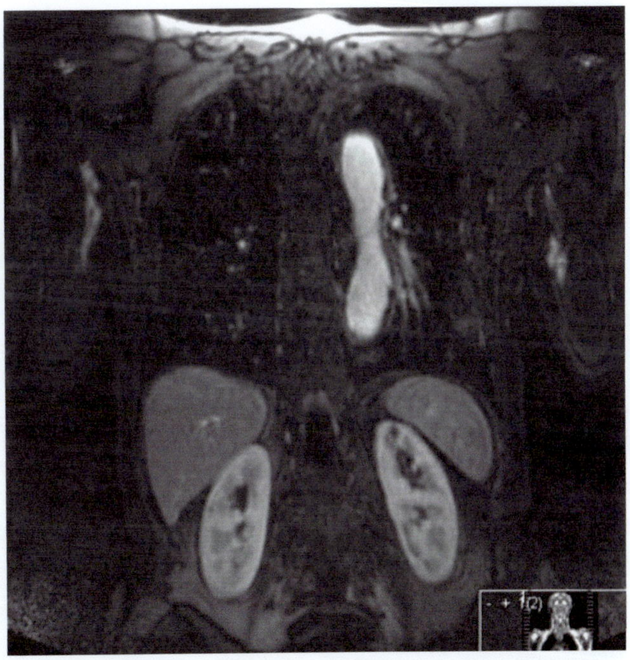

Fig. 12.25 GRE MRI after Gadolinium injection shows mild enhancement

Cardiac Sarcoidosis

Clinical History

A 30-year-old male patient was referred to our institution because of suspected cardiac involvement of a newly diagnosed sarcoidosis. Coronary angiography excluded coronary artery disease and showed a severely reduced left ventricular function. A CT of the chest demonstrated bihilar lymphadenopathy. Subsequently, the patient was transferred to our institution to confirm cardiac involvement of the sarcoidosis by PET/MR.

Imaging Technique

To suppress physiological glucose uptake of the myocardium the patient was put on a low-carbohydrate diet for 1 day and had to fast 12 h prior to the scan. PET/MR images were acquired 64 min after iv injection of 238 MBq 18F-FDG. Furthermore, myocardial perfusion was assessed at resting conditions by slow bolus iv injection over 30 s of 219 MBq 13N-ammonia. MR: T1 VIBE Dixon for attenuation correction, True-FISP CINE (wall motion), T1 IR 15 min. 40 ml of Gd-DTPA were injected.

Findings

Bihilar lymphadenopathy with increased FDG uptake in the lymph nodes confirms the diagnosis of sarcoidosis. Areas in the left ventricle with increased FDG uptake and reduced perfusion indicate active inflammation and reveal cardiac involvement of the sarcoidosis. Also, a severely reduced left ventricular ejection fraction with severe hypokinesis of the lateral wall demonstrates dilated cardiomyopathy (DCM) as a consequence of cardiac sarcoidosis. Furthermore, areas demonstrating late gadolinium enhancement (LGE) indicate myocardial infiltration and scarring.

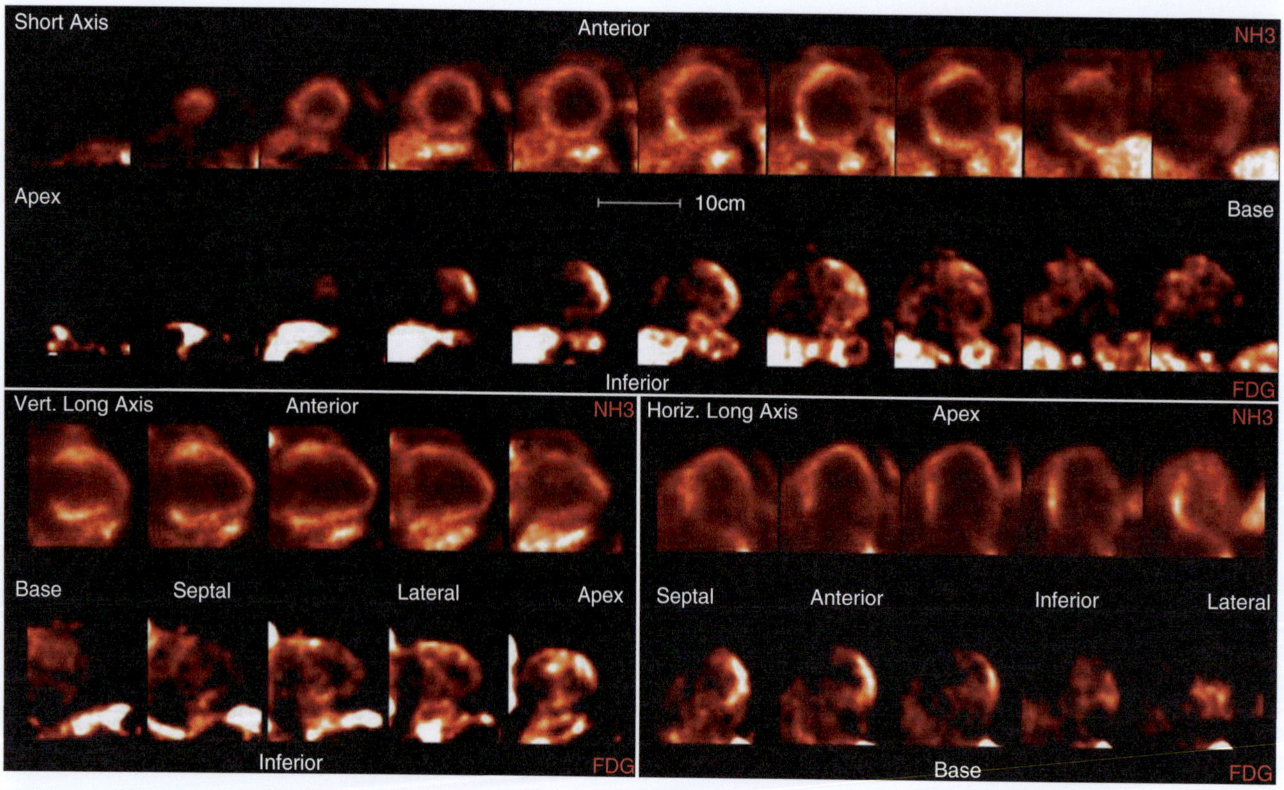

Fig. 12.26 Illustration of short axis and vertical/horizontal long axis images of the myocardial perfusion (*top rows*) and inflammation (*bottom rows*). Both reduced 13N-ammonia and upregulated 18F-FDG uptake is clearly depicted in the anteriolateral and lateral wall as a sign of active cardiac sarcoidosis in these regions

Teaching Points

Late gadolinium enhancement appears predominantly in epicardial regions of the myocardium when cardiac involvement of sarcoidosis is present and only rarely spreads to the endocardium. Areas of LGE represent fibrotic changes as a consequence of fibroganulomatous replacement of the myocardium.

Different patterns of perfusion and glucose metabolism in PET in the case of cardiac involvement of sarcoidosis are known. Normal perfusion and active inflammation represent an early stage of the disease, while reduced perfusion and active inflammation indicates an advanced stage. Finally, reduced or absent perfusion and no inflammation indicates end-stage cardiac sarcoidosis.

The integrated information of PET and MR allow exact assessment of the stage and inflammatory state of the disease and therapy monitoring.

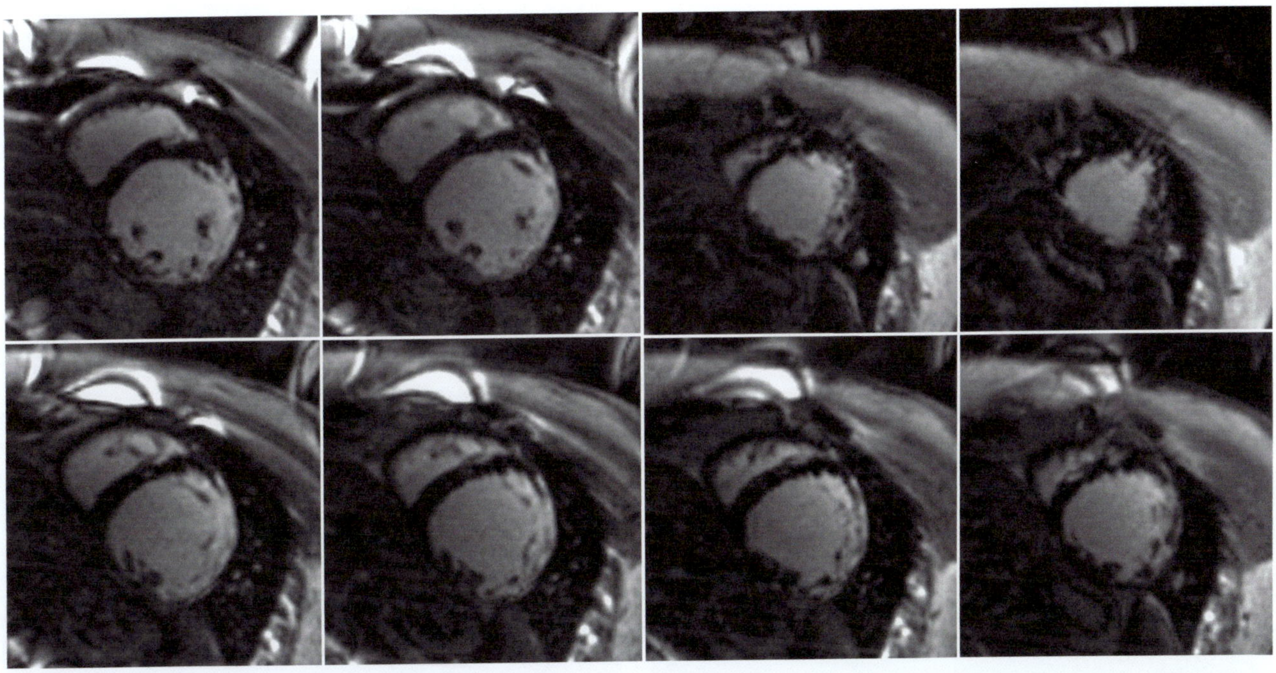

Fig. 12.27 LGE short axis images of the left ventricle. Large areas of the anterolateral and lateral wall show predominantly epicardial LGE indicating myocardial infiltration and scarring

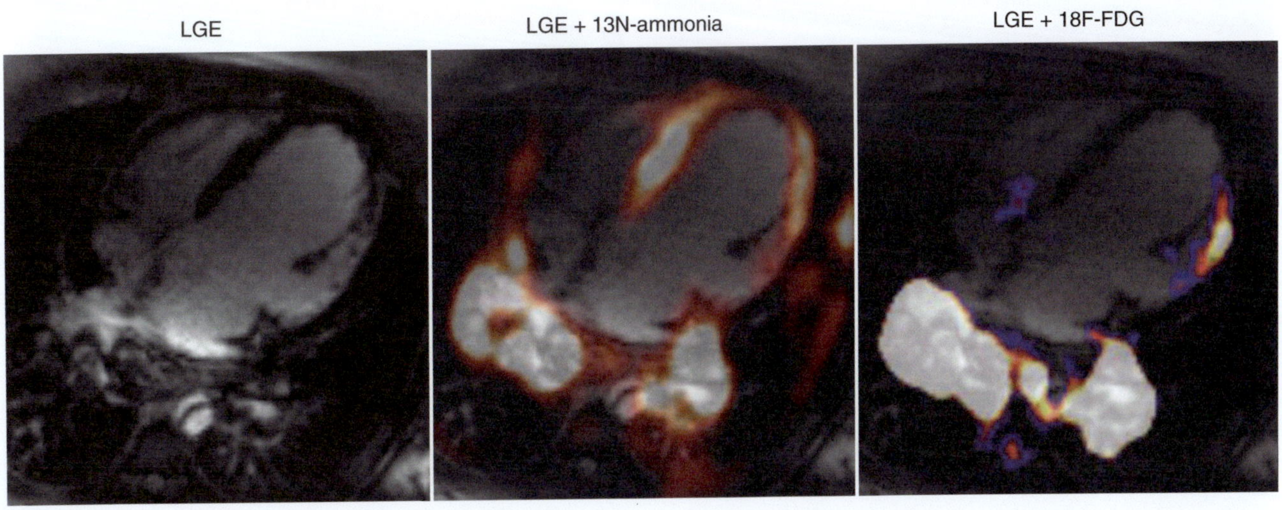

Fig. 12.28 Four chamber view shows an area of transmural LGE in the lateral wall (*left*). Here clearly reduced perfusion (*middle*) and upregulated glucose metabolism (*right*) is observed as a sign of active inflammation. Note both increased 13N-ammonia and 18F-FDG uptake in bilateral hilar lymph nodes

Frontotemporal Dementia (FTD)

Clinical History

Forty-nine-year-old patient with behavioural deficits and increasing memory loss. Study requested for differential diagnosis of possible neurodegenerative dementia.

Imaging Technique

PET measurement started 62 min after injection of 151 MBq [18F]FDG. Simultaneous acquisition of MRI sequences (Dixon and 3D T1).

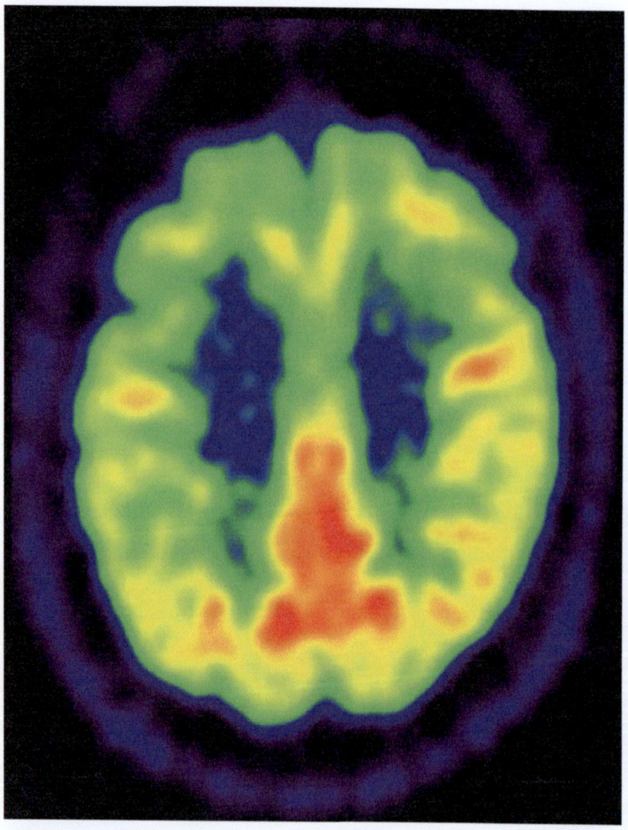

Fig. 12.29 Patient with frontotemporal dementia (FTD) known as Pick's Disease, a frontal form of fronto-temporal-lobe degenerations. Axial [18F]FDG PET image showing the characteristic regional deficits with reduced bihemispheric [18F]FDG tracer uptake in the frontal lobe and relative sparing of posterior brain regions

Findings

Transaxial PET image shows a pattern of reduced bihemispheric [18F]FDG tracer uptake in the frontal lobe and relative sparing of posterior brain regions, especially the percutaneous. The fusion images (Fig. 12.32) [18F]FDG-PET/T1w MRI in 3 projections shows that the regions of reduced [18F]FDG tracer uptake correspond to the regions with most pronounced brain atrophy (frontal lobe). Finally, coronal T1w MRI (below) shows no signs of hippocampal atrophy.

Teaching Points

The combination of functional [18F]FDG-PET and structural MR information leads to the most likely diagnosis of frontotemporal dementia (FTD). The main differential diagnosis behavioural atypical variant of Alzheimer's Disease (AD) is unlikely due to normal metabolism in the precuneus/posterior cingulate region and due to lack of hippocampal atrophy.

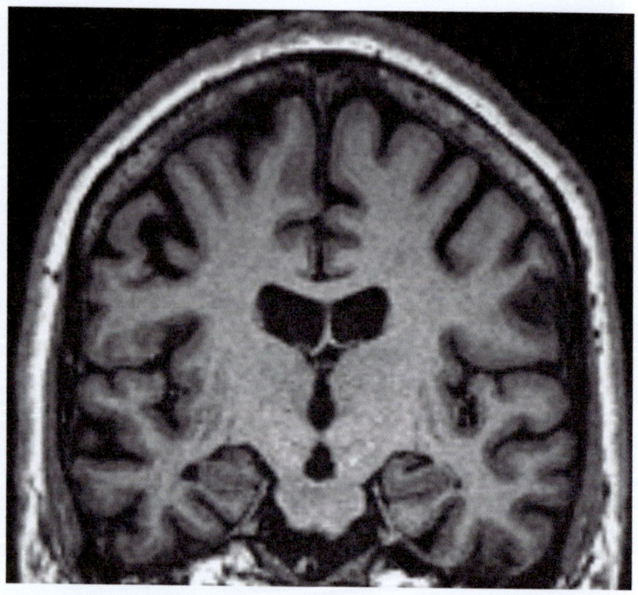

Fig. 12.30 Coronal T1w MRI showing no signs of hippocampal atrophy

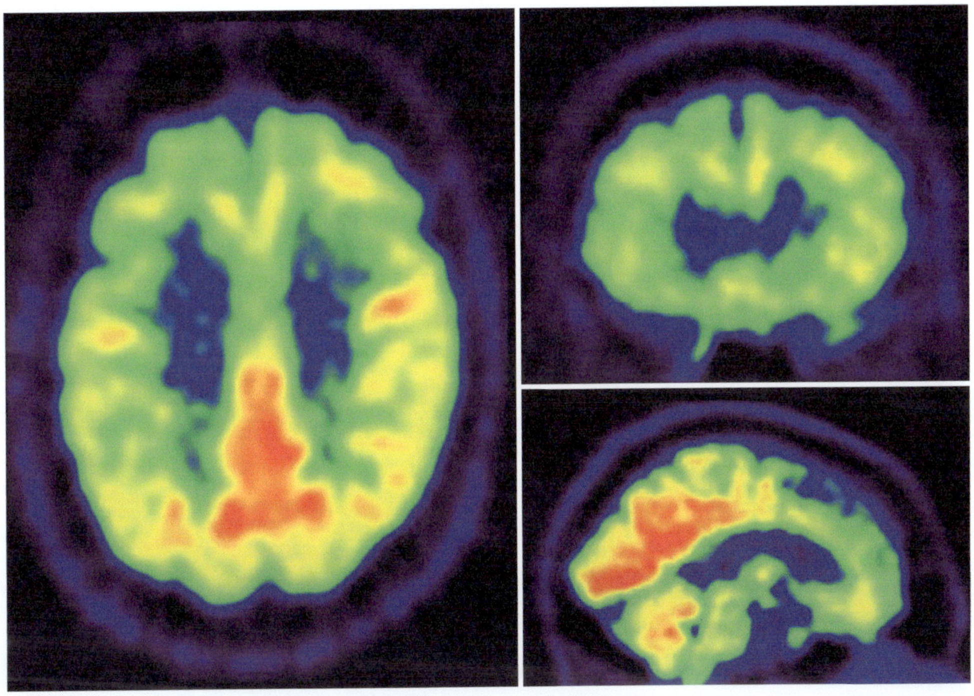

Fig. 12.31 Multi-planar reformatted PET images show the characteristic regional deficits in FDG uptake in a patient with Pick's Disease with reduced bihemispheric FDG tracer uptake in the frontal lobe and relative sparing of posterior brain regions

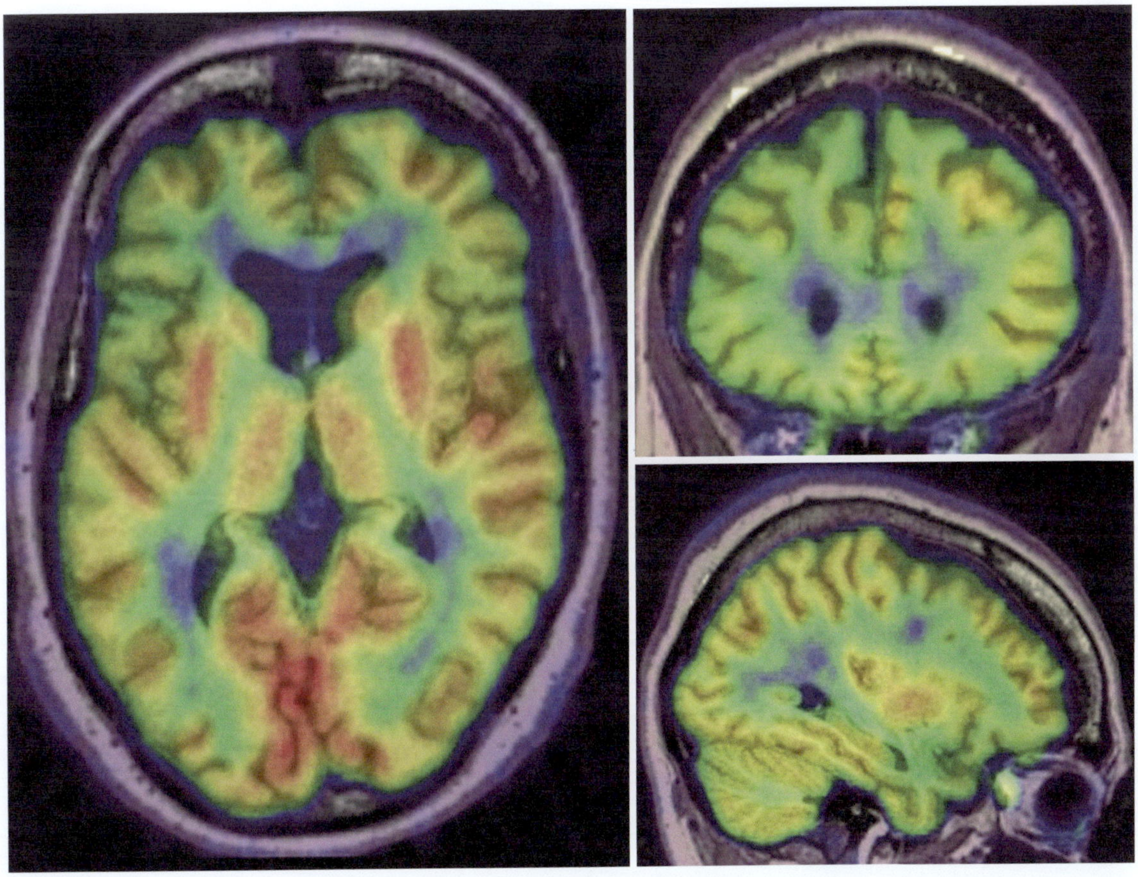

Fig. 12.32 Fused axial (*left*) coronal (*middle*) and sagittal (*right*) of PET and T1W MRI images showing the characteristic regional deficits in FDG uptake reduction and atrophy

Alzheimer's Disease (AD)

Clinical History

Seventy-three-year-old male subject with slowly progressing memory deficits since 4 years. Study requested for differential diagnosis of neurodegenerative dementia.

Imaging Technique

[18F]FDG-PET measurement started 57 min after injection of 155 MBq [18F]FDG. Simultaneous acquisition of MRI sequences (Dixon, 3D T1 and coronal T2).

Findings

Parietal hypometabolism in [18F]FDG-PET images is indicative of AD. MRI data including volumetric T1w sequence showing severe global brain atrophy as well as hippocampal atrophy in T2 w coronal sequence confirms the diagnosis.

Teaching Points

The combination of functional and structural information strengthens the diagnosis of Alzheimer's Disease.

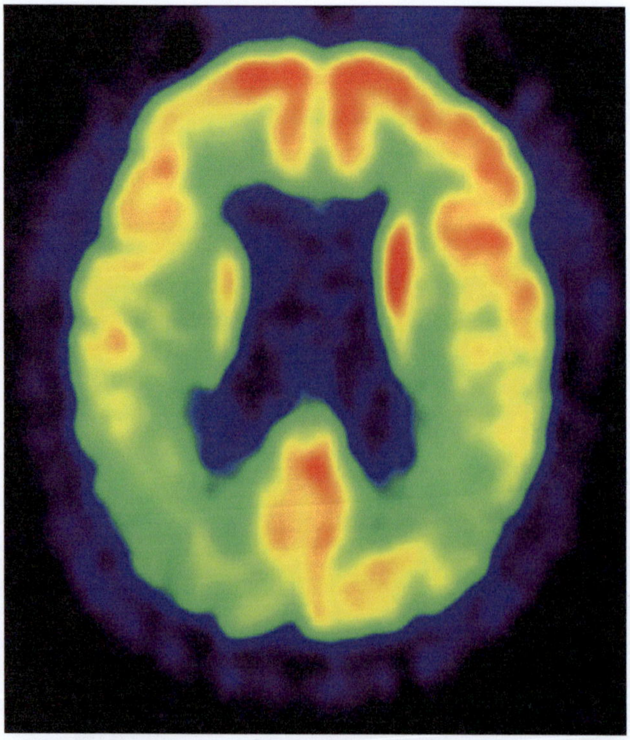

Fig. 12.33 [18F]FDG-PET in axial projection shows a symmetrically reduced tracer uptake in the bilateral dorsolateral parietal cortex as well as decreased uptake in the right precuneus/posterior cingulate cortex

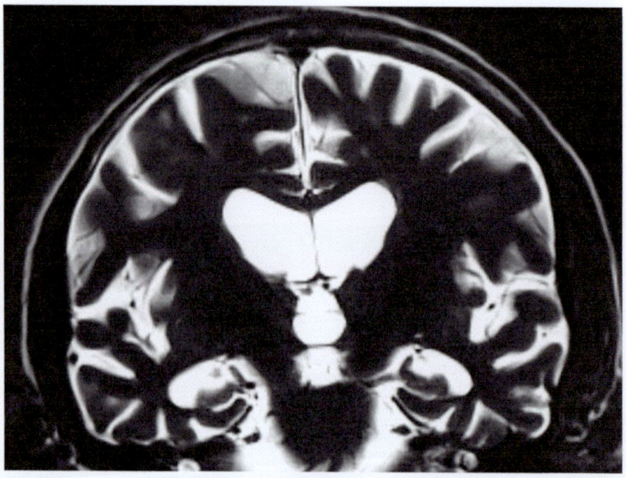

Fig. 12.34 T2w MRI in coronal orientation demonstrates severe bilateral hippocampal atrophy

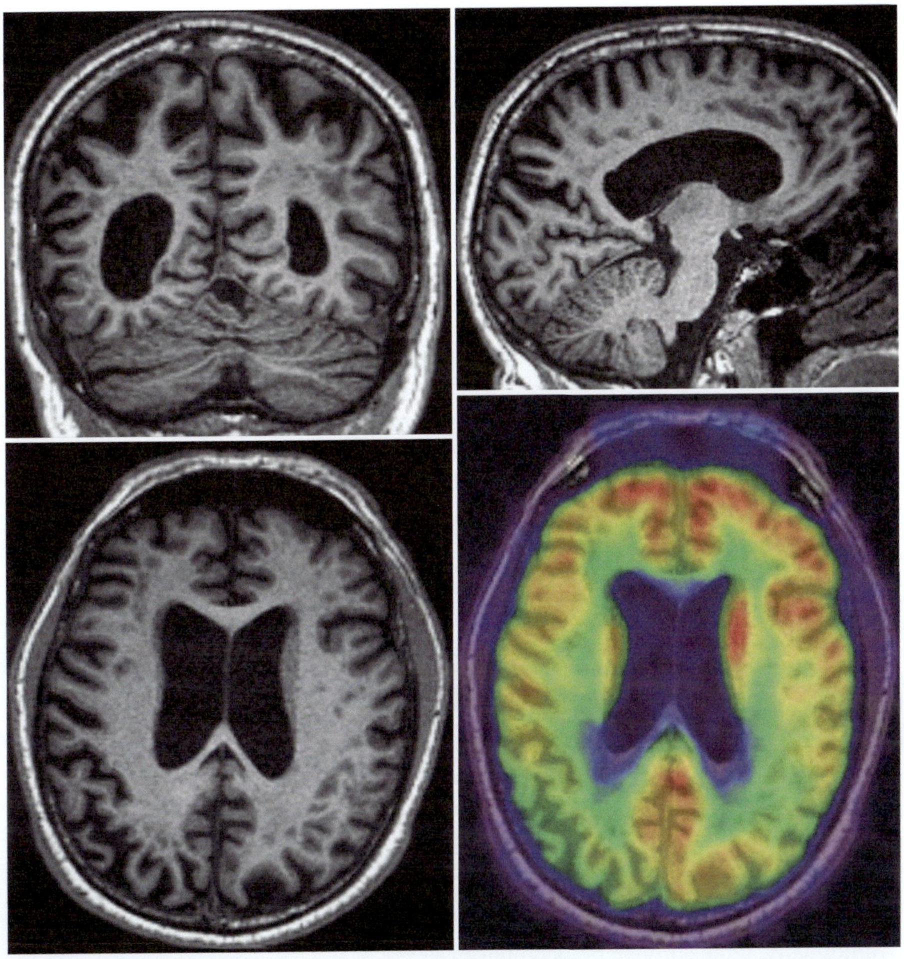

Fig. 12.35 T1w structural MRI in 3 projections shows a parietal-emphasized global atrophy. The image on the *bottom right* demonstrates a fusion with FDG-PET that highlights a spatial overlap between lateral parietal hypometabolism and cortical atrophy

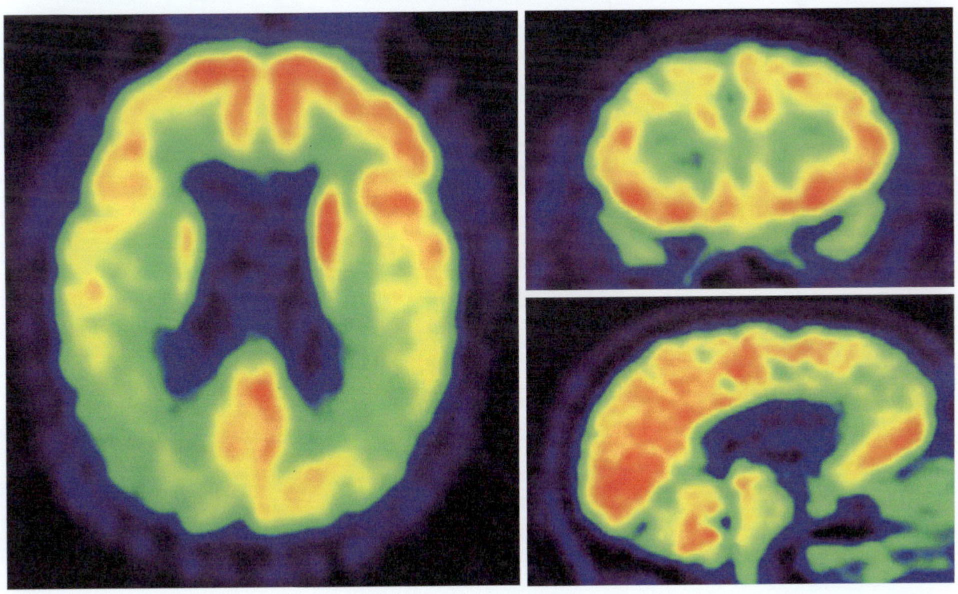

Fig. 12.36 Multi-planar reformatting (MPR) of FDG-PET images showing a characteristic symmetrically reduced tracer uptake in the bilateral dorsolateral parietal cortex and in the right precuneus/posterior cingulate cortex

Posterior Cortical Atrophy

Clinical History

Sixty-eight-year-old patient with predominant visuo-spatial deficits as well as cognitive decline. Neurodegenerative dementia? DD? Structural abnormality?

Imaging Technique

Two separate studies were performed with different tracers: F18-FDG and C11-PIB. FDG-PET measurement started 60 min after injection of 151 MBq F18-FDG. PiB-PET measurement started 41 min after injection of 371 MBq C11-PiB. Simultaneous acquisition of MRI sequences (Dixon, 3D T1).

Findings

Transaxial FDG-PET images (Fig. 12.37) show a asymmetrically reduced parietal and temporo-occipital FDG tracer uptake predominantly in the right occipital lobe extending from the cortex into the white matter including a photopenic lesion without any FDG uptake. The fusion images FDG-PET/T1w MRI in 3 projections (Fig. 12.38) show that the photopenic lesion without any FDG tracer uptake corresponds to an irregular dorsal extension of the right ventricle. Additionally, reduced bilateral occipital FDG tracer uptake and the respective occipital cortical atrophy is seen. PiB-PET image (Fig. 12.39) shows diffusely increased PiB tracer uptake in bilateral cortical regions peaking in the precuneus as well as increased subcortical PiB tracer uptake in bilateral striatum.

Teaching Points

Although information provided by PET alone would already favour diagnosis of AD, structural MR information helps in further differentiating the etiology by clarifying the asymmetrical hypometabolic/photopenic lesion in the right occipital lobe and in detecting the distinct bilateral occipital cortical atrophy, suggesting posterior cortical atrophy as final diagnosis.

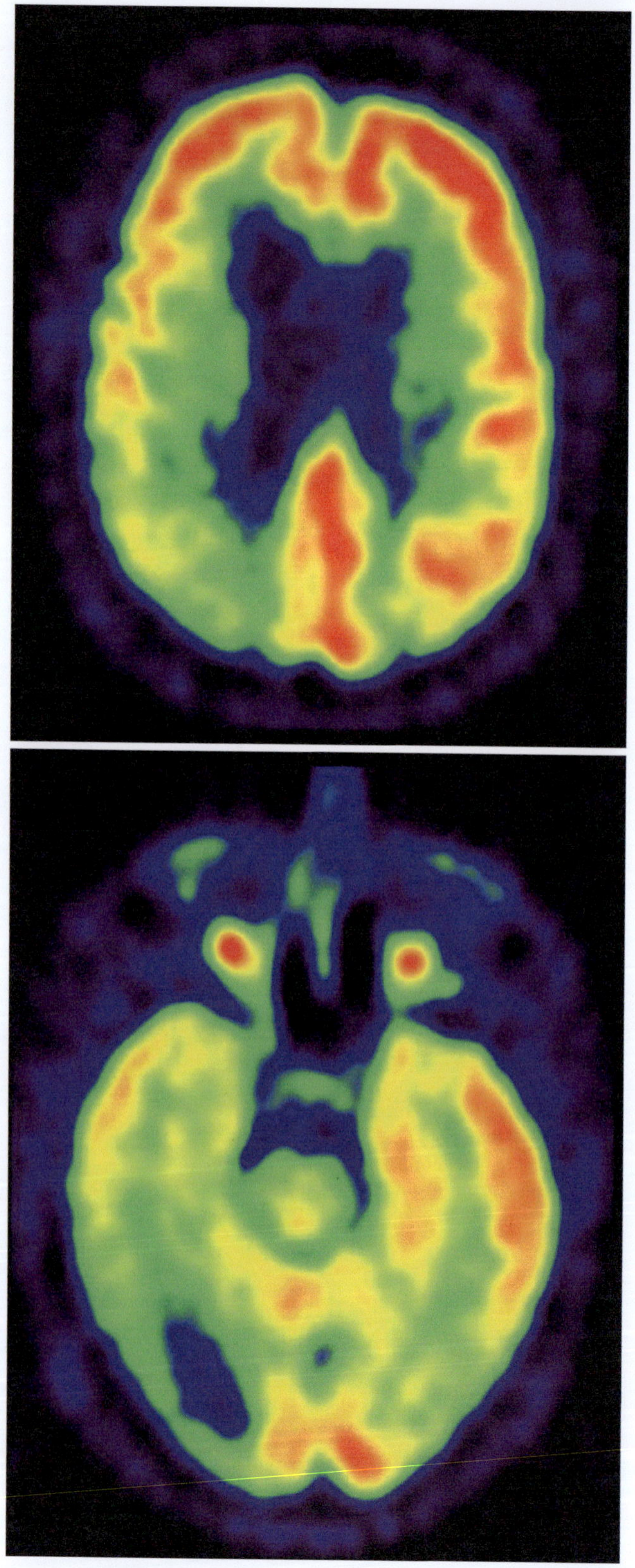

Fig. 12.37 Two axial PET images showing asymmetrically reduced parietal and temporo-occipital FDG tracer uptake predominantly in the right occipital lobe extending from the cortex into the white matter

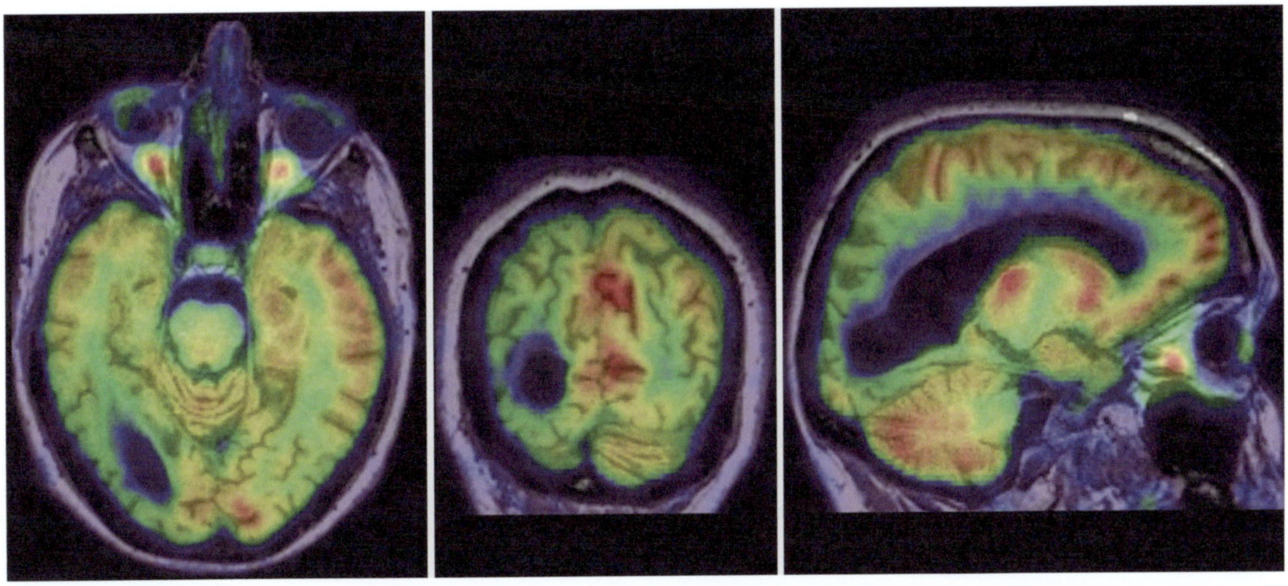

Fig. 12.38 Multiplanar reformatted (MPR) FDG PET images fused with axial (*left*) coronal (*middle*) and sagittal (*right*) of T1W MRI images show that the photopenic lesion without any FDG tracer uptake corresponds to an irregular dorsal extension of the right ventricle. Additionally reduced occipital FDG uptake and occipital cortical atrophy can be appreciated

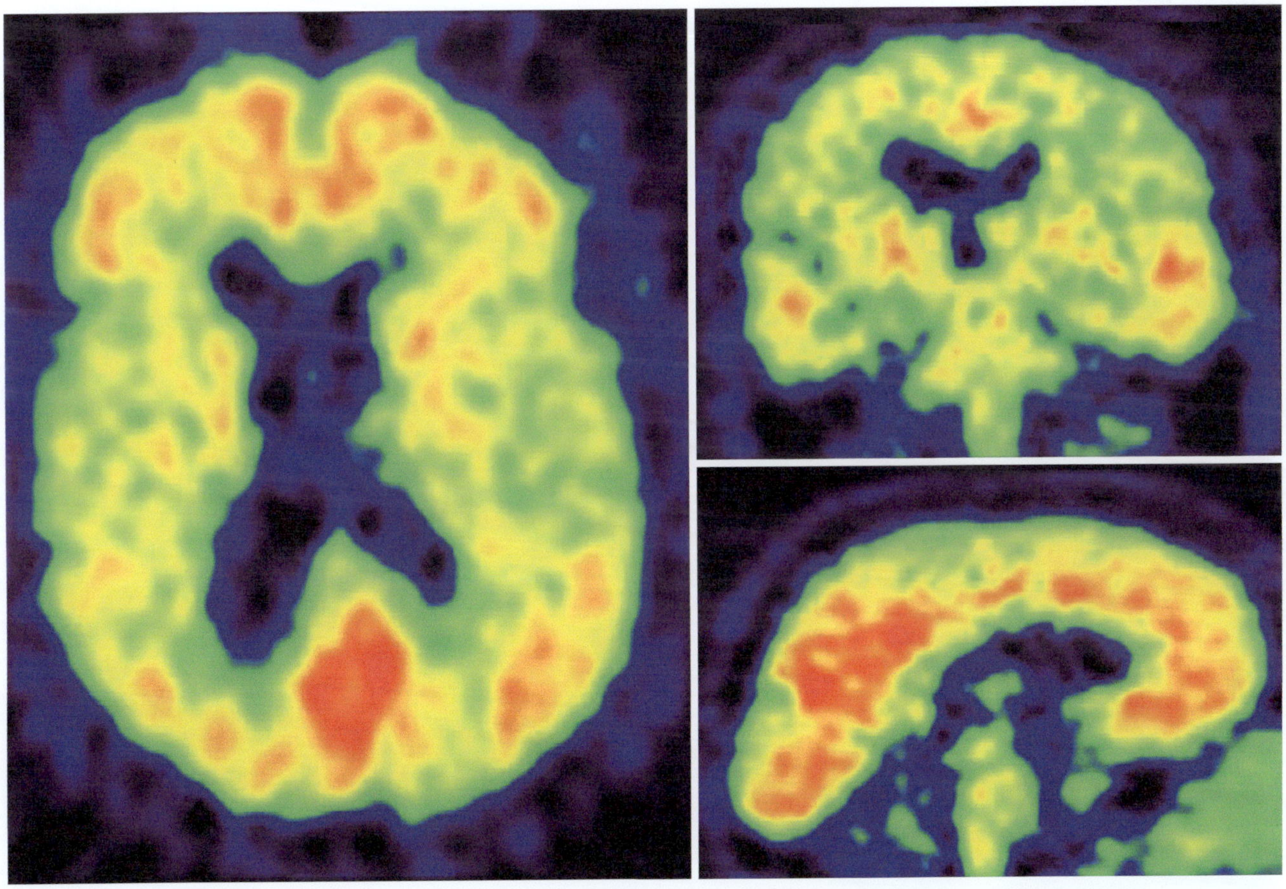

Fig. 12.39 Multiplanar reformatted images in axial, coronal and sagittal planes of C11-PIB PET images shows diffusely increased PiB tracer uptake in bilateral cortical regions peaking in the precuneus as well as increased subcortical PiB tracer uptake in bilateral striatum

References

1. Balink H, Collins J, Bruyn GA, Bruyn G, Gemmel F (2009) F-18 FDG PET/CT in the diagnosis of fever of unknown origin. Clin Nucl Med 34:862–868
2. Basu S, Kumar R, Alavi A (2010) PET and PET/CT imaging in infection and inflammation: its critical role in assessing complications related to therapeutic interventions in patients with cancer. Indian J Cancer 47:371–379
3. Yokota S, Kikuchi M, Nozawa T, Kizawa T, Kanetaka T, Kadota K, Miyamae T, Mori M (2012) Febrile responses in patients with pediatric rheumatic diseases. Nihon Rinsho Meneki Gakkai Kaishi 35:511–519
4. Temma T, Saji H (2012) Radiolabelled probes for imaging of atherosclerotic plaques. Am J Nucl Med Mol Imaging 2:432–447
5. Dweck MR, Chow MWL, Joshi NV, Williams MC, Jones C, Fletcher AM, Richardson H, White A, McKillop G, van Beek EJR, Boon NA, Rudd JHF, Newby DE (2012) Coronary arterial 18F-sodium fluoride uptake: a novel marker of plaque biology. J Am Coll Cardiol 59:1539–1548
6. Hermann S, Starsichova A, Waschkau B, Kuhlmann M, Wenning C, Schober O, Schäfers M (2012) Non-FDG imaging of atherosclerosis: will imaging of MMPs assess plaque vulnerability? J Nucl Cardiol 19:609–617
7. Arnaldi D, Morbelli S, Morrone E, Campus C, Nobili F (2012) Cognitive impairment in degenerative parkinsonisms: role of radionuclide brain imaging. Q J Nucl Med Mol Imaging 56:55–67
8. de Souza LC, Lehéricy S, Dubois B, Stella F, Sarazin M (2012) Neuroimaging in dementias. Curr Opin Psychiatry 25:473–479
9. Lopez OL, McDade E, Riverol M, Becker JT (2011) Evolution of the diagnostic criteria for degenerative and cognitive disorders. Curr Opin Neurol 24:532–541
10. Heiss W-D, Zimmermann-Meinzingen S (2012) PET imaging in the differential diagnosis of vascular dementia. J Neurol Sci 322:268–273
11. Lopez OL, McDade E, Riverol M, Becker JT (2011) Evolution of the diagnostic criteria for degenerative and cognitive disorders. Curr Opin Neurol 24:532–541

MIX
Papier aus verantwortungsvollen Quellen
Paper from responsible sources
FSC® C105338

If you have any concerns about our products,
you can contact us on
ProductSafety@springernature.com

In case Publisher is established outside the EU,
the EU authorized representative is:
Springer Nature Customer Service Center GmbH
Europaplatz 3, 69115 Heidelberg, Germany

Printed by Libri Plureos GmbH
in Hamburg, Germany